Genomics in Rheumatic Diseases

Editors

S. LOUIS BRIDGES, Jr.
CARL D. LANGEFELD

RHEUMATIC DISEASE CLINICS OF NORTH AMERICA

www.rheumatic.theclinics.com

Consulting Editor
MICHAEL H. WEISMAN

August 2017 • Volume 43 • Number 3

ELSEVIER

1600 John F. Kennedy Boulevard ● Suite 1800 ● Philadelphia, Pennsylvania, 19103-2899
http://www.theclinics.com

RHEUMATIC DISEASE CLINICS OF NORTH AMERICA Volume 43, Number 3
August 2017 ISSN 0889-857X, ISBN 13: 978-0-323-53255-6

Editor: Lauren Boyle
Developmental Editor: Casey Potter

Rheumatic Disease Clinics of North America (ISSN 0889-857X) is published quarterly by Elsevier Inc., 360 Park Avenue South, New York, NY 10010-1710. Months of issue are February, May, August, and November. Business and editorial offices: 1600 John F. Kennedy Boulevard, Suite 1800, Philadelphia, PA 19103-2899. Periodicals postage paid at New York, NY and additional mailing offices. Subscription prices are USD 335.00 per year for US individuals, USD 659.00 per year for US institutions, USD 100.00 per year for US students and residents, USD 395.00 per year for Canadian individuals, USD 823.00 per year for Canadian institutions, USD 465.00 per year for international individuals, USD 823.00 per year for international institutions, and USD 230.00 per year for Canadian and foreign students/residents. To receive student/resident rate, orders must be accompanied by name of affiliated institution, date of term, and the *signature* of program/residency coordinator on institution letterhead. Orders will be billed at individual rate until proof of status received. Foreign air speed delivery is included in all *Clinics* subscription prices. All prices are subject to change without notice. **POSTMASTER:** Send address changes to *Rheumatic Disease Clinics of North America,* Elsevier Health Sciences Division, Subscription Customer Service, 3251 Riverport Lane, Maryland Heights, MO 63043. **Customer Service: 1-800-654-2452 (US and Canada). From outside of the US and Canada: 314-447-8871. Fax: 314-447-8029. For print support,** e-mail: **JournalsCustomerService-usa@elsevier.com**. **For online support, e-mail: JournalsOnline Support-usa@elsevier.com**.

Reprints. For copies of 100 or more of articles in this publication, please contact the Commercial Reprints Department, Elsevier Inc., 360 Park Avenue South, New York, New York, 10010-1710; Tel.: +1-212-633-3874, Fax: +1-212-633-3820, and E-mail: reprints@elsevier.com.

Rheumatic Disease Clinics of North America is covered in *MEDLINE/PubMed (Index Medicus), Current Contents/Clinical Medicine, Science Citation Index, ISI/BIOMED,* and *EMBASE/Excerpta Medica.*

Contributors

CONSULTING EDITOR

MICHAEL H. WEISMAN, MD
Cedars-Sinai Chair in Rheumatology, Director, Division of Rheumatology, Professor of Medicine, Cedars-Sinai Medical Center, Distinguished Professor, David Geffen School of Medicine, University of California, Los Angeles, Los Angeles, California

EDITORS

S. LOUIS BRIDGES, Jr., MD, PhD
Anna Lois Waters Professor of Medicine, Director, Division of Clinical Immunology and Rheumatology, Director, Comprehensive Arthritis, Musculoskeletal, Bone and Autoimmunity Center, School of Medicine, University of Alabama at Birmingham, Birmingham, Alabama

CARL D. LANGEFELD, PhD
Public Health Genomics, Department of Biostatistical Sciences, Division of Public Health Sciences, Wake Forest School of Medicine, Wake Forest University, Winston-Salem, North Carolina

AUTHORS

GRETCHEN BANDOLI, PhD
Department of Pediatrics, University of California, San Diego, La Jolla, California

ANNE BARTON, FRCP, PhD
Professor, Division of Musculoskeletal and Dermal Sciences, Arthritis Research UK Centre for Genetics and Genomics, Centre for Musculoskeletal Research, Manchester Academic Health Science Centre, The University of Manchester, NIHR Manchester Musculoskeletal Biomedical Research Unit, Central Manchester NHS Foundation Trust, Manchester Academic Health Science Centre, Manchester, United Kingdom

JAMES BLUETT, MBBS, PhD
Division of Musculoskeletal and Dermal Sciences, Arthritis Research UK Centre for Genetics and Genomics, Centre for Musculoskeletal Research, Manchester Academic Health Science Centre, The University of Manchester, Manchester, United Kingdom

S. LOUIS BRIDGES, Jr., MD, PhD
Anna Lois Waters Professor of Medicine, Director, Division of Clinical Immunology and Rheumatology, Director, Comprehensive Arthritis, Musculoskeletal, Bone and Autoimmunity Center, School of Medicine, University of Alabama at Birmingham, Birmingham, Alabama

MATTHEW A. BROWN, MBBS, MD, FRACP, FAHMS, FAA
Professor, Institute of Health and Biomedical Innovation, Translational Research
Institute, Princess Alexandra Hospital, Queensland University of Technology, Brisbane,
Queensland, Australia

CHRISTINA D. CHAMBERS, PhD, MPH
Department of Pediatrics, University of California, San Diego, La Jolla, California

JAKE Y. CHEN, PhD
Professor of Genetics, Associate Director and Chief Bioinformatics Officer, Informatics
Institute, School of Medicine, University of Alabama at Birmingham, Birmingham,
Alabama

CHELSEY J. FORBESS SMITH, MD
Department of Rheumatology, University of California, San Diego, La Jolla, California

AMRIE C. GRAMMER, PhD
AMPEL BioSolutions and RILITE Research Institute, Charlottesville, Virginia

AIMEE HANSON, BSc (Hons)
Research Fellow, Translational Research Institute, Princess Alexandra Hospital,
University of Queensland Diamantina Institute, Brisbane, Queensland, Australia

AIMEE O. HERSH, MD
Assistant Professor of Pediatrics, Pediatric Rheumatology, University of Utah School of
Medicine, Salt Lake City, Utah

LINDA T. HIRAKI, MD, FRCPC, ScD
Clinician Scientist, Division of Rheumatology, SickKids Hospital, Scientist Track
Investigator, SickKids Research Institute, Division of Epidemiology, Dalla Lana School of
Public Health, Assistant Professor, Department of Paediatrics, University of Toronto,
Toronto, Ontario, Canada

JUN HIRATA, MS
Department of Statistical Genetics, Osaka University Graduate School of Medicine, Suita,
Osaka, Japan; Department of Human Genetics and Disease Diversity, Graduate School of
Medical and Dental Sciences, Tokyo Medical and Dental University, Pharmaceutical
Discovery Research Laboratories, Teijin Pharma Limited, Tokyo, Japan

JOSEPH HOLOSHITZ, MD
Department of Internal Medicine, University of Michigan, Ann Arbor, Michigan

TOM W.J. HUIZINGA, MD, PhD
Professor and Head of Department of Rheumatology, Leiden University Medical Center,
Leiden, The Netherlands

DANIEL L. KASTNER, MD, PhD
Inflammatory Disease Section, Intramural Research Program, Metabolic, Cardiovascular
and Inflammatory Disease Genomics Branch, National Human Genome Research
Institute, National Institutes of Health, Bethesda, Maryland

TOSHIHIRO KISHIKAWA, MD
Departments of Statistical Genetics, and Otorhinolaryngology–Head and Neck Surgery,
Osaka University Graduate School of Medicine, Suita, Osaka, Japan

RACHEL KNEVEL, MD, PhD
Research Fellow, Raychaudhuri Lab, Division of Genetics, Brigham and Women's Hospital, Post-Doctoral Research Fellow, Harvard Medical School, Boston, Massachusetts; The Broad Institute, Cambridge, Massachusetts; Clinical Fellow in Rheumatology, Leiden University Medical Center, Leiden, The Netherlands

FINA KURREEMAN, PhD
Assistant Professor, Leiden University Medical Center, Leiden, The Netherlands

CARL D. LANGEFELD, PhD
Public Health Genomics, Department of Biostatistical Sciences, Division of Public Health Sciences, Wake Forest School of Medicine, Wake Forest University, Winston-Salem, North Carolina

VINCENT A. LAUFER, BA
MD/PhD Student, Division of Clinical Immunology and Rheumatology, School of Medicine, University of Alabama at Birmingham, Birmingham, Alabama

PETER E. LIPSKY, MD
AMPEL BioSolutions and RILITE Research Institute, Charlottesville, Virginia

TONY MERRIMAN, PhD
Department of Biochemistry, University of Otago, Dunedin, New Zealand

HIROTSUGU ODA, MD, PhD
Inflammatory Disease Section, Intramural Research Program, Metabolic, Cardiovascular and Inflammatory Disease Genomics Branch, National Human Genome Research Institute, National Institutes of Health, Bethesda, Maryland; Department of Pediatrics, Kitano Hospital, Tazuke Kofukai Medical Research Institute, Osaka, Japan

YUKINORI OKADA, MD, PhD
Department of Statistical Genetics, Osaka University Graduate School of Medicine, Suita, Osaka, Japan

KRISTIN PALMSTEN, ScD
Department of Pediatrics, University of California, San Diego, La Jolla, California

SAMPATH PRAHALAD, MD, MS
Marcus Professor and Chief of Pediatric Rheumatology, Departments of Pediatrics and Human Genetics, Children's Healthcare of Atlanta, Emory University School of Medicine, Atlanta, Georgia

PAULA S. RAMOS, PhD
Assistant Professor, Division of Rheumatology and Immunology, Departments of Medicine, and Public Health Sciences, Medical University of South Carolina, Charleston, South Carolina

SAORI SAKAUE, MD
Department of Statistical Genetics, Osaka University Graduate School of Medicine, Suita, Osaka, Japan; Department of Allergy and Rheumatology, Graduate School of Medicine, The University of Tokyo, Tokyo, Japan

EARL D. SILVERMAN, MD, FRCPC
Division of Rheumatology, SickKids Hospital, Associate Scientist Emeritus, SickKids Research Institute, Professor Emeritus, Departments of Paediatrics and Medicine, University of Toronto, Toronto, Ontario, Canada

VINCENT VAN DRONGELEN, PhD
Department of Internal Medicine, University of Michigan, Ann Arbor, Michigan

Contents

Human genetic diversity is the result of population genetic forces. This genetic variation influences disease risk and contributes to health disparities. Natural selection is an important influence on human genetic variation. Because immune and inflammatory function genes are enriched for signals of positive selection, the prevalence of rheumatic disease-risk alleles seen in different populations is partially the result of differing selective pressures (eg, due to pathogens). This review summarizes the genetic regions associated with susceptibility to different rheumatic diseases and concomitant evidence for natural selection, including known agents of selection exerting selective pressure in these regions.

The monogenic autoinflammatory diseases are a group of illnesses with prominent rheumatic manifestations that are characterized by genetically determined recurrent sterile inflammation and are thus inborn errors of innate immunity. Molecular targeted therapies against inflammatory cytokines, such as interleukin 1 and tumor necrosis factor, and intracellular cytokine signaling pathways have proved effective in many cases. Emerging next-generation sequencing technologies have accelerated the identification of previously unreported genes causing autoinflammatory diseases. This review covers several of the prominent recent advances in the field of autoinflammatory diseases, including gene discoveries, the elucidation of new pathogenic mechanisms, and the development of effective targeted therapies.

Genetics in rheumatoid arthritis (RA) has moved from the finding of HLA-shared epitope decades ago toward the understanding of the role of HLA in RA and the findings of ~100 additional genetic risk variants for disease susceptibility as well as several risk variants for severe disease. These findings increased our understanding of RA abnormality. Still, the mechanisms by which many of the variants exhibit their effect are not yet understood.

Vincent van Drongelen and Joseph Holoshitz

The cause and pathogenesis of rheumatoid arthritis (RA) are influenced by environmental and genetic risk factors. Shared epitope-coding human leukocyte antigen (HLA)-DRB1 alleles increase RA risk and severity; however, the underlying mechanisms of action remain unclear. In contrast, several other DRB1 alleles protect against RA. Additionally, genome-wide association studies suggest that RA associates with other, HLA and non-HLA, genes; but the relative contributions of such risk loci to RA are incompletely understood. Future research challenges include integrating the epidemiologic and genomic data into validated arthritogenic pathways and determining the mechanisms of interaction between RA risk genes and environmental influences.

James Bluett and Anne Barton

Treatment of rheumatoid arthritis (RA) has substantially improved in recent years because of the development of novel drugs. However, response is not universal for any of the treatment options, and selection of an effective therapy is currently based on a trial-and-error approach. Delayed treatment response increases the risk of progressive joint damage and resultant disability and also has a significant impact on quality of life for patients. For many drugs, the patient's genetic background influences response to therapy, and understanding the genetics of response to therapy in RA may allow for targeted personalized health care.

Tony Merriman

Genome-wide association studies (GWAS) have identified nearly 30 loci associated with urate concentrations that also influence the subsequent risk of gout. The ABCG2 Q141 K variant is highly likely to be causal and results in internalization of ABCG2, which can be rescued by drugs. Three other GWAS loci contain uric acid transporter genes, which are also highly likely to be causal. However identification of causal genes at other urate loci is challenging. Finally, relatively little is known about the genetic control of progression from hyperuricemia to gout. Only 4 small GWAS have been published for gout.

Aimee Hanson and Matthew A. Brown

Ankylosing spondylitis (AS) is a common inflammatory arthritis in which genetic factors are the primary determinants of disease risk and severity. Substantial progress has been made in identifying genetic pathways involved in the disease, and in translating those discoveries to drug discovery programs. Recently discovered novel disease pathways include those involved in control of DNA methylation, bacterial sensing, and mucosal immunity. Additional pathways are likely to be identified as a higher proportion of the genetic risk of AS is determined.

Linda T. Hiraki and Earl D. Silverman

Systemic lupus erythematosus (SLE) is a systemic, autoimmune, multi-system disease with a heterogeneous clinical phenotype. Genome-wide association studies have identified multiple susceptibility loci, but these explain a fraction of the estimated heritability. This is partly because within the broad spectrum of SLE are monogenic diseases that tend to cluster in patients with young age of onset, and in families. This article highlights insights into the pathogenesis of SLE provided by these monogenic diseases. It examines genetic causes of complement deficiency, abnormal interferon production, and abnormalities of tolerance, resulting in monogenic SLE with overlapping clinical features, autoantibodies, and shared inflammatory pathways.

Aimee O. Hersh and Sampath Prahalad

Juvenile idiopathic arthritis (JIA) affects approximately 1 in 1000 US children. The cause of JIA is most likely multifactorial and due to an interplay of genetics and environmental factors. This article summarizes the known genetic risk factors for JIA that have been identified, and in some cases replicated, using a variety of methods, including genomewide association and candidate gene association studies. A brief discussion regarding pharmacogenomics and studies to data linking genetics to treatment response and outcomes is included.

Vincent A. Laufer, Jake Y. Chen, Carl D. Langefeld, and S. Louis Bridges, Jr.

The use of high-throughput omics may help to understand the contribution of genetic variants to the pathogenesis of rheumatic diseases. We discuss the concept of missing heritability: that genetic variants do not explain the heritability of rheumatoid arthritis and related rheumatologic conditions. In addition to an overview of how integrative data analysis can lead to novel insights into mechanisms of rheumatic diseases, we describe statistical approaches to prioritizing genetic variants for future functional analyses. We illustrate how analyses of large datasets provide hope for improved approaches to the diagnosis, treatment, and prevention of rheumatic diseases.

Amrie C. Grammer and Peter E. Lipsky

Rheumatic Autoimmune Inflammatory Diseases such as Sjögren's and lupus lack modern treatments. Less than 5% of drugs approved by the

FDA from 2014 to mid-2016 had a RAID indication. Many RAID standard-of-care drugs were repurposed based on serendipitous observations, similarity-of-disease categorization, and/or off-target effects. Recently, drug repurposing has become more intentional, relying on an evolving awareness of molecular underpinnings, as well as a better understanding of drug-target interactions by computational modeling. Understanding mechanisms of disease pathogenesis can be synergistic in identifying new drug candidates and target pathways using unbiased Big-Data repositioning approaches as genomics, PheWAS (disease mechanism-of-action), GWAS and/or epigenetic-profiling.

Yukinori Okada, Toshihiro Kishikawa, Saori Sakaue, and Jun Hirata

Recent developments in human genome genotyping and sequencing technologies, such as genome-wide association studies and whole-genome sequencing analyses, have successfully identified several risk genes of rheumatic diseases. Fine-mapping studies using the HLA imputation method revealed that classical and non-classical HLA genes contribute to the risk of rheumatic diseases. Integration of human disease genomics with biological, medical, and clinical databases should contribute to the elucidation of disease pathogenicity and novel drug discovery. Disease risk genes identified by large-scale genetic studies are considered to be promising resources for novel drug discovery, including drug repositioning and biomarker microRNA screening for rheumatoid arthritis.

Special Article

Gretchen Bandoli, Kristin Palmsten, Chelsey J. Forbess Smith, and Christina D. Chambers

The evidence to date regarding corticosteroid exposure in pregnancy and select pregnancy and birth outcomes is limited and inconsistent. The authors provide a narrative review of published literature summarizing the findings for oral clefts, preterm birth, birth weight, preeclampsia, and gestational diabetes mellitus. Whenever possible, the results are limited to oral or systemic administration with a further focus on use in autoimmune disease. Although previous studies of corticosteroid exposure in pregnancy reported an increased risk of oral clefts in the offspring, more recent studies have not replicated these findings.

RHEUMATIC DISEASE CLINICS OF NORTH AMERICA

THE CLINICS ARE AVAILABLE ONLINE!
Access your subscription at:
www.theclinics.com

Foreword

Genomics in Rheumatic Diseases

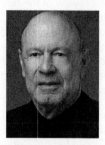

Michael H. Weisman, MD
Consulting Editor

The current issue is one of a kind, bringing together basic, clinical, translational, and computational scientists into one space to address the role of genomics in Rheumatology. Lou Bridges and Carl Langefeld have done a remarkable job in accomplishing this feat.

Paula Ramos discusses the role of population genetics as a tool to understand the emergence of our diseases from past events of selection. Rachel Knevel and colleagues address genetic challenges where the disease is phenotypically heterogeneous and we have limited data on the functional significance of the findings. Van Drongelen and Holoshitz focus on the HLA alleles' discovery and its impact on our understanding of the connection between genetic susceptibility and environmental triggers in rheumatoid arthritis (RA). Tony Merriman addresses the role of genetic discovery and its impact on urate metabolism and clinical gout, emerging fields of great interest in a disease for which we know a great deal yet have little impact on its frequency and severity in the real world. Hiraki and Silverman give us the pediatric perspective on genes and lupus by examining the clues to its pathogenesis from observations made in young-onset systemic lupus erythematosus from consanguineous marriages or in subjects with particularly severe disease. Hanson and Brown remind us that despite the remarkable heritability of ankylosing spondylitis and the old and new discoveries of HLA and non-HLA associations, we are still short in our knowledge about how these discoveries affect the pathogenesis of disease. Hersh and Prahalad remind us how much more we need to know about genetic risk for juvenile idiopathic arthritis, a remarkably heterogeneous collection of phenotypes.

Bluett and Barton address the gap in our understanding of how we can employ genetic data to aid treatment decisions in RA, otherwise known as the concept of personalized medicine. Okada and colleagues discuss the recent developments in human genome genotyping as we try to integrate large clinical and biological databases to promote novel drug discovery in the rheumatic diseases. Grammer and Lipsky are

Rheum Dis Clin N Am 43 (2017) xiii–xiv
http://dx.doi.org/10.1016/j.rdc.2017.05.002
0889-857X/17/© 2017 Published by Elsevier Inc.

rheumatic.theclinics.com

at the forefront of the emerging field of drug repositioning, and they discuss the multiple approaches to this major collaborative effort taking place among scientists from diverse fields. Oda and Kastner bring us up-to-date with their descriptions of how emerging genomic technologies contribute to the advancements in understanding of the autoinflammatory diseases. Laufer and colleagues get right to the heart of the dilemma of how to translate genetic discovery into practice in their review of the relationship between initiation and perpetuation of chronic rheumatic diseases.

Finally, as a bonus for this issue, we were able to include an excellent discussion of the clinical dilemma facing patients and their doctors regarding safety risks when corticosteroids are administered in pregnancy for disease control. This article simply did not arrive to production soon enough to be included in the previous excellent issue, highly recommended, on reproductive health in the rheumatic diseases.

Michael H. Weisman, MD
Division of Rheumatology
Cedars-Sinai Medical Center
David Geffen School of Medicine at UCLA
8700 Beverly Boulevard
Los Angeles, CA 90024, USA

E-mail address:
Michael.Weisman@cshs.org

Preface

Genomics in Rheumatic Diseases: Hope for the Future

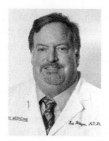
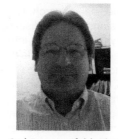

S. Louis Bridges, Jr., MD, PhD   Carl D. Langefeld, PhD
Editors

The more I learn, the more I realize how much I don't know.

This quote, attributed to Albert Einstein, is an apt way to begin this issue. The field of genomics seems to constantly expand and now includes genome sequence, functional and comparative genomic analyses, bioinformatics, epigenomics/epigenetics, gene expression, gene regulation (including microRNAs), and metagenomics. Concomitant with these advances, comprehending human biology through understanding the genetic material present in a cell or organism and how it works seems to become more formidable. However, through reductionist approaches, incremental gains provide optimism for better understanding of human diseases and their diagnosis, prevention, and treatment.

If one takes a "splitter" approach rather than a "lumper" approach, there are more than 100 rheumatic diseases, which include inflammatory conditions such as rheumatoid arthritis, autoimmune diseases such as systemic lupus erythematosus, metabolic diseases such as gout, and degenerative conditions such as osteoarthritis. A variety of phenotypes have been addressed using genomic approaches, including disease susceptibility, analysis of subphenotypes/clinical subsets, disease severity, treatment response (pharmacogenomics), and so forth. While genomics plays a role in almost all human diseases, much of the influence on development of rheumatic diseases is nongenetic, which encompasses environmental, lifestyle, diet, and random factors, which are exceedingly difficult to accurately measure and interpret.

In this issue, we address a selected subset of topics relevant to genomics in rheumatic diseases, in addition to the traditional discussion of associations between genes/loci and disease states. This includes focus on population genetics and natural selection; influences on disease severity and treatment response, the role of the major

Rheum Dis Clin N Am 43 (2017) xv–xvi
http://dx.doi.org/10.1016/j.rdc.2017.05.001
0889-857X/17/© 2017 Published by Elsevier Inc.

histocompatibility complex locus, drug repositioning strategies, and integrative approaches. Diseases that are discussed include rheumatoid arthritis, systemic lupus erythematosus, gout, ankylosing spondylitis, autoinflammatory diseases (which are typically monogenic), and juvenile idiopathic arthritis. We chose not to include several topics (scleroderma, osteoarthritis, psoriatic arthritis, inflammatory myositis, vasculitis, others) because of excellent recent reviews elsewhere in the medical literature, a paucity of high-quality data upon which to write a review, or page limitations in this issue.

Looking at recent trends in biomedical research, two underlying themes that have emerged as ways to better understand human disease seem antithetical: big data analysis (computational biology, systems biology, integrative biology, and so forth) and the emergence of single-cell technologies. While this issue does not address single-cell approaches per se, one article focuses on the use of integrative approaches to stratify pathologic genetic variants, and another focuses on the use of large datasets to identify new uses for existing drugs.

In summary, genome-based approaches can be incorporated into research designed to dissect how various elements work together to affect the human body in both health and disease. New findings help to focus on which questions to ask as well as on how to answer them. Genomics research can potentially lead to improved diagnostic tests, more effective strategies for disease management, and better decision-making tools for both health care providers and patients. We are hopeful that the question is not if, but when, we will cross the threshold of integrating results of genomics research in everyday practice of medicine.

We are very grateful to this issue's authors, who are leaders in the field of rheumatic diseases research. Their contributions have helped to greatly advance the field, and their perspectives have resulted in outstanding, informative articles.

S. Louis Bridges, Jr., MD, PhD
Division of Clinical Immunology and Rheumatology
Comprehensive Arthritis, Musculoskeletal, Bone
and Autoimmunity Center
University of Alabama at Birmingham
1720 Second Avenue South, SHEL 178
Birmingham, AL 35294-2182, USA

Carl D. Langefeld, PhD
Public Health Genomics and
Department of Biostatistical Sciences
Division of Public Health Sciences
Wake Forest School of Medicine
Winston-Salem, NC 27157, USA

E-mail addresses:
LBridges@uab.edu (S.L. Bridges, Jr.)
clangefe@wakehealth.edu (C.D. Langefeld)

Population Genetics and Natural Selection in Rheumatic Disease

Paula S. Ramos, PhD[a,b,*]

KEYWORDS

- Rheumatic diseases • Population genetics • Natural selection • Genetic variation
- Genetic disease association • Genetic diversity • Adaptation • Genetic disease risk

KEY POINTS

- If untreated, rheumatic diseases can diminish reproductive potential and impair the ability to raise offspring that successfully reproduce. Thus, it is likely that the frequency of disease-risk alleles seen in populations around the world is influenced by population-specific natural selection.
- Both autoimmune and nonautoimmune rheumatic disorders show genetic associations in regions with signatures of selection.
- The prevalence of rheumatic disease may result, at least partially, from past events of selection that increased host resistance to infection.
- Many of the complexities of gene effects in different rheumatic diseases can be explained by population genetics phenomena.

INTRODUCTION

Rheumatic diseases are a family of more than 100 chronic, and often disabling, illnesses characterized by inflammation and loss of function, especially in the joints, tendons, ligaments, bones, and muscles. They collectively affect more than 20% of US adults, with osteoarthritis, rheumatoid arthritis (RA), spondylarthritides, gout,

Disclosure Statement: The author has nothing to disclose.
Conflict of Interest: The authors declare no conflict of interest.
This study was supported by the US National Institute of Arthritis and Musculoskeletal and Skin Diseases of the National Institutes of Health (NIH) under Award Numbers K01 AR067280, R03 AR065801, and P60 AR062755. The content is solely the responsibility of the author and does not necessarily represent the official views of NIH.
[a] Division of Rheumatology and Immunology, Department of Medicine, Medical University of South Carolina, 96 Jonathan Lucas Street, Suite 816, Charleston, SC 29425, USA; [b] Department of Public Health Sciences, Medical University of South Carolina, Charleston, SC, USA
* Division of Rheumatology and Immunology, Department of Medicine, Medical University of South Carolina, 96 Jonathan Lucas Street, Suite 816, Charleston, SC 29425.
E-mail address: ramosp@musc.edu

and fibromyalgia being the most prevalent.[1,2] Patients often endure lifelong debilitating symptoms, reduced productivity at work, and high medical expenses. Arthritis and related illnesses, as well as back or spine problems, are major causes of disability.[3] Importantly, because many rheumatic diseases present before or during a woman's reproductive years, they can have effects on fetal and maternal outcomes,[4] such as pregnancy loss in women with systemic lupus erythematosus (SLE)[4,5] and vasculitis,[4] and infertility in women with RA.[5]

Most rheumatic diseases exhibit marked gender and ethnic disparities. Most predominately afflict women (eg, RA, SLE, systemic sclerosis, fibromyalgia), but spondyloarthropathies and gout are more common in men.[6] African American individuals are at higher risk than European American individuals for SLE and systemic sclerosis, which they tend to develop earlier in life and experience more severe disease.[7] Despite the variation in prevalence, incidence, and disease severity that are known to vary among ethnic groups, little is known about the genetic etiology of these diseases in the different populations and the reasons for the ethnic disparities remain elusive.

Left untreated, most rheumatic diseases can affect the ability to raise offspring that successfully reproduce and result in reduced reproductive fitness. Thus, alternative forces must exist that permit the relative high frequency of risk alleles. Because immune and inflammatory responses can be highly sensitive to environmental change,[8] evolutionary adaptation to specific environments might have driven selection on immune-related genetic variants, impacting variant frequencies and leaving signatures of selection in the genome. Given that infectious organisms are strong agents of natural selection,[9,10] it is plausible that alleles selected for protection against infection confer increased risk of autoimmune and inflammatory diseases, as the "hygiene hypothesis"[11] postulates. It is thought that the adaptation to pathogen pressure through functional variation in immune-related genes conferred a specific selective advantage for host survival, including protection from pathogens and tolerance to microbiota.[12] However, the emergence of such variation conferring resistance to pathogens is also influencing immune and inflammatory disease risk in specific populations.

In the past decade, multiple genome scans for signatures of selection on common variation have identified many immune-related loci.[13–17] Similarly, 90 genome-wide association studies (GWAS) (**Table 1**) have established rheumatic disease–associated alleles. There is also growing evidence that autoimmune and inflammatory disease–associated variants are under selection.[17–21] This review expands on our previous work[22] and summarizes the evidence for rheumatic disease–associated loci under selection and the candidate selective pressures. Given that genomic variation can have clinically important consequences,[23] elucidating the patterns of variation and the functional role of the selective pressure might contribute to a better understanding of disease etiology and the development of new therapies for improved disease management.

SHARED GENETIC ETIOLOGY IN RHEUMATIC DISEASES

The family of rheumatic diseases is remarkable for its heterogeneity and similar underlying mechanisms. The genetic heritability of rheumatic diseases is extremely variable, ranging from very high in ankylosing spondylitis (AS) to almost negligible in systemic sclerosis.[24] GWAS have proved particularly powerful for autoimmune diseases,[25] including many autoimmune rheumatic diseases, which might be due to their immune and inflammatory genetic etiology. **Table 1** summarizes the rheumatic diseases with published GWAS and the number of disease-associated loci uncovered from these GWAS.

The common genetic etiology is exemplified by the sharing of associated loci among rheumatic diseases, such as the Human Leukocyte Antigen (*HLA*), *STAT4*,

Table 1
Rheumatic diseases with published genome-wide association studies (GWAS) and respective number of associated loci

Rheumatic Disease	Number of	
	GWAS	Loci
ANCA-associated vasculitis (AAV)	1	18
Ankylosing spondylitis (AS)	3	21
Behçet disease (BD)	5	9
Dermatomyositis (DM)	1	1
Gout	4	14
Granulomatosis with polyangiitis (GPA)	1	6
Juvenile idiopathic arthritis (JIA)	3	6
Kawasaki disease (KD)	6	16
Osteoarthritis (OA)	9	16
Osteoporosis (OP)	3	3
Paget disease (PD)	2	9
Psoriasis (PS)	11	60
Psoriatic arthritis (PsA)	2	4
Rheumatoid arthritis (RA)	19	129
Sjögren's syndrome (SS)	1	4
Systemic lupus erythematosus (SLE)	16	124
Systemic sclerosis (SScl)	3	10

Numbers compiled from the NHGRI-EBI Catalog of Published Genome-Wide Association Studies (https://www.ebi.ac.uk/gwas). Accessed October 24, 2016.[46]

TNIP1, TNFAIP3, and *BLK*.[26] This sharing of risk loci is greater among the groups of diseases characterized by the presence of particular serum autoantibodies (seropositive; such as RA, SLE) than it is between the seropositive and seronegative diseases (those typically characterized as not having associated serum autoantibodies).[26] This supports the consensus that there is a common genetic background predisposing to autoimmunity and inflammation, and that further combinations of more serologically defined and disease-specific variation at *HLA* and non-*HLA* genes, in interaction with epigenetic and environmental factors, contribute to disease and its clinical manifestations. It has been suggested that different population genetic factors (eg, natural selection with coevolution with pathogens, random mutation, isolations, migrations, and interbreeding) in similar or distinct environments led to the establishment of the current plethora of loci that predispose to autoimmunity.[27] It is thus plausible that population-level phenomena are a reason behind the complexity of gene effects in different autoimmune and rheumatic diseases.

POPULATION GENETICS, NATURAL SELECTION, AND ADAPTATION

The genetic basis of disease is influenced by individual and population variation. Population-level phenomena, such as mutation, migration, genetic drift, and natural selection, have left an imprint on genetic variation that is likely to influence phenotypic expression in specific populations.[23] Given its role in driving genetic variation, population genetics can help elucidate human genetic diversity and, consequently, disease etiology.

Natural selection is the process by which a trait becomes either more or less common in a population depending on the differential reproductive success of those with the trait. Natural selection drives *adaptation*, the evolutionary process whereby over generations the members of a population become better suited to survive and reproduce in that environment. N*egative (or purifying) selection* is the most common mechanism of selection, usually associated with rare Mendelian disorders. *Positive selection* increases the prevalence of adaptive traits by increasing the frequency of favorable alleles and is often associated with common complex traits.[28] The enrichment for signals of positive selection among genes associated with complex traits is well documented.[14,29–31] *Balancing selection* favors genetic diversity by retaining variation in the population as a result of heterozygote advantage and frequency-dependent advantage. Despite rarer, a pertinent example is the *HLA* (also known as major histocompatibility complex (*MHC*)) region,[32,33] where highly polymorphic loci play a central role in the recognition and presentation of antigens to the immune system. The high levels of polymorphism are the results of pathogen-driven balancing selection.[34] The heterozygote advantage against multiple pathogens contributes to the evolution of HLA diversity, which in turn confers resistance against multiple pathogens and explains the persistence of alleles conferring susceptibility to disease.[35] Nevertheless, there is also recent evidence that positive selection might be acting on specific HLA alleles in a local population due to unique environmental pressures.[36]

Natural selection leaves a distinctive molecular signature in the targeted genomic region, and different statistical methods have been developed to detect signatures of selection.[12] It has been hypothesized by Klironomos and colleagues[37] that, in addition to genetic (sequence) variation, heritable epigenetic modifications can affect rates of fitness increase, as well as patterns of genotypic and phenotypic change during adaptation. However, the role of epigenetic variation in the response to natural selection has not been formally assessed, as the methodology to test signatures of natural selection on epigenetic variation is just emerging.[38]

NATURAL SELECTION IN RHEUMATIC DISEASE

Given that, if untreated, rheumatic diseases can diminish reproductive potential and impair the ability to raise offspring that successfully reproduce, some evolutionary process must sustain the relative high frequency of risk alleles seen in current populations around the world. Because the human genome is shaped by adaptation to environmental pressures at the population level, one plausible reason for the higher frequency of disease-risk alleles may be the direct effect of population-specific natural selection. This hypothesis is supported by the experimental evidence for MHC heterozygote superiority against multiple pathogens, a mechanism that would contribute to the evolution of HLA diversity and explain the persistence of alleles conferring susceptibility to disease.[35]

There is compelling evidence that natural selection is acting on a significant fraction of the human genome.[15,39–43] Immune function genes and pathways are consistently reported in tests for natural selection. As a result of several genome-wide scans, more than 300 immune-related genes have been suggested as putative targets of positive selection.[13–17] Although the challenge in validating the true signals remains,[44] several genes involved in immune-related functions have been shown to be under selection.[20,45]

A total of 61 regions with evidence for selection and association with at least one rheumatic disease are shown in **Table 2**. This table includes 35 regions previously

Table 2
Rheumatic disease regions with evidence for selection and implicated agents of selection

Gene Region	Position	Rheumatic Disease Association	References for Evidence of Natural Selection	Population	Selective Pressure	References for Pathogen-Driven Selection
TNFRSF14, MMEL1*	1p36.32	RA		YRI		
IL23R	1p31.3	AS	18		Protozoa	53
MAGI3, PTPN22*	1p13.2	RA, SLE	19,20	YRI	Protozoa	53
FCGR2B	1q23.3	SLE	57		Plasmodium falciparum	57
TNFSF4	1q25.1	RA, SS, SLE	19			
NCF2, RGL1*	1q25.3	SLE		ASI		
CR1	1q32	SLE	65		Plasmodium falciparum	65
TLR5	1q41-q42	SLE	20	YRI	Salmonella enterica ser. Typhimurium and other exposures	20
PELI1*	2p14	KD		ASI		
ALMS1P, DGUOK*	2p13.1	SLE	19	CEU		
PARD3B*	2q33.3	OA	20	CEU		
CNTN6*	3p26.3	SLE		ASI		
XCR1, CCR3*	3p21.31	BD		YRI		
CCDC66, ARHGEF3	3p14.3	RA	20	YRI		
BTLA	3q13.2	RA		ASI		
ARHGAP31, CD80	3q13.33	JIA, SLE	21	YRI		
MRPS22*	3q23	KD	20	ASI		
SLC2A9*	4p16.1	Gout		YRI		
KCNIP4*	4p15.2	RA	20	CEU, YRI		
TECRL*	4q13.1	KD		CEU		
ANTRX2	4q21	AS	21			

(continued on next page)

Table 2
(continued)

Gene Region	Position	Rheumatic Disease Association	References for Evidence of Natural Selection	Population	Selective Pressure	References for Pathogen-Driven Selection
IL2, IL21*	4q27	RA	21,47	YRI		
Intergenic*	4q28.3	SLE		ASI		
PTGER4	5p13.1	AS	21,53		Protozoa	53
COMMD10, SEMA6A*	5q23.1	GPA		ASI, CEU		
ALDH7A1*	5q23.2	OP		CEU		
TNIP1	5q33.1	SLE, SScl, PsA	19			
PTTG1	5q33.3	SLE	19			
IRF4*	6p25.3	RA		CEU		
ITPR3	6p21.31	SLE	20	YRI		
HLA*	6p22.1- 6p21.32	AAV, AS, BD, GPA, JIA, KD, OA, PS, PsA, RA, SS, SLE, SScl	20,21,66-69	ASI, CEU, YRI	Bacterial infection	34,54,55
SNRPC, UHRF1BP1*	6p21.31	SLE	19-21	CEU	Mycobacterium tuberculosis	70
VARS, LSM2	6p21	SLE	21			
CCDC167, MIR4462*	6p21.2	SLE		YRI		
PRDM1, ATG5*	6q21	RA, SLE		YRI		
TRAF3IP2*	6q21	PS, PsA		YRI		
IKZF1	7p12.2	SLE	19			
GTF2I*	7q11.23	SS	20	ASI		
HIP1*	7q11.23	SLE	21	YRI		
LSMEM1, NPM1P14*	7q31.1	OA		ASI		
XKR6, BLK*	8p23.1	KD, RA, SS, SLE, SSc	19,20	ASI		
GRHL2*	8q22.3	RA		CEU		

Gene(s)	Cytoband	Disease	References	Infectious disease	Population
KDM4C*	9p24.1	SLE			ASI
NTNG2, SETX*	9q34.13	SLE	20		CEU
FAM171A1*	10p13	SLE			ASI
CTNNA3*	10q21.3	PsA			CEU
CD5	11q12.2	RA	71		
GRM5*	11q14.3	RA			CEU
OSBPL8*	12q21.2	SLE			CEU
SH2B3, NAA25	12q24.12-q24.13	RA	21,56	Bacterial infection[56]	
KIAA0391*	14q23.1	PS			ASI
PRKCH, HIF1A*	14q23.1	RA	20		CEU, YRI
CLEC16A, CIITA	16p13.13	RA, SLE	19,21,72		
ITGAM, ITGAX	16p11.2	SLE	19,20		
PRSS54*	16q21	SLE			YRI
WWOX	16q23.2	OA	20		CEU
IRF8	16q24.1	RA, SScl	73		
RABEP1, NUP88*	17p13.2	RA			CEU
BCAS3, NACA2*	17q23.2	Gout, OA	20		ASI
TYK2	19p13.2	RA, SLE	53	Protozoa[53]	
PAK7*	20p12.2	PS			YRI

Rheumatic disease associations were reported in the literature (column "references for evidence of natural selection"), and/or in the NHGRI-EBI GWAS Catalog accessed on October 24, 2016. In addition to the disease-associated regions with evidence for selection reported in the literature, rheumatic disease-associated loci from the GWAS catalog with evidence of recent positive selection from HapMap phase II data (assessed by the presence of at least 2 single-nucleotide polymorphisms within approximately 200 kb with an absolute integrated Haplotype Score value in the top 0.1% of the genome-wide distribution in one population) are also included and denoted by the asterisk. See **Table 1** for disease abbreviations.

Abbreviations: ASI, Asian; CEU, European; YRI, African populations.

reported as being under selection in the literature,[22] plus rheumatic disease–associated loci from current GWAS (in **Table 1**) and evidence of recent positive selection from HapMap phase II data.[15] Specifically, a region published in the GWAS Catalog[46] as associated with a rheumatic disease was considered as exhibiting evidence for natural selection if it contained at least 2 single-nucleotide polymorphisms (SNPs) within 200 kb with an absolute integrated Haplotype Score (iHS) value in the top 0.1% of the genome-wide distribution in one population (Asian, European, or African). A total of 39 regions that met these criteria are included in **Table 2**, 14 of which were previously reported. These 39 regions with evidence for selection represent approximately 10% of all regions associated with a rheumatic disease in a GWAS: 13% for SLE, 9% for RA, 7% for psoriasis (PS), and 5% for AS. This fraction of disease-associated loci with concomitant evidence for selection is higher than previous reports focusing on SNPs instead of regions. Notably, when using the top 1% of iHS variants, Raj and colleagues[21] reported that inflammatory diseases (which included AS, RA, and SLE) have 5% of SNPs targeted by positive selection. Limiting comparisons to SNPs instead of regions might miss regions with both evidence for disease association and selection at different SNPs. The numbers of GWAS-associated loci, including those with and without concomitant evidence for recent positive selection, are illustrated in **Fig. 1**. Among all regions in **Table 2**, a higher number of signals of selection were found in European (36%), followed by Asian (32%) and African (32%) populations. This is consistent with previous reports of enrichment of inflammatory disease SNPs targeted by positive selection in subjects of European ancestry.[21,47]

AGENTS OF SELECTION

The wide variety of environments inhabited by human populations is likely exerting different selective pressures that lead to adaptation through natural selection. Climatic factors, such as altitude, latitude, UV radiation levels, and temperature, as well as diet

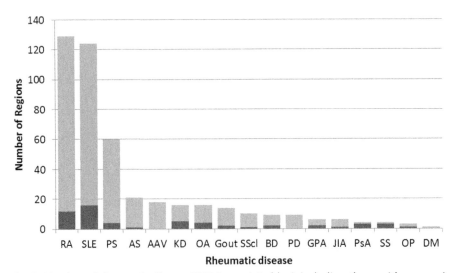

Fig. 1. Number of rheumatic disease GWAS-associated loci, including those with concomitant evidence for recent positive selection (*dark shaded area*). See **Table 1** for disease abbreviations.

and pathogens, have been reported as agents of selection driving adaptations to these environments and lifestyles. As recently reviewed,[22] some relevant examples include signals of natural selection driven by annual photoperiod variation reported for restless leg syndrome risk variants,[48] correlation between climate variables and SNPs involved in immune response, as well as pathways related to UV radiation, infection and immunity, and cancer,[49] and correlations between worldwide migration trajectories and variants associated with, among others, SLE and systemic sclerosis.[50] Interestingly, expression quantitative trait loci (eQTLs) (see Vincent A. Laufer and colleagues' article, "Integrative Approaches to Understanding the Pathogenic Role of Genetic Variation in Rheumatic Diseases," in this issue for definition) from immune function and metabolism genes are enriched in signals of environmental adaptation,[51] which highlights the importance of regulatory variations in local adaptation.

Nevertheless, the strongest effect of climate is in shaping the spatial pattern and species diversity of human pathogens,[9] which is directly relevant to immune and inflammatory disease predisposition. As recently reviewed,[52] in the constant coevolutionary battle between host and pathogen, pathogens that diminish reproductive potential, either through death or poor health, drive selection on genetic variants that affect pathogen resistance. As Hancock and colleagues[49] suggested, it is likely that selection signals in immune-related loci may implicate variants evolving under a model of antagonistic pleiotropy, where the selective pressure was pathogen resistance, and the inflammatory disorder is a pleiotropic consequence of the resistance allele. This could hence be a mechanism explaining the prevalence of immune risk alleles that are common in the population.

Indeed, pathogens have been the main selective pressure through human evolution.[10] In an analysis that included climate, diet regimes, and pathogen loads, Fumagalli and colleagues[10] showed that the diversity of the local pathogenic environment is the predominant driver of local adaptation, and that climate conditions only played a relatively minor role. In addition, they reported an enrichment of genes associated to SLE, RA, and AS, which supports the hypothesis that some susceptibility alleles for rheumatic diseases may be maintained in human population due to past selective processes.[10] The enrichment for signals of positive selection in inflammatory disease susceptibility loci has been recently corroborated.[21] Reviews of selection signatures left by pathogen-exerted pressure, including immune-related genes, can be found elsewhere.[52,53]

Genetic regions associated with susceptibility to different rheumatic diseases and evidence of selection that has been attributed to host-pathogen coevolution are shown in **Table 2**. In a fraction of the regions with evidence for selection and disease association, known pathogens have been implicated as the selective pressure. Variation in the *HLA* and *SH2B3* has been reported as a protective factor against bacterial infection.[34,54–56] Resistance to protozoa and tuberculosis infection has been implicated as the selective pressure for *PTPN22* and *UHRF1BP1*, respectively. Interestingly, the SLE susceptibility allele in *UHRF1BP1* is associated with decreased *UHRF1BP1* RNA expression in different cell subsets, suggesting that the disease-risk allele under selection has a regulatory effect.[21] In the context of SLE predisposing loci, Clatworthy and colleagues[57] have shown that *FCGR2B* is important in controlling the immune response to *Plasmodium falciparum*, the parasite responsible for the most severe form of malaria, and suggests that the higher frequency of human *FCGR2B* polymorphisms predisposing to SLE in Asian and African individuals may be maintained because these variants reduce susceptibility to malaria. Grossman and colleagues[20] implicated *Salmonella typhimurium* and other exposures that directionally drive selection of the Toll-like receptor 5 (TLR5) gene,[58] which is involved in recognition of flagellated bacteria. Unlike endosomal TLRs, such as TLR7 and TLR8, that have been subject to purifying selection, cell-surface TLRs involved in pathogen recognition experienced more relaxed constraints.[59] The nonsynonymous variant in PTPN22 shows complex signatures of selection, increasing the risk of SLE, RA, and other autoimmune diseases, but being protective against Crohn disease.[60] Karlsson and colleagues[61] recently reported that cholera has exerted strong selective pressure on proinflammatory pathways.

Despite the modest number of examples that offer clear functional hypotheses (eg, SH2B3, TRL5), collectively this list supports the hypothesis that the increased prevalence of rheumatic disease may result, at least partially, from past events of selection that increased host resistance to infection.[62]

SUMMARY

This review summarizes the genetic regions associated with susceptibility to different rheumatic diseases and concomitant evidence for selection, including known agents of selection exerting selective pressure in these regions. Uncovering these rheumatic disease–associated loci under selection underscores the importance of population genetics and how the understanding of human genetic diversity is crucial to understanding disease etiology or treatment response at both the population and individual levels.

A combination of population-level phenomena, including possibly bottlenecks, migration, admixture, natural selection, and random genetic drift, are likely contributors to this complexity of gene effects in different rheumatic diseases. Given the complex history of selective pressures acting on humans, unequal selective pressures and a diverse spectrum of plausible evolutionary models are expected to be exerted on susceptibility loci for rheumatic diseases.[28] It is likely that several pathogens have exerted pressure on the same loci and that selection can vary in form, intensity, time, and space, which is consistent with the observation that both risk and protective alleles for rheumatic diseases increased in frequency due to selection.[17] For most regions, the exact selective pressure leaving the signature of selection is unclear. Clearly, these signatures are not necessarily the result of adaptation, but might be a consequence of random genetic drift. In any case, regardless of the population phenomenon shaping current human genetic diversity, this genetic variation is the basis of clinically relevant traits at both the individual and population levels.[23]

An important next step to delineate the selective advantage conferred by these rheumatic disease-risk variants are functional studies using in vitro experiments and model organisms to identify the underlying functional variants and quantify the phenotypic consequences of the candidate adaptive alleles. Human-pathogen coevolution is ongoing and, despite the emergence of new pathogens (eg, human immunodeficiency virus), potential pathogens driving these host-specific adaptations are expected to have long-standing relationships with humans, including those that cause malaria, smallpox, cholera, tuberculosis, and leprosy,[63] as well as the human microbiome.[64] Regardless of the agent of selection and the reasons for the emergence of both common and rare rheumatic disease–causing alleles, incorporating population genetics to understand human genetic diversity will lead to a better understanding of the causes of health disparities, identification of functional variants and discovery of cellular mechanisms, and contribute to the development of new therapies.

REFERENCES

1. Helmick CG, Felson DT, Lawrence RC, et al. Estimates of the prevalence of arthritis and other rheumatic conditions in the United States. Part I. Arthritis Rheum 2008;58(1):15–25.
2. Lawrence RC, Felson DT, Helmick CG, et al. Estimates of the prevalence of arthritis and other rheumatic conditions in the United States. Part II. Arthritis Rheum 2008;58(1):26–35.
3. CDC. Prevalence and most common causes of disability among adults—United States, 2005. MMWR Morb Mortal Wkly Rep 2009;58:421–6. Available at: https://www.cdc.gov/mmwr/preview/mmwrhtml/mm5816a2.htm.
4. Ostensen M, Andreoli L, Brucato A, et al. State of the art: reproduction and pregnancy in rheumatic diseases. Autoimmun Rev 2015;14(5):376–86.
5. Clowse ME, Chakravarty E, Costenbader KH, et al. Effects of infertility, pregnancy loss, and patient concerns on family size of women with rheumatoid arthritis and systemic lupus erythematosus. Arthritis Care Res 2012;64(5):668–74.
6. NIH. Arthritis and Rheumatic Diseases. National Institutes of Health Publication No. 14–4999. 2014. Available at: http://www.niams.nih.gov/Health_Info/Arthritis/arthritis_rheumatic.pdf.
7. NIH. Progress in Autoimmune Diseases Research. National Institutes of Health Publication No. 05-514. 2005. Available at: www.niaid.nih.gov/topics/autoimmune/documents/adccfinal.pdf.
8. Okin D, Medzhitov R. Evolution of inflammatory diseases. Curr Biol 2012;22(17):R733–40.
9. Guernier V, Hochberg ME, Guegan JF. Ecology drives the worldwide distribution of human diseases. PLoS Biol 2004;2(6):e141.
10. Fumagalli M, Sironi M, Pozzoli U, et al. Signatures of environmental genetic adaptation pinpoint pathogens as the main selective pressure through human evolution. PLoS Genet 2011;7(11):e1002355.
11. Strachan DP. Hay fever, hygiene, and household size. BMJ 1989;299(6710):1259–60.
12. Quintana-Murci L, Clark AG. Population genetic tools for dissecting innate immunity in humans. Nature reviews. Immunology 2013;13(4):280–93.
13. Pickrell JK, Coop G, Novembre J, et al. Signals of recent positive selection in a worldwide sample of human populations. Genome Res 2009;19(5):826–37.
14. Sabeti PC, Varilly P, Fry B, et al. Genome-wide detection and characterization of positive selection in human populations. Nature 2007;449(7164):913–8.
15. Voight BF, Kudaravalli S, Wen X, et al. A map of recent positive selection in the human genome. PLoS Biol 2006;4(3):e72.
16. Barreiro LB, Laval G, Quach H, et al. Natural selection has driven population differentiation in modern humans. Nat Genet 2008;40(3):340–5.
17. Barreiro LB, Quintana-Murci L. From evolutionary genetics to human immunology: how selection shapes host defence genes. Nat Rev Genet 2010;11(1):17–30.
18. Jostins L, Ripke S, Weersma RK, et al. Host-microbe interactions have shaped the genetic architecture of inflammatory bowel disease. Nature 2012;491(7422):119–24.
19. Ramos PS, Shaftman SR, Ward RC, et al. Genes associated with SLE are targets of recent positive selection. Autoimmune Dis 2014;2014:203435.
20. Grossman SR, Andersen KG, Shlyakhter I, et al. Identifying recent adaptations in large-scale genomic data. Cell 2013;152(4):703–13.

21. Raj T, Kuchroo M, Replogle JM, et al. Common risk alleles for inflammatory diseases are targets of recent positive selection. Am J Hum Genet 2013;92(4): 517–29.
22. Ramos PS, Shedlock AM, Langefeld CD. Genetics of autoimmune diseases: insights from population genetics. J Hum Genet 2015;60(11):657–64.
23. Torkamani A, Pham P, Libiger O, et al. Clinical implications of human population differences in genome-wide rates of functional genotypes. Front Genet 2012;3:211.
24. Selmi C, Lu Q, Humble MC. Heritability versus the role of the environment in autoimmunity. J Autoimmun 2012;39(4):249–52.
25. Hu X, Daly M. What have we learned from six years of GWAS in autoimmune diseases, and what is next? Curr Opin Immunol 2012;24(5):571–5.
26. Kirino Y, Remmers EF. Genetic architectures of seropositive and seronegative rheumatic diseases. Nature reviews. Rheumatology 2015;11(7):401–14.
27. Ramos PS, Criswell LA, Moser KL, et al. A comprehensive analysis of shared loci between systemic lupus erythematosus (SLE) and sixteen autoimmune diseases reveals limited genetic overlap. PLoS Genet 2011;7(12):e1002406.
28. Di Rienzo A. Population genetics models of common diseases. Curr Opin Genet Dev 2006;16(6):630–6.
29. Bustamante CD, Fledel-Alon A, Williamson S, et al. Natural selection on protein-coding genes in the human genome. Nature 2005;437(7062):1153–7.
30. Blekhman R, Man O, Herrmann L, et al. Natural selection on genes that underlie human disease susceptibility. Curr Biol 2008;18(12):883–9.
31. Torgerson DG, Boyko AR, Hernandez RD, et al. Evolutionary processes acting on candidate cis- regulatory regions in humans inferred from patterns of polymorphism and divergence. PLoS Genet 2009;5(8):e1000592.
32. Andres AM, Hubisz MJ, Indap A, et al. Targets of balancing selection in the human genome. Mol Biol Evol 2009;26(12):2755–64.
33. Gineau L, Luisi P, Castelli EC, et al. Balancing immunity and tolerance: genetic footprint of natural selection in the transcriptional regulatory region of HLA-G. Genes Immun 2015;16(1):57–70.
34. Prugnolle F, Manica A, Charpentier M, et al. Pathogen-driven selection and worldwide HLA class I diversity. Curr Biol 2005;15(11):1022–7.
35. McClelland EE, Penn DJ, Potts WK. Major histocompatibility complex heterozygote superiority during coinfection. Infect Immun 2003;71(4):2079–86.
36. Kawashima M, Ohashi J, Nishida N, et al. Evolutionary analysis of classical HLA class I and II genes suggests that recent positive selection acted on DPB1*04:01 in Japanese population. PLoS One 2012;7(10):e46806.
37. Klironomos FD, Berg J, Collins S. How epigenetic mutations can affect genetic evolution: model and mechanism. BioEssays 2013;35(6):571–8.
38. Wang J, Fan C. A neutrality test for detecting selection on DNA methylation using single methylation polymorphism frequency spectrum. Genome Biol Evol 2015; 7(1):154–71.
39. Eberle MA, Rieder MJ, Kruglyak L, et al. Allele frequency matching between SNPs reveals an excess of linkage disequilibrium in genic regions of the human genome. PLoS Genet 2006;2(9):e142.
40. Sabeti PC, Reich DE, Higgins JM, et al. Detecting recent positive selection in the human genome from haplotype structure. Nature 2002;419(6909):832–7.
41. Smith JM, Haigh J. The hitch-hiking effect of a favourable gene. Genet Res 1974; 23(1):23–35.
42. Williamson SH, Hubisz MJ, Clark AG, et al. Localizing recent adaptive evolution in the human genome. PLoS Genet 2007;3(6):e90.

43. Gulko B, Hubisz MJ, Gronau I, et al. A method for calculating probabilities of fitness consequences for point mutations across the human genome. Nat Genet 2015;47(3):276–83.

44. Akey JM. Constructing genomic maps of positive selection in humans: where do we go from here? Genome Res 2009;19(5):711–22.

45. Fumagalli M, Cagliani R, Pozzoli U, et al. Widespread balancing selection and pathogen-driven selection at blood group antigen genes. Genome Res 2009; 19(2):199–212.

46. Hindorff LA, MacArthur J, Morales J, et al. A catalog of published genome-wide association studies. Available at: https://www.ebi.ac.uk/gwas. Accessed October 24, 2016.

47. Brinkworth JF, Barreiro LB. The contribution of natural selection to present-day susceptibility to chronic inflammatory and autoimmune disease. Curr Opin Immunol 2014;31:66–78.

48. Forni D, Pozzoli U, Cagliani R, et al. Genetic adaptation of the human circadian clock to day-length latitudinal variations and relevance for affective disorders. Genome Biol 2014;15(10):499.

49. Hancock AM, Witonsky DB, Alkorta-Aranburu G, et al. Adaptations to climate-mediated selective pressures in humans. PLoS Genet 2011;7(4):e1001375.

50. Corona E, Chen R, Sikora M, et al. Analysis of the genetic basis of disease in the context of worldwide human relationships and migration. PLoS Genet 2013;9(5): e1003447.

51. Ye K, Lu J, Raj SM, et al. Human expression QTLs are enriched in signals of environmental adaptation. Genome Biol Evol 2013;5(9):1689–701.

52. Karlsson EK, Kwiatkowski DP, Sabeti PC. Natural selection and infectious disease in human populations. Nat Rev Genet 2014;15(6):379–93.

53. Cagliani R, Sironi M. Pathogen-driven selection in the human genome. Int J Evol Biol 2013;2013:204240.

54. Hughes AL, Nei M. Pattern of nucleotide substitution at major histocompatibility complex class I loci reveals overdominant selection. Nature 1988;335(6186): 167–70.

55. Qutob N, Balloux F, Raj T, et al. Signatures of historical demography and pathogen richness on MHC class I genes. Immunogenetics 2012;64(3):165–75.

56. Zhernakova A, Elbers CC, Ferwerda B, et al. Evolutionary and functional analysis of celiac risk loci reveals SH2B3 as a protective factor against bacterial infection. Am J Hum Genet 2010;86(6):970–7.

57. Clatworthy MR, Willcocks L, Urban B, et al. Systemic lupus erythematosus-associated defects in the inhibitory receptor FcgammaRIIb reduce susceptibility to malaria. Proc Natl Acad Sci U S A 2007;104(17):7169–74.

58. Hawn TR, Wu H, Grossman JM, et al. A stop codon polymorphism of Toll-like receptor 5 is associated with resistance to systemic lupus erythematosus. Proc Natl Acad Sci U S A 2005;102(30):10593–7.

59. Barreiro LB, Ben-Ali M, Quach H, et al. Evolutionary dynamics of human Toll-like receptors and their different contributions to host defense. PLoS Genet 2009;5(7): e1000562.

60. Parkes M, Cortes A, van Heel DA, et al. Genetic insights into common pathways and complex relationships among immune-mediated diseases. Nat Rev Genet 2013;14(9):661–73.

61. Karlsson EK, Harris JB, Tabrizi S, et al. Natural selection in a Bangladeshi population from the cholera-endemic Ganges River Delta. Sci Transl Med 2013;5(192): 192ra186.

62. Sironi M, Clerici M. The hygiene hypothesis: an evolutionary perspective. Microbes Infect 2010;12(6):421–7.
63. Anderson RM, May RM. Coevolution of hosts and parasites. Parasitology 1982; 85(Pt 2):411–26.
64. Honda K, Littman DR. The microbiome in infectious disease and inflammation. Annu Rev Immunol 2012;30:759–95.
65. Cockburn IA, Mackinnon MJ, O'Donnell A, et al. A human complement receptor 1 polymorphism that reduces *Plasmodium falciparum* rosetting confers protection against severe malaria. Proc Natl Acad Sci U S A 2004;101(1):272–7.
66. Cagliani R, Riva S, Pozzoli U, et al. Balancing selection is common in the extended MHC region but most alleles with opposite risk profile for autoimmune diseases are neutrally evolving. BMC Evol Biol 2011;11:171.
67. Black FL, Hedrick PW. Strong balancing selection at HLA loci: evidence from segregation in South Amerindian families. Proc Natl Acad Sci U S A 1997; 94(23):12452–6.
68. Liu X, Fu Y, Liu Z, et al. An ancient balanced polymorphism in a regulatory region of human major histocompatibility complex is retained in Chinese minorities but lost worldwide. Am J Hum Genet 2006;78(3):393–400.
69. Tan Z, Shon AM, Ober C. Evidence of balancing selection at the HLA-G promoter region. Hum Mol Genet 2005;14(23):3619–28.
70. Barreiro LB, Tailleux L, Pai AA, et al. Deciphering the genetic architecture of variation in the immune response to *Mycobacterium tuberculosis* infection. Proc Natl Acad Sci U S A 2012;109(4):1204–9.
71. Carnero-Montoro E, Bonet L, Engelken J, et al. Evolutionary and functional evidence for positive selection at the human CD5 immune receptor gene. Mol Biol Evol 2012;29(2):811–23.
72. Swanberg M, Lidman O, Padyukov L, et al. MHC2TA is associated with differential MHC molecule expression and susceptibility to rheumatoid arthritis, multiple sclerosis and myocardial infarction. Nat Genet 2005;37(5):486–94.
73. Choudhury A, Hazelhurst S, Meintjes A, et al. Population-specific common SNPs reflect demographic histories and highlight regions of genomic plasticity with functional relevance. BMC Genomics 2014;15:437.

Genomics, Biology, and Human Illness
Advances in the Monogenic Autoinflammatory Diseases

Hirotsugu Oda, MD, PhD[a,b,*], Daniel L. Kastner, MD, PhD[c]

KEYWORDS

- Haploinsufficiency of A20 (HA20) • Otulipenia • Deficiency of ADA2 (DADA2)
- Interferonopathy • CANDLE/PRAAS • SAVI • NLRC4 inflammasome
- Pyrin inflammasome

KEY POINTS

- Two deubiquitinase (DUB) deficiencies, haploinsufficiency of A20 (HA20) and otulipenia, derive from the impairment of the negative regulation in immune signaling.
- Deficiency of adenosine deaminase 2 (DADA2) results in clinical manifestations, including recurrent lacunar strokes, polyarteritis nodosa (PAN)-like vasculitis, hypogammaglobulinemia, Diamond-Blackfan anemia, and bone marrow failure.
- Stimulator of interferon genes (STING)-associated vasculopathy with onset in infancy (SAVI) is characterized by severe dermatologic and pulmonary lesions.
- Clinical features of NLRC4-related autoinflammatory syndromes vary from cold-induced fever to chronic central nervous system inflammation or macrophage activation syndrome (MAS).
- RhoA GTPase suppresses the pyrin inflammasome by stimulating pyrin phosphorylation, which in turn favors the binding of inhibitory 14-3-3 proteins to pyrin. Certain bacterial toxins inactivate RhoA and thereby derepress the pyrin inflammasome. Mutations in *MEFV*, encoding pyrin, and *MVK*, encoding mevalonate kinase, predispose to autoinflammatory disease (AID) by decreasing 14-3-3 interaction with pyrin.

Disclosure Statement: This work is supported by the Intramural Research Program of the NHGRI, and Dr H. Oda is supported by JSPS Postdoctoral Fellowships for Research Abroad.
[a] Inflammatory Disease Section, Intramural Research Program, Metabolic, Cardiovascular and Inflammatory Disease Genomics Branch, National Human Genome Research Institute, National Institutes of Health, Building 10, Room B3-4129, Bethesda, MD 20892, USA; [b] Department of Pediatrics, Kitano Hospital, Tazuke Kofukai Medical Research Institute, 2-4-20, Ohgimachi, Kita-ku, Osaka 530-8480, Japan; [c] Inflammatory Disease Section, Intramural Research Program, Metabolic, Cardiovascular and Inflammatory Disease Genomics Branch, National Human Genome Research Institute, National Institutes of Health, Building 50, Room 5222, Bethesda, MD 20892, USA
* Corresponding author.
E-mail address: hirotsugu.oda@nih.gov

INTRODUCTION

Autoinflammatory diseases (AID) are a group of disorders characterized by seemingly unprovoked inflammation that may be recurrent or sometimes nearly continuous. The term, *autoinflammatory*, first appeared in the literature in 1999 to describe 2 monogenic disorders with recurrent fevers and episodes of systemic inflammation without high-titer autoantibodies or antigen-specific T cells: familial Mediterranean fever (FMF) and the then newly described TNF receptor–associated periodic syndrome.[1] At present more than 20 monogenic AID have been reported. The clinical manifestations of AID are typically driven by genetically determined dysregulation of innate immunity, which results in overproduction of inflammatory cytokines, such as interleukin (IL)-1β, IL-6, IL-18, tumor necrosis factor (TNF), and type I interferon (IFN). Specific treatments targeting these cytokine signaling pathways have proved effective in many AID patients, highlighting the importance of accurate genetic diagnosis and detailed molecular pathophysiology.

This article reviews some of the recent advances in the field of AID over the past 3 years, including the discovery of several newly identified monogenic disorders (**Table 1**). It also focuses on recent insights into the pathogenesis of FMF to demonstrate how genetics and basic biology have synergized to demystify one important mechanism of host-pathogen interaction.

THE DEUBIQUITINASE DEFICIENCIES

NF-κB denotes a group of transcription factors that regulate the expression of genes involved in the cell cycle, immune response, differentiation, and DNA repair. This signaling pathway is in part regulated by ubiquitination, a protein post-transcriptional modification process.[2,3] The DUBs are a group of enzymes that specifically remove ubiquitin (Ub) moieties from target proteins, and their dysregulation has been reported to result in various human diseases.[4] Several DUBs, including A20, CYLD, OTULIN, and OTUD7B (Cezanne), act as negative regulators of NF-κB signaling.[2] Prior to 2016, CYLD was the only DUB for which germline mutations had been implicated in a Mendelian human disease.[5]

Haploinsufficiency of A20

A20 is a DUB that plays a key inhibitory role in the NF-κB proinflammatory pathway. The inhibitory function of A20 is coordinately effected by its N-terminal ovarian tumor (OTU) domain-mediated DUB activity and by its C-terminal zinc finger-mediated E3 Ub ligase activity. Thus, A20 removes lysine 63 (K63)-linked Ub chains from proinflammatory signaling complexes, leading to their disassembly, and then conjugates the constituent proteins with lysine 48 (K48)-linked Ub chains, marking them for proteasomal degradation. Hence, the net effect of A20 is anti-inflammatory and a deficiency of A20 is predicted to cause unchecked inflammation.

In 2016, Zhou and colleagues[6] reported 6 families with dominantly inherited truncating mutations in the *TNFAIP3* gene, which encodes A20. Clinical manifestations included early-onset fevers, arthralgia, oral and genital ulcers, and ocular inflammation, in some cases resembling Behçet disease. Five of the mutations were in the OTU domain, whereas 1 was in a zinc finger domain. Mutant A20 demonstrated no inhibitory effect on the NF-κB pathway, whereas a mixture of wild-type and mutant A20 had substantial inhibitory activity, suggesting that the mutant proteins are likely to act through haploinsufficiency rather than a dominant-negative effect. In vitro reconstitution experiments showed accumulation of K63-Ub on RIPK1, one of the A20 substrates, an effect that was also confirmed in patients' cells. Patients'

Table 1
Newly identified monogenic autoinflammatory disorders

Disease	Gene	Protein	Phenotypes	Disease Mechanism
HA20	TNFAIP3	A20	• Fever, arthralgia, ulcers (oral and genital), and ocular inflammation	HA20 leads to exacerbated NF-κB signaling and NLRP3 inflammasome activation
Otulipenia/OTULIN-related autoinflammatory syndrome	OTULIN	OTULIN	• Fever, neutrophilic dermatosis, lipodystrophy, arthralgia, diarrhea, and failure to thrive	Loss of OTULIN leads to impaired removal of linear Ub from proinflammatory signaling complexes
DADA2	CECR1	ADA2	• Fever • Lacunar strokes • Livedo racemosa, ulceration, myalgia • Hepatosplenomegaly, lymphadenopathy • Renal hypertension, aneurysm • Portal hypertension • Anemia, thrombocytopenia, hypogammaglobulinemia	Reduced serum level of ADA2 resulting in: • Polarization of macrophages toward M1 (proinflammatory) subsets over M2 (anti-inflammatory) • Abnormal neutrophil activation • Impaired endothelial development • Impaired B-cell differentiation
SAVI	TMEM173	STING	• Fever • Skin lesions (rash, skin nodules, gangrenous lesions leading to amputation, nail dystrophy/loss, and nasal septum perforation) • Interstitial lung disease with inflammatory infiltrate, fibrosis, emphysematous changes	Gain-of-function in STING leads to the constitutive activation of IFN-β signaling
CANDLE	PSMB8 PSMB4 PSMA3 PSMB9 POMP	β5i β7 α7 β1i POMP	• Fever, panniculitis, chilblains, lipodystrophy, arthropathy, and brain calcification	Defects in proteasome formation, also associated with up-regulation of type I IFN
NLRC4-related autoinflammatory syndromes	NLRC4	NLRC4	• Fever, enterocolitis, splenomegaly, and MAS (NLRC4-MAS) • Cold-induced fever and urticaria (FCAS-like) • Fever, rash, arthralgia, chronic meningitis, brain atrophy, and sensorineural hearing loss (NOMID-like)	Gain-of-function in NLRC4 leads to abnormal activation of NLRC4 inflammasome, resulting in aberrant production of IL-1β and IL-18, and dysregulation of pyroptotic cell death

peripheral blood mononuclear cells and fibroblasts also demonstrated strong phosphorylation of IκBα, IKKα/β, and p38 with and without TNF stimulation, consistent with constitutive NF-κB activity. Spontaneous NLRP3 inflammasome activation leading to IL-1β release was observed in peripheral blood mononuclear cells, and 1 of the patients showed a good clinical response to IL-1β inhibition, consistent with previous reports suggesting the role of A20 as a negative regulator of the NLRP3 inflammasome in mice.[7,8] Zhou and colleagues dubbed this novel Mendelian disease, HA20 (**Fig. 1A**).

Recent studies suggest an essential role of A20 in the development and appropriate regulation of immune cells, and its dysregulation has been linked to various human diseases. Common nucleotide variants in TNFAIP3 have been associated with multiple autoimmune diseases, including systemic lupus erythematosus (SLE), type I diabetes, inflammatory bowel disease, ankylosing arthritis, Sjögren syndrome, and rheumatoid arthritis.[9] Furthermore, somatic loss-of-function mutations in A20 have been described in B-cell lymphoma, which suggests its role as a tumor-suppressor gene.[10] Complete loss of A20 in mice (Tnfaip3$^{-/-}$) resulted in early lethality due to persistent NF-κB activation and severe multiorgan inflammation,[11] whereas immune cell–specific ablation resulted in autoimmunity, such as SLE.[12] One of the reported HA20 cases initially carried the diagnosis of SLE,[6] and recently a new case of HA20 from Japan was reported to have autoimmune lymphoproliferative syndrome.[13] Together, these reports underscore the importance of A20 in immune regulation, and suggest that further study is needed to define the full clinical spectrum of HA20.

Otulipenia/OTULIN-Related Autoinflammatory Syndrome

Linear (or methionine 1–linked) ubiquitination is catalyzed by the linear Ub assembly complex (LUBAC),[14,15] consisting of HOIL-1, HOIP, and SHARPIN. LUBAC plays a critical role in the activation of NF-κB signaling by ligating linear Ub to its target proteins, which include NEMO and RIPK1. OTULIN (FAM105B) is a DUB that, as a cysteine protease, exclusively hydrolyzes linear Ub, prevents baseline accumulation of linear Ub on LUBAC components, and restricts ubiquitination of LUBAC target proteins (**Fig. 1B**).[16–18] OTULIN has an N-terminal PUB-interacting site, through which it interacts with HOIP,[19] and a C-terminal OTU domain that mediates its DUB activity.

Zhou and colleagues[20] and Damgaard and colleagues[21] independently reported that homozygous mutations of OTULIN cause a novel systemic autoinflammatory disorder. Patients with biallelic mutations were characterized by neonatal-onset fever, neutrophilic dermatosis, panniculitis, lipodystrophy, joint swelling, diarrhea, and failure to thrive. Due to their dermatologic findings, 2 patients were initially diagnosed with chronic atypical neutrophilic dermatosis with lipodystrophy and elevated temperature (CANDLE). Two of the mutations were missense substitutions that were predicted to be damaging and the other was a frameshift mutation. Indeed, protein expression of OTULIN was severely reduced in all the patients, suggesting the instability of the mutant proteins. Zhou and colleagues further demonstrated that patients' cells showed enhanced phosphorylation of IκBα and linear Ub accumulation on NEMO after cytokine stimulation. Overproduction of inflammatory cytokines, including TNF, IL-1β, IL-6, IL-17, IL-18, and IFN-γ, was detected in patients' serum samples. Anti-TNF therapy was effective in controlling disease activity as well as suppressing inflammatory markers in the blood.

OTULIN-null mice (gumby/gumby) are embryonic lethal due to defects in angiogenesis.[18] Damgaard and colleagues[21] generated mice with an inducible system of immune cell-specific OTULIN ablation. Strikingly, the immune cell-specific OTULIN ablation resulted in rapid weight loss and systemic inflammation, which was completely reversed by anti-TNF treatment. These investigators further tested the effects of lineage-specific OTULIN deletion in multiple cell types. Only OTULIN disruption in the myeloid cell lineage led to inflammatory phenotypes, which included enlargement of lymphoid organs, immune cell infiltration in the liver, and the elevation of serum inflammatory cytokines. T-cell–specific or B-cell–specific OTULIN ablation did not result in an overt phenotype. HOIP and SHARPIN expression levels, however, were strongly reduced, presumably due to LUBAC destabilization, which suggests a possible unexpected mechanism of lineage-specific LUBAC regulation.

Although loss of OTULIN leads to excessive inflammation through accumulation of linear Ub, germline deficiencies of LUBAC also result in autoinflammation. Boisson and colleagues[22,23] reported 3 RBCK1 (HOIL-1)–deficient and one RNF31 (HOIP)–deficient patients, characterized by immunodeficiency, rash, gastrointestinal manifestations, myopathy, and systemic autoinflammation. The patients' fibroblasts showed less linear Ub accumulation and reduced NF-κB signaling, relative to controls, whereas patients' monocytes were hyperactive on IL-1β stimulation. Furthermore, loss of SHARPIN in mice is responsible for the paradoxic phenotypes of the chronic proliferative dermatitis mouse, in which systemic multiorgan inflammation coexists with immunodeficiency.[24–26] These reports underscore the importance of linear ubiquitination in both proinflammatory and anti-inflammatory pathways.

DEFICIENCY OF ADENOSINE DEAMINASE 2

In 2014 Zhou and colleagues[27] and Navon Elkan and colleagues[28] identified biallelic loss-of-function CECR1 mutations in patients presenting with fevers and early-onset strokes and/or with vasculitis resembling PAN, a systemic necrotizing vasculitis typically affecting medium-sized muscular arteries.[29] Zhou and her colleagues reported 9 patients with fevers, early-onset (<5 year old) lacunar strokes, livedoid rash, hepatosplenomegaly, cytopenia, and systemic vasculopathy, including 2 patients with PAN and 1 with small-vessel vasculitis; 8 of the 9 patients had histories of lacunar strokes mainly affecting the deep-brain nuclei and the brain stem. Several strokes were hemorrhagic or underwent hemorrhagic transformation, leading to long-term disability. Most of the strokes occurred during episodes of systemic inflammation. These patients also presented with various sequelae of systemic vascular disease, including livedo racemosa, myositis, portal hypertension, and ophthalmologic complications. Biopsy samples from skin, liver, and brain exhibited vasculopathic changes, including impaired endothelial integrity, endothelial cellular activation, and inflammation. Four patients had hypogammaglobulinemia, and 2 of them had multiple episodes of bacterial and viral infections.

Simultaneously and independently, Navon Elkan and colleagues[28] reported 24 patients with PAN with biallelic CECR1 mutations, 19 of whom were of Georgian Jewish ancestry. Among them, 18 presented with childhood-onset PAN (<10 years old), including 6 who received the diagnosis during infancy (<1 year old). Most of the patients had cutaneous involvement, most commonly livedo racemosa. Five patients had episodes of either strokes or intracranial hemorrhage, whereas 10 had signs of peripheral neuropathy. Aneurysm formation in visceral arteries was observed in 6 patients, with associated renal hypertension and gastrointestinal manifestations.

CECR1 encodes ADA2, which can convert adenosine to inosine and 2'-deoxyadenosine to 2'-deoxyinosine.[30] Although ADA2 has partial structural homology with ADA (ADA1), the deficiency of which causes human severe combined immunodeficiency (SCID) through the intracellular accumulation of toxic nucleotides, these 2 enzymes differ in many aspects.[30] Whereas ADA1 acts as a monomer and is primarily localized intracellularly, ADA2 acts as a dimer and is secreted into the extracellular space. The

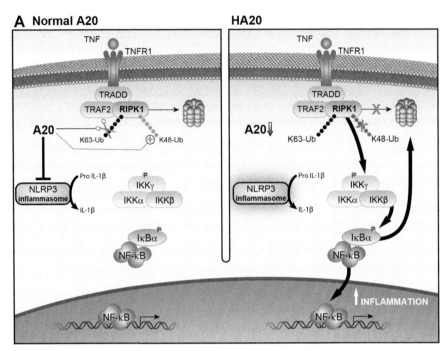

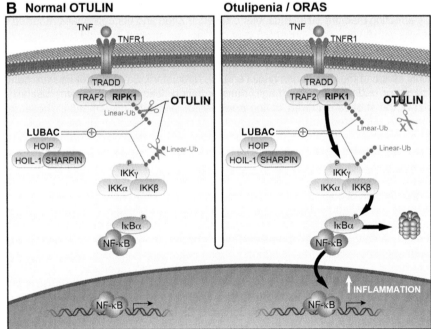

Fig. 1. Proposed mechanisms of pathogenesis in DUB deficiencies. (*A*) After binding TNF, a signaling complex is recruited to the TNF receptor. The addition of K63-linked Ub chains to RIPK1 stabilizes its signaling complex and leads to phosphorylation of the IKK complex, degradation of IκBα, and translocation of the NF-κB heterodimer into the nucleus. Under normal conditions (*left*), A20 removes K63-linked Ub chains from the RIPK1 complex and

patients described in both reports had a marked reduction of ADA2 protein concentrations and ADA2-specific enzymatic activity in the blood, suggesting that the detected mutations were loss of function. In the structural analysis, the missense mutations were predicted to affect the catalytic and dimerization domains or protein stability. Knock-down of *cecr1b* in zebrafish embryos resulted in intracranial hemorrhages and neutropenia, which were rescued by coinjection with human wild-type *CECR1* (but not mutant *CECR1*), establishing the pathogenicity of the mutations. Zhou and colleagues, therefore, proposed the term, *DADA2*, to denote the human disease.

ADA2 is expressed in the myeloid lineage and, once secreted, it induces differentiation of monocytes into macrophages, possibly by binding proteoglycan-like structures on the cellular surface.[31] DADA2 patient monocytes showed impaired differentiation toward the anti-inflammatory (M2) macrophage population under standard culture conditions, thus leading to polarized differentiation toward the proinflammatory (M1) macrophage subset.[27] A recent transcriptome-wide analysis using DADA2 patients' blood samples displayed a strong up-regulation of neutrophil-related genes as well as a moderate IFN signature, and the investigators also reported the accumulation of myeloperoxidase in patients' polymorphonuclear cells.[32] Zhou and colleagues[27] further reported that the DADA2 patients' brain and skin samples showed substantial endothelial activation and damage, and up-regulation of inflammatory cytokines. Coculture of patients' monocytes with a human primary endothelial cell layer led to considerable disruption of its integrity. These studies suggest that the deficiency of ADA2 results in vascular damage at least in part mediated by skewed monocytic differentiation and neutrophil activation.

All the Georgian Jewish patients in the report from Navon Elkan and colleagues[28] were homozygous for a mutation encoding a p.Gly47Arg substitution. The carrier frequency of this mutation in the endogamous Georgian Jewish population was 0.102, which is consistent with the apparently high prevalence of this disease in this population. Conserved haplotypes were detected around several missense mutations, including p.Gly47Arg, suggesting the existence of a possible founder effect.[27] A heterozygous p.Tyr453Cys *CECR1* mutation was identified in 2 siblings with late-onset lacunar strokes in the Siblings with Ischemic Stroke Study.[27,33] Although no genome-wide association study loci for stroke have been identified in the *CECR1* gene region, the effect of this gene on non-Mendelian cases of stroke and other vascular diseases should be further pursued.

Recent reports have broadened the clinical spectrum of DADA2 beyond the typical clinical picture of systemic inflammation presented in the first articles. *CECR1* mutations have been demonstrated in patients with autoimmunity, lymphoproliferation, and a combined immunodeficiency[34] as well as patients presenting primarily with common variable immunodeficiency.[35] The lymphoproliferative picture is shared by

---

instead conjugates its constituent proteins with K48-linked Ub chains to mark them for proteasomal degradation. In HA20, heterozygous loss of function of A20 results in the impaired suppressive function of A20, leading to excessive activation of NF-κB signaling (*right*). (*B*) LUBAC conjugates linear Ub to targets, including NEMO and RIPK1, which potentiate NF-κB signaling. OTULIN restricts this signaling by hydrolyzing linear Ub on LUBAC and its target proteins (*left*). In otulipenia/OTULIN-related autoinflammatory syndrome (ORAS), biallelic loss of function of OTULIN results in loss of this suppressive function, leading to accentuated activation of NF-κB signaling (*right*). For the sake of simplicity, ubiquitination on TRAF2 and TNFR1 are not shown in these figures.

a mutation-positive patient who was diagnosed with Castleman disease and responded to anti–IL-6 treatment.[36] Biallelic *CECR1* mutations have also been found in patients presenting with anemia, thrombocytopenia, and splenomegaly, leading to the initial clinical diagnosis of Diamond-Blackfan anemia or storage disease.[37] Recently, a biallelic 770-kb deletion of chromosome 22q11.1 encompassing both *CECR1* and *IL17RA* (encoding the IL-17 receptor A) was reported in 2 siblings with a history of both mucocutaneous infection and early-onset systemic vasculitis.[38] This finding, taken together with the 28-kb deletion in the *CECR1* locus reported by Zhou and colleagues,[27] indicates the importance of structural genomic analysis in the genetic diagnosis of DADA2.

Given the specter of stroke, vasculitis, and the other possible manifestations of DADA2, treatment strategies have been the subject of intense investigation. In many cases, corticosteroids, methotrexate, cyclophosphamide, azathioprine, and IL-1 inhibitors have been ineffective. Navon Elkan and colleagues[28] reported the use of anti-TNF agents in 10 DADA2 vasculitis patients, among which 8 demonstrated a complete response. This strategy has been further supported by a recent report from Ombrello and colleagues,[39] demonstrating that anti-TNF treatment has completely prevented the recurrence of strokes in 15 DADA2 patients with a previous history of stroke. Hematopoietic stem cell transplantation (HSCT) is another possible therapeutic strategy, because the pathogenesis of DADA2 seems to derive mainly from the myeloid cell lineage. The effectiveness of HSCT was initially reported by Van Eyck and colleagues,[40] followed by several articles[37,41] in which HSCT normalized the plasma level of ADA2 and suppressed disease manifestations. It will be important to establish the risk-benefit ratios for anti-TNF, HSCT, and other potential therapies in various clinical settings across the widening spectrum of DADA2.

Lastly, although the zebrafish data of Zhou and colleagues[27] clearly establish the importance of *CECR1* in vascular and myeloid development, the field has been hampered by the lack of an obvious murine *CECR1* orthologue that would permit the development of a mouse model. Whether through the development of alternative animal models or through the more detailed study of leukocyte and endothelial biology in DADA2 patients, there is still much to be learned about the basic biology of this disease.

TYPE I INTERFERONOPATHIES

Type I IFNs (mainly IFN-α and IFN-β) are a group of cytokines that play an important role in host defense. Binding of type I IFN to the IFN-α/β receptor induces the transcription of hundreds of genes called IFN-stimulated genes (ISGs) by activating the Janus kinase (JAK)-STAT signaling pathway. The overproduction of type I IFN leads to a group of Mendelian inherited diseases called type I interferonopathies. For example, Aicardi-Goutières syndrome derives from either loss-of-function mutations in cytoplasmic nucleic acid metabolism or gain-of-function mutations in pattern recognition receptors, such as MDA5 (encoded by the *IFIH1* gene), leading to severe encephalopathy and systemic autoimmunity resembling SLE (see Linda T. Hiraki and Earl D. Silverman's article, "Genomics of Systemic Lupus Erythematosus (SLE): Insights Gained by Studying Monogenic Young-Onset SLE," in this issue for further discussion of Aicardi-Goutières syndrome). Up-regulation of ISGs in the peripheral blood (IFN signature) was proposed as a screening method for interferonopathy, analogous to the up-regulation of type I IFN signaling in SLE patients.[42–44]

Stimulator of Interferon Genes–Associated Vasculopathy with Onset in Infancy

Recently the cyclic GMP-AMP synthase (cGAS)–cyclic GMP-AMP (cGAMP)–STING pathway was identified as the mechanism for the detection of cytoplasmic double-stranded DNA (dsDNA).[45] On recognition and binding of cytoplasmic dsDNA, cGAS synthesizes cGAMP as a second messenger, which then activates STING, an endoplasmic reticulum (ER)-resident adapter molecule. cGAMP induces the translocation of STING from the ER to the ER-Golgi intermediate compartment (ERGIC) to recruit TANK-binding kinase 1 and IFN regulatory factor 3, resulting in up-regulation of type I IFN transcription (**Fig. 2**).

In 2014 Liu and colleagues[46] identified de novo germline or somatic mosaic gain-of-function mutations in *TMEM173,* encoding STING, in 6 patients with early-onset autoinflammatory disorders manifesting dermatologic and pulmonary involvement. Skin lesions were seen in all 6 patients, with telangiectatic, pustular, or blistering rashes and gangrenous lesions, the latter of which were exacerbated by cold exposure and even required surgical amputations. Microscopically these skin lesions were characterized by marked vascular inflammation around capillaries with fibrin and immune complex deposition. Concomitantly various degrees of interstitial lung disease were observed in 5 of 6 patients. Lung biopsies showed a scattered lymphocytic inflammatory infiltrate, interstitial fibrosis, and emphysematous changes. Strong IFN signatures as well as constitutive phosphorylation of signal transducer and activator of transcription (STAT) 1 in patients' lymphocytes were observed, consistent with the constitutive activity of mutant STING in an in vitro assay. Patients' vascular endothelial cell layers

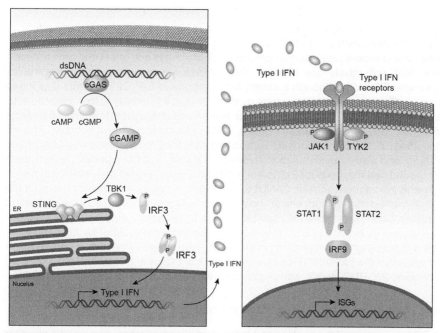

Fig. 2. The STING–type I IFN pathway. Cytosolic sensing of dsDNA by cGAS leads to the production of cGAMP as a second messenger, which then activates STING in the ER and further up-regulates type I IFN transcription via the recruitment of TANK-binding kinase 1 (TBK1) and IFN regulatory factor 3 (IRF3). The binding of type I IFN molecules to their receptors initiates the transcription of hundreds of ISGs via the activation of the JAK-STAT pathway.

from lesional skin samples expressed markers of endothelial inflammation and activation. These investigators proposed the term, SAVI, to denote this condition.

To date, more than 20 patients from multiple pedigrees have been reported with gain-of-function mutations in TMEM173.[46–54] Most of the mutations encode amino acid substitutions located close to the dimerization site of STING, and 2 recombinant mutants (p.N154S and p.V155M) were reported to form a stable homodimer.[46] Dobbs and colleagues[55] recently demonstrated that disease-associated STING mutants trafficked to the ERGIC without cGAMP stimulation and also that these active mutants were less susceptible to degradation, both of which could explain the constitutively active characteristics of STING mutants in SAVI. Melki and colleagues[54] identified 3 novel missense mutations in STING (p.C206Y, p.R281Q, and p.R284G), all of which lie outside the linker region important for homodimerization. The precise molecular mechanism of STING mutants in SAVI remains to be defined.

Although therapies, such as corticosteroids and disease-modifying antirheumatic drugs, or various inhibitors of TNF, IL-1, and IL-6, have been reported to elicit minimal clinical responses, accumulating evidence suggests the effectiveness of JAK inhibition in SAVI. Ex vivo treatment with any of 3 JAK inhibitors blocked the constitutive phosphorylation of STAT1 in a patient's B and CD4$^+$ T cells.[46] Recently 2 articles reported the clinical efficacy of JAK inhibitors in SAVI,[52,56] with reduction in febrile episodes and almost complete resolution of dermatologic lesions. Early genetic diagnosis and treatment may prevent the eventual need for surgical amputations and the irreversible pulmonary damage of SAVI.

Chronic Atypical Neutrophilic Dermatosis with Lipodystrophy and Elevated Temperature/Proteasome-Associated Autoinflammatory Syndrome

CANDLE, characterized by fever, panniculitis, and brain calcification, is another form of type I interferonopathy with biallelic loss-of-function mutations in PSMB8, which encodes the inducible proteasome component β5i.[57–60] It is one of several clinical conditions that collectively are denoted the proteasome-associated autoinflammatory syndrome (PRAAS). Although a strong IFN signature in CANDLE patients suggested the association between proteasome dysfunction and IFN signaling, the direct molecular mechanism had not been well defined. Brehm and colleagues[61] reported 8 patients with mutations in 4 proteasome genes, PSMA3 (encoding the α7 subunit), PSMB4 (encoding β7), PSMB9 (encoding β1i), and encoding the proteasome maturation protein (POMP), and also 1 novel mutation in PSMB8. Of note, 6 of the reported patients were compound heterozygous for 2 different genes (discussed previously), which suggested a digenic inheritance model in CANDLE. In addition, 1 patient was heterozygous for the POMP frameshift mutation, which likely causes haploinsufficiency, suggesting a novel autosomal-dominant mode of inheritance. The investigators also demonstrated that proteasome inhibition in fibroblasts from healthy individuals, either by knockdown or pharmacologic inhibition, resulted in strong up-regulation of IFN-related genes, which recapitulated the patients' IFN signature. A clinical trial of a JAK inhibitor for CANDLE is ongoing (NCT01724580), with promising preliminary results.[62]

NLRC4-RELATED AUTOINFLAMMATORY SYNDROMES

NLRC4, a member of the nucleotide-binding and oligomerization domain–like receptor family, assembles with neuronal apoptosis inhibitory protein (NAIP) and apoptosis associated speck-like protein containing a caspase recruitment domain (ASC) to form an inflammasome complex on the intracellular entry of ligands, such as bacterial flagellin or components of the bacterial type 3 secretion system. As a result, the NLRC4 inflammasome mediates the autocatalysis of procaspase-1 to the enzymatically active caspase-1, which subsequently catalyzes the cleavage of pro–IL-1β and to their biologically active mature forms and also induces a rapid lytic cell death, called pyroptosis.

In 2014 Canna and colleagues[63] and Romberg and colleagues[64] independently reported that heterozygous gain-of-function mutations of *NLRC4* (p.T337S and p.V341A, respectively) caused an AID. The phenotypes of these patients were characterized by early-onset multiple fever episodes, enterocolitis, splenomegaly, MAS-like flares, and persistent serum IL-18 elevation. In both reports, in vitro overexpression of mutant NLRC4 protein led to increased cleavage of caspase-1, and patients' macrophages exhibited increased production of IL-1β and IL-18, more frequent formation of ASC specks, and increased susceptibility to cell death, suggesting that these mutations result in constitutive activation of the NLRC4 inflammasome.

Concurrently, Kitamura and colleagues[65] reported that another mutation in *NLRC4* (p.H443P) caused a somewhat milder phenotype with cold-induced fever and urticaria, which resembled familial cold autoinflammatory syndrome (FCAS). Transgenic mice expressing this mutant *NLRC4* allele developed severe inflammatory infiltrates in the skin and joints, erosion of bones, splenomegaly, and elevated levels of IL-1β, IL-17A, and granulocyte colony-stimulating factor in the blood. Hypercytokinemia could be induced by adoptive transfer of bone marrow from mutant mice into wild-type recipients. Cold exposure of mutant mice augmented the cutaneous inflammation, which recapitulated the patients' phenotype.

Recently, a fourth mutation of *NLRC4* (p.T177A) was reported in a patient with periodic fever, rash, arthralgia, sensorineural hearing loss, chronic meningitis, and cerebral atrophy, all of which are consistent with neonatal-onset multisystem inflammatory disease (NOMID).[66] In this article, multiple induced pluripotent stem cell (iPSC)-derived monocytic lineage cells from the patient showed a differential pattern of inflammasome activation, and whole-exome sequencing between these normal and inflammatory groups of iPSCs identified the *NLRC4* p.T177A mutation, suggesting that the patient had somatic mosaicism of this *NLRC4* mutation.

A structural study showed that ADP-bound NLRC4 is in an autoinhibited state that is achieved by an ADP-mediated intramolecular interaction.[67] Disruption of this interaction by ligand binding may facilitate conformational changes and attenuate ADP binding, both of which could result in NLRC4 inflammasome activation. All the mutations identified in human NLRC4-related autoinflammatory syndromes are in close proximity to the ADP-binding site and p.Thr177 and p.His443 individually form a hydrogen bond to the ADP molecule. This clustering of disease-causing mutations in the nucleotide-binding domain, as well as the phenotypic variability and the presence of somatic mosaicism discussed previously, all suggest the similarities between NLRC4-related autoinflammatory syndromes and cryopyrin-associated periodic syndrome caused by *NLRP3* mutations.

Hemophagocytic disorders, such as MAS and hemophagocytic lymphohistiocytosis (HLH), are life-threatening sepsis-like conditions notable for acute cytopenias, hyperferritinemia, coagulopathy, and multiple organ damage, and, if not promptly treated, they are associated with high mortality rates. In addition to *NLRC4*-MAS, several conditions, such as familial HLH and systemic-onset juvenile idiopathic arthritis, are predisposed to MAS. During the flares, serum total IL-18 and free IL-18 are extraordinarily high, although its role in the pathogenesis of MAS/HLH remains controversial.[68] Recently administration of recombinant human IL-18 binding protein successfully rescued a patient with NLRC4-MAS, who did not respond to a combination of immunosuppressive drugs, anti-IL-1, anti-TNF, and $\alpha_4\beta_7$ integrin inhibitory therapies.[69] This not only substantiates a proinflammatory role for IL-18 in MAS but also raises a possible new treatment option for various MAS/HLH-inducing clinical conditions.

RECENT ADVANCES IN FAMILIAL MEDITERRANEAN FEVER AND THE PYRIN INFLAMMASOME

FMF is the longest-recognized and one of the most extensively studied hereditary autoinflammatory disorders. It is characterized by recurrent 1-day to 3-day febrile attacks accompanied by serositis, synovitis, and/or cutaneous inflammation. Two independent consortia identified *MEFV*, the gene mutated in FMF, by positional cloning in 1997.[70,71] Since that time, the mechanism by which mutations in pyrin, the encoded protein, cause FMF has been the topic of intense investigation. Although at first FMF was hypothesized as an autosomal recessive disease deriving from biallelic loss-of-function mutations mainly in exon 10 of *MEFV* (encoding the B30.2 domain of pyrin), subsequent reports of 30% to 40% of FMF patients carrying only 1 mutated allele of *MEFV*, coupled with the conspicuous absence of null mutations, raised the possibility that FMF is caused by gain-of-function mutations in *MEFV*.

Human pyrin consists of an N-terminal PYRIN domain (PYD), a B-box zinc finger domain, a coiled-coil domain, and a C-terminal approximately 200–amino acid B30.2 domain (also known as the rfp/PRY/SPRY domain). As discussed previously, a majority of FMF-causing mutations are located in the B30.2 domain.[72] The PYD interacts with ASC through a homotypic PYD-PYD interaction.[73] Chae and colleagues[74] reported in 2011 that homozygous knockin mice harboring any 1 of 3 human B30.2 domains with an FMF mutation showed constitutive activation of caspase-1 in macrophages and IL-1β secretion after lipopolysaccharide stimulation (without a second signal), which was completely dependent on ASC and caspase-1 but not on NLRP3. This article also demonstrated that this prominent inflammatory phenotype was not induced by knockout of the murine *Mefv* gene, and crosses between knockin and knockout mice supported the hypothesis that FMF-associated mutations are gain-of-function with a gene-dosage effect.

In 2014 Xu and colleagues[75] published a breakthrough article that shed considerable light on the mechanism by which pyrin contributes to host defense. These investigators demonstrated that pyrin inflammasome activation is induced by modifications of host RhoA by certain bacterial toxins. RhoA inactivation is a shared mechanism of bacterial virulence that prevents the reorganization of the host actin cytoskeleton and thus inhibits leukocyte migration, phagocytosis, and degranulation. These pyrin inflammasome-activating modifications of RhoA include monoglucosylation, adenylation, ADP-ribosylation, and deamidation, occurring on different residues. Thus, it was hypothesized that pyrin would recognize these RhoA modifications by sensing a downstream effect, although the molecular details were at the time unknown.

In 2016 Park and colleagues[76] elucidated the molecular mechanism by which RhoA inactivation leads to pyrin inflammasome activation (**Fig. 3**). Under physiologic conditions RhoA induces the phosphorylation of pyrin on its residues p.Ser208 and p.Ser242 through 2 effector kinases, protein kinase N (PKN) 1 and PKN2. Pyrin phosphorylation on these residues permits its interaction with 14-3-3, a regulatory protein, that in turn inhibits pyrin inflammasome formation. The binding of 14-3-3 and PKN1/2 to FMF-associated mutant pyrin is substantially reduced, and the constitutive activation of the pyrin inflammasome in FMF knockin mice as well as FMF patient cells is inhibited by pharmacologic PKN activation. Bacterial inactivation of RhoA diminishes PKN activity and thus favors the dephosphorylated form of pyrin that can assemble an inflammasome. This paradigm, sometimes termed, *the guard mechanism*,[76] by which microbial products activate innate immunity through their indirect biologic effects on

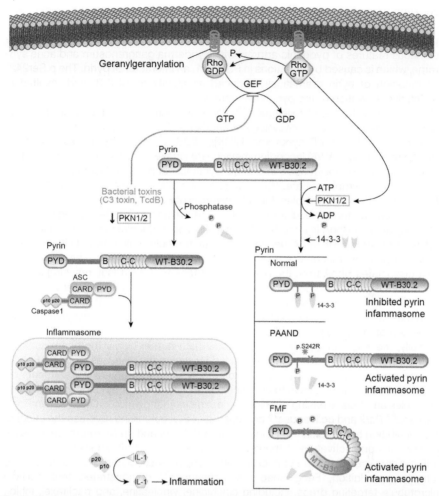

Fig. 3. Mechanism of pyrin inflammasome regulation and the diseases caused by pyrin dysregulation. In the resting state Rho family guanosine triphosphate hydrolases (GTPases) are activated by GEF. This in turn activates PKN1/2-mediated inactivation of pyrin through its phosphorylation and the recruitment of 14-3-3, a regulatory protein. During certain bacterial infections, RhoA inactivation by bacterial toxins leads to the downstream activation of the pyrin inflammasome by preventing the activation of PKN1/2, with the resultant dephosphorylation of pyrin and dissociation of 14-3-3. In PAAND and FMF, mutations of pyrin diminish the binding of 14-3-3 to pyrin and lead to spontaneous or more easily triggered activation of the pyrin inflammasome.

the cell, is common among plants, but the pyrin inflammasome represents one of the first documented examples of the guard mechanism in the animal kingdom.

The importance of pyrin p.Ser242 phosphorylation was further highlighted by the recent identification of a novel pyrin-related disorder distinct from FMF, called pyrin-associated autoinflammation with neutrophilic dermatosis (PAAND). In 2016 Masters and colleagues[77] reported the heterozygous p.Ser242Arg mutation in a group of patients with neutrophilic dermatosis (severe acne, sterile skin abscess, and pyoderma gangrenosum), recurrent long-lasting fever episodes, arthralgia, and myalgia/myositis, associated with the up-regulation of systemic inflammatory markers. The prominent dermatologic manifestations of these patients resemble the cutaneous features of pyogenic arthritis with pyoderma gangrenosum and acne syndrome, which is caused by mutations in PSTPIP1, an interactor of pyrin. The p.Ser242-Arg mutation of pyrin dramatically reduced its affinity to 14-3-3, and resulted in constitutive activation of the pyrin inflammasome.

Unexpectedly, Park and colleagues'[76] report also demonstrated a role for the pyrin inflammasome in the pathophysiology of another AID, mevalonate kinase deficiency (also known as hyper-IgD syndrome [HIDS]). HIDS is caused by recessive loss-of-function mutations in *MVK*, encoding mevalonate kinase, an enzyme that is important both in cholesterol biosynthesis and in the synthesis of nonsterol isoprenes, such as geranylgeranyl pyrophosphate. Pharmacologic inhibition of cholesterol synthesis by statins, which mimics the molecular pathogenesis of HIDS, had been shown to induce IL-1β release, but the molecular mechanism was unknown.[78,79] Reasoning that geranylgeranylation of RhoA is important for its trafficking to the plasma membrane,[80] and that the impairment of RhoA geranylgeranylation would inhibit its activity and thus result in pyrin inflammasome activation, Park and colleagues showed that statin treatment dissociates RhoA from the plasma membrane to the cytosol, resulting in IL-1β production. This IL-1β production is blocked by supplementation of geranylgeranyl pyrophosphate or pharmacologic activation of PKNs, is dependent only on the pyrin inflammasome (but not on NLRP3, NLRC4, or AIM2), and is associated with decreased binding of pyrin to 14-3-3 proteins.

Finally, these recent genetic and functional data further clarify the pharmacologic mechanism of colchicine, a medication used for rheumatic diseases (such as Behçet disease) and is also one of the most commonly used and effective treatments for FMF.[81,82] Colchicine is known to enhance the activity of RhoA by depolymerizing microtubules and thus releasing guanine nucleotide exchange factor (GEF)-H1, an RhoA activator.[83] Park and colleagues[76] demonstrated that colchicine reverses the effect of RhoA inhibition by C3 toxin from *Clostridium botulinum* and, furthermore, suppresses the spontaneous activation of the pyrin inflammasome in FMF knockin mice and in FMF patients' cells but not in the cells from cryopyrin-associated periodic syndrome patients. In addition, Feng Shao and colleagues[84] demonstrated that multiple microtubule-targeting drugs, including colchicine, vinblastine, and paclitaxel, inhibit pyrin inflammasome-mediated ASC aggregation. These data are consistent with the clinical response of FMF patients to colchicine treatment and the exquisite specificity of colchicine for FMF among the hereditary periodic fever syndromes.

SUMMARY

Recent genomic technologies, including next-generation sequencing, have substantially contributed to the advancement of the field of AID by catalyzing the discovery of new causative genes and pathways in AID patients. Some of these patients did not present with classic symptoms of AID, underscoring the heterogeneity of the clinical manifestations of AID. Also, the wide spectrum of clinical symptoms deriving from mutations in a single gene as exemplified by DADA2 highlights the importance of further clinical studies and the elucidation of pathogenic mechanisms. Conversely, the broad range of effects of A20 mutations from low to high penetrance and even somatic changes exemplifies the importance of comprehensive genetic approaches. The success of novel targeted therapies for previously uncontrollable AID patients emphasizes the importance of promoting translational research in this field. Exciting challenges remain to deliver rapid and accurate genetic diagnosis and effective treatments to currently undiagnosed AID patients.

REFERENCES

1. McDermott MF, Aksentijevich I, Galon J, et al. Germline mutations in the extracellular domains of the 55 kDa TNF receptor, TNFR1, define a family of dominantly inherited autoinflammatory syndromes. Cell 1999;97(1):133–44.
2. Zinngrebe J, Montinaro A, Peltzer N, et al. Ubiquitin in the immune system. EMBO Rep 2014;15(1):28–45.
3. Panday A, Inda ME, Bagam P, et al. Transcription Factor NF-kappaB: an update on intervention strategies. Arch Immunol Ther Exp (Warsz) 2016;64(6):463–83.
4. Hanpude P, Bhattacharya S, Dey AK, et al. Deubiquitinating enzymes in cellular signaling and disease regulation. IUBMB Life 2015;67(7):544–55.
5. Rajan N, Ashworth A. Inherited cylindromas: lessons from a rare tumour. Lancet Oncol 2015;16(9):e460–9.
6. Zhou Q, Wang H, Schwartz DM, et al. Loss-of-function mutations in TNFAIP3 leading to A20 haploinsufficiency cause an early-onset autoinflammatory disease. Nat Genet 2016;48(1):67–73.
7. Vande Walle L, Van Opdenbosch N, Jacques P, et al. Negative regulation of the NLRP3 inflammasome by A20 protects against arthritis. Nature 2014;512(7512): 69–73.
8. Duong BH, Onizawa M, Oses-Prieto JA, et al. A20 restricts ubiquitination of pro-interleukin-1beta protein complexes and suppresses NLRP3 inflammasome activity. Immunity 2015;42(1):55–67.
9. Zhang M, Peng LL, Wang Y, et al. Roles of A20 in autoimmune diseases. Immunol Res 2016;64(2):337–44.
10. Kato M, Sanada M, Kato I, et al. Frequent inactivation of A20 in B-cell lymphomas. Nature 2009;459(7247):712–6.
11. Lee EG, Boone DL, Chai S, et al. Failure to regulate TNF-induced NF-kappaB and cell death responses in A20-deficient mice. Science 2000;289(5488):2350–4.
12. Ma A, Malynn BA. A20: linking a complex regulator of ubiquitylation to immunity and human disease. Nat Rev Immunol 2012;12(11):774–85.
13. Takagi M, Ogata S, Ueno H, et al. Haploinsufficiency of TNFAIP3 (A20) by germline mutation is involved in autoimmune lymphoproliferative syndrome. J Allergy Clin Immunol 2016. [Epub ahead of print].
14. Sasaki K, Iwai K. Roles of linear ubiquitinylation, a crucial regulator of NF-kappaB and cell death, in the immune system. Immunol Rev 2015;266(1):175–89.
15. Kirisako T, Kamei K, Murata S, et al. A ubiquitin ligase complex assembles linear polyubiquitin chains. EMBO J 2006;25(20):4877–87.
16. Keusekotten K, Elliott PR, Glockner L, et al. OTULIN antagonizes LUBAC signaling by specifically hydrolyzing Met1-linked polyubiquitin. Cell 2013; 153(6):1312–26.
17. Fiil BK, Damgaard RB, Wagner SA, et al. OTULIN restricts Met1-linked ubiquitination to control innate immune signaling. Mol Cell 2013;50(6):818–30.
18. Rivkin E, Almeida SM, Ceccarelli DF, et al. The linear ubiquitin-specific deubiquitinase gumby regulates angiogenesis. Nature 2013;498(7454):318–24.
19. Schaeffer V, Akutsu M, Olma MH, et al. Binding of OTULIN to the PUB domain of HOIP controls NF-kappaB signaling. Mol Cell 2014;54(3):349–61.

20. Zhou Q, Yu X, Demirkaya E, et al. Biallelic hypomorphic mutations in a linear deubiquitinase define otulipenia, an early-onset autoinflammatory disease. Proc Natl Acad Sci U S A 2016;113(36):10127–32.

21. Damgaard RB, Walker JA, Marco-Casanova P, et al. The Deubiquitinase OTULIN is an essential negative regulator of inflammation and autoimmunity. Cell 2016; 166(5):1215–30.e20.

22. Boisson B, Laplantine E, Prando C, et al. Immunodeficiency, autoinflammation and amylopectinosis in humans with inherited HOIL-1 and LUBAC deficiency. Nat Immunol 2012;13(12):1178–86.

23. Boisson B, Laplantine E, Dobbs K, et al. Human HOIP and LUBAC deficiency underlies autoinflammation, immunodeficiency, amylopectinosis, and lymphangiectasia. J Exp Med 2015;212(6):939–51.

24. Tokunaga F, Nakagawa T, Nakahara M, et al. SHARPIN is a component of the NF-kappaB-activating linear ubiquitin chain assembly complex. Nature 2011; 471(7340):633–6.

25. Ikeda F, Deribe YL, Skanland SS, et al. SHARPIN forms a linear ubiquitin ligase complex regulating NF-kappaB activity and apoptosis. Nature 2011;471(7340): 637–41.

26. Gerlach B, Cordier SM, Schmukle AC, et al. Linear ubiquitination prevents inflammation and regulates immune signalling. Nature 2011;471(7340):591–6.

27. Zhou Q, Yang D, Ombrello AK, et al. Early-onset stroke and vasculopathy associated with mutations in ADA2. N Engl J Med 2014;370(10):911–20.

28. Navon Elkan P, Pierce SB, Segel R, et al. Mutant adenosine deaminase 2 in a polyarteritis nodosa vasculopathy. N Engl J Med 2014;370(10):921–31.

29. Forbess L, Bannykh S. Polyarteritis nodosa. Rheum Dis Clin North Am 2015;41(1): 33–46, vii.

30. Zavialov AV, Engstrom A. Human ADA2 belongs to a new family of growth factors with adenosine deaminase activity. Biochem J 2005;391(Pt 1):51–7.

31. Zavialov AV, Yu X, Spillmann D, et al. Structural basis for the growth factor activity of human adenosine deaminase ADA2. J Biol Chem 2010;285(16):12367–77.

32. Belot A, Wassmer E, Twilt M, et al. Mutations in CECR1 associated with a neutrophil signature in peripheral blood. Pediatr Rheumatol Online J 2014;12:44.

33. Meschia JF, Brown RD Jr, Brott TG, et al. The Siblings With Ischemic Stroke Study (SWISS) protocol. BMC Med Genet 2002;3:1.

34. Van Eyck L Jr, Hershfield MS, Pombal D, et al. Hematopoietic stem cell transplantation rescues the immunologic phenotype and prevents vasculopathy in patients with adenosine deaminase 2 deficiency. J Allergy Clin Immunol 2015;135(1): 283–7.e5.

35. Schepp J, Bulashevska A, Mannhardt-Laakmann W, et al. Deficiency of adenosine deaminase 2 causes antibody deficiency. J Clin Immunol 2016;36(3): 179–86.

36. Van Eyck L, Liston A, Wouters C. Mutant ADA2 in vasculopathies. N Engl J Med 2014;371(5):480.

37. Van Montfrans JM, Hartman EA, Braun KP, et al. Phenotypic variability in patients with ADA2 deficiency due to identical homozygous R169Q mutations. Rheumatology (Oxford) 2016;55(5):902–10.

38. Fellmann F, Angelini F, Wassenberg J, et al. IL-17 receptor A and adenosine deaminase 2 deficiency in siblings with recurrent infections and chronic inflammation. J Allergy Clin Immunol 2016;137(4):1189–96.e1–2.

39. Amanda K, Ombrello KB, Hoffmann P, et al. The Deficiency of Adenosine Deaminase Type 2 (DADA2)-Results of Anti-TNF Treatment in a Cohort of Patients with a

History of Stroke. Paper presented 2016 ACR/ARHP Annual Meeting. Washington, DC, September 28, 2016.

40. Van Eyck L, Liston A, Meyts I. Mutant ADA2 in vasculopathies. N Engl J Med 2014;371(5):478–9.
41. van Montfrans J, Zavialov A, Zhou Q. Mutant ADA2 in vasculopathies. N Engl J Med 2014;371(5):478.
42. Ytterberg SR, Schnitzer TJ. Serum interferon levels in patients with systemic lupus erythematosus. Arthritis Rheum 1982;25(4):401–6.
43. Gota C, Calabrese L. Induction of clinical autoimmune disease by therapeutic interferon-alpha. Autoimmunity 2003;36(8):511–8.
44. Bennett L, Palucka AK, Arce E, et al. Interferon and granulopoiesis signatures in systemic lupus erythematosus blood. J Exp Med 2003;197(6):711–23.
45. Tao J, Zhou X, Jiang Z. cGAS-cGAMP-STING: The three musketeers of cytosolic DNA sensing and signaling. IUBMB Life 2016;68(11):858–70.
46. Liu Y, Jesus AA, Marrero B, et al. Activated STING in a vascular and pulmonary syndrome. N Engl J Med 2014;371(6):507–18.
47. Jeremiah N, Neven B, Gentili M, et al. Inherited STING-activating mutation underlies a familial inflammatory syndrome with lupus-like manifestations. J Clin Invest 2014;124(12):5516–20.
48. Munoz J, Rodiere M, Jeremiah N, et al. Stimulator of interferon genes-associated vasculopathy with onset in infancy: a mimic of childhood granulomatosis with polyangiitis. JAMA Dermatol 2015;151(8):872–7.
49. Omoyinmi E, Melo Gomes S, Nanthapisal S, et al. Stimulator of interferon genes-associated vasculitis of infancy. Arthritis Rheum 2015;67(3):808.
50. Picard C, Thouvenin G, Kannengiesser C, et al. Severe pulmonary fibrosis as the first manifestation of interferonopathy (TMEM173 Mutation). Chest 2016;150(3): e65–71.
51. Konig N, Fiehn C, Wolf C, et al. Familial chilblain lupus due to a gain-of-function mutation in STING. Ann Rheum Dis 2017;76(2):468–72.
52. Fremond ML, Rodero MP, Jeremiah N, et al. Efficacy of the Janus kinase 1/2 inhibitor ruxolitinib in the treatment of vasculopathy associated with TMEM173-activating mutations in 3 children. J Allergy Clin Immunol 2016;138(6):1752–5.
53. Clarke SL, Pellowe EJ, de Jesus AA, et al. Interstitial lung disease caused by STING-associated vasculopathy with onset in infancy. Am J Respir Crit Care Med 2016;194(5):639–42.
54. Melki I, Rose Y, Uggenti C, et al. Disease-associated mutations identify a novel region in human STING necessary for the control of type I interferon signaling. J Allergy Clin Immunol 2017. [Epub ahead of print].
55. Dobbs N, Burnaevskiy N, Chen D, et al. STING activation by translocation from the ER is associated with infection and autoinflammatory disease. Cell Host Microbe 2015;18(2):157–68.
56. Seo J, Kang JA, Suh DI, et al. Tofacitinib relieves symptoms of stimulator of interferon genes (STING)-associated vasculopathy with onset in infancy caused by 2 de novo variants in TMEM173. J Allergy Clin Immunol 2016;139:1396–9.e12.
57. Liu Y, Ramot Y, Torrelo A, et al. Mutations in proteasome subunit beta type 8 cause chronic atypical neutrophilic dermatosis with lipodystrophy and elevated temperature with evidence of genetic and phenotypic heterogeneity. Arthritis Rheum 2012;64(3):895–907.
58. Kitamura A, Maekawa Y, Uehara H, et al. A mutation in the immunoproteasome subunit PSMB8 causes autoinflammation and lipodystrophy in humans. J Clin Invest 2011;121(10):4150–60.

59. Arima K, Kinoshita A, Mishima H, et al. Proteasome assembly defect due to a proteasome subunit beta type 8 (PSMB8) mutation causes the autoinflammatory disorder, Nakajo-Nishimura syndrome. Proc Natl Acad Sci U S A 2011;108(36): 14914–9.

60. Agarwal AK, Xing C, DeMartino GN, et al. PSMB8 encoding the beta5i proteasome subunit is mutated in joint contractures, muscle atrophy, microcytic anemia, and panniculitis-induced lipodystrophy syndrome. Am J Hum Genet 2010;87(6): 866–72.

61. Brehm A, Liu Y, Sheikh A, et al. Additive loss-of-function proteasome subunit mutations in CANDLE/PRAAS patients promote type I IFN production. J Clin Invest 2015;125(11):4196–211.

62. Sanchez GAM, Reinhardt AL, Brogan P, et al. Chronic Atypical Neutrophilic Dermatosis With Lipodystrophy and Elevated Temperatures (CANDLE): clinical characterization and initial response to janus kinase inhibition with baricitinib. Arthritis Rheum 2013;65:S758–9.

63. Canna SW, de Jesus AA, Gouni S, et al. An activating NLRC4 inflammasome mutation causes autoinflammation with recurrent macrophage activation syndrome. Nat Genet 2014;46(10):1140–6.

64. Romberg N, Al Moussawi K, Nelson-Williams C, et al. Mutation of NLRC4 causes a syndrome of enterocolitis and autoinflammation. Nat Genet 2014;46(10): 1135–9.

65. Kitamura A, Sasaki Y, Abe T, et al. An inherited mutation in NLRC4 causes autoinflammation in human and mice. J Exp Med 2014;211(12):2385–96.

66. Kawasaki Y, Oda H, Ito J, et al. Identification of a high-frequency somatic NLRC4 mutation as a cause of autoinflammation by pluripotent cell-based phenotype dissection. Arthritis Rheum 2017;69(2):447–59.

67. Hu Z, Zhou Q, Zhang C, et al. Structural and biochemical basis for induced self-propagation of NLRC4. Science 2015;350(6259):399–404.

68. Bracaglia C, Prencipe G, De Benedetti F. Macrophage Activation Syndrome: different mechanisms leading to a one clinical syndrome. Pediatr Rheumatol Online J 2017;15(1):5.

69. Canna SW, Girard C, Malle L, et al. Life-threatening NLRC4-associated hyperinflammation successfully treated with IL-18 inhibition. J Allergy Clin Immunol 2016. [Epub ahead of print].

70. Ancient missense mutations in a new member of the RoRet gene family are likely to cause familial Mediterranean fever. The International FMF Consortium. Cell 1997;90(4):797–807.

71. French FMF Consortium. A candidate gene for familial Mediterranean fever. Nat Genet 1997;17(1):25–31.

72. Manukyan G, Aminov R. Update on pyrin functions and mechanisms of familial mediterranean fever. Front Microbiol 2016;7:456.

73. Richards N, Schaner P, Diaz A, et al. Interaction between pyrin and the apoptotic speck protein (ASC) modulates ASC-induced apoptosis. J Biol Chem 2001; 276(42):39320–9.

74. Chae JJ, Cho YH, Lee GS, et al. Gain-of-function Pyrin mutations induce NLRP3 protein-independent interleukin-1beta activation and severe autoinflammation in mice. Immunity 2011;34(5):755–68.

75. Xu H, Yang J, Gao W, et al. Innate immune sensing of bacterial modifications of Rho GTPases by the Pyrin inflammasome. Nature 2014;513(7517):237–41.

76. Park YH, Wood G, Kastner DL, et al. Pyrin inflammasome activation and RhoA signaling in the autoinflammatory diseases FMF and HIDS. Nat Immunol 2016; 17(8):914–21.
77. Masters SL, Lagou V, Jeru I, et al. Familial autoinflammation with neutrophilic dermatosis reveals a regulatory mechanism of pyrin activation. Sci Transl Med 2016;8(332):332ra345.
78. Kuijk LM, Beekman JM, Koster J, et al. HMG-CoA reductase inhibition induces IL-1beta release through Rac1/PI3K/PKB-dependent caspase-1 activation. Blood 2008;112(9):3563–73.
79. Mandey SH, Kuijk LM, Frenkel J, et al. A role for geranylgeranylation in interleukin-1beta secretion. Arthritis Rheum 2006;54(11):3690–5.
80. Garcia-Mata R, Boulter E, Burridge K. The 'invisible hand': regulation of RHO GTPases by RHOGDIs. Nat Rev Mol Cell Biol 2011;12(8):493–504.
81. Goldfinger SE. Colchicine for familial Mediterranean fever. N Engl J Med 1972; 287(25):1302.
82. Mandhare A, Banerjee P. Therapeutic use of colchicine and its derivatives: a patent review. Expert Opin Ther Pat 2016;26:1–18.
83. Krendel M, Zenke FT, Bokoch GM. Nucleotide exchange factor GEF-H1 mediates cross-talk between microtubules and the actin cytoskeleton. Nat Cell Biol 2002; 4(4):294–301.
84. Gao W, Yang J, Liu W, et al. Site-specific phosphorylation and microtubule dynamics control Pyrin inflammasome activation. Proc Natl Acad Sci U S A 2016; 113(33):E4857–66.

Genomic Influences on Susceptibility and Severity of Rheumatoid Arthritis

Rachel Knevel, MD, PhD[a,b,c,d,*], Tom W.J. Huizinga, MD, PhD[c],
Fina Kurreeman, PhD[c]

KEYWORDS

- Genomics • Genetics • Rheumatoid arthritis • Severity • Phenotype

KEY POINTS

- Genetic studies have increased our understanding of rheumatoid arthritis (RA), pointing out the importance of HLA-DRB1 HLA-B and HLA-DPB1, JAK-STAT signaling, NF-kB, and T-cell receptor signaling.
- The genetics of RA severity is challenging because of the variability of the phenotype, the large amount of data needed, and the interactions with environment.
- The heterogeneity within RA hampers the findings of strong genetic associations.
- The combination of genetic risk factors into a Genetic Risk Scores creates a fairly good predictive model, but its clinical applicability is yet limited.
- Future studies are needed that focus on the functional understanding of the found genetic variants as well as on the development of methods that can encompass with the complexity of RA development.

INTRODUCTION

Rheumatoid arthritis (RA) is widely considered the most common chronic inflammatory arthritis. RA is characterized by symmetric polyarthritis of the small hand and feet joints, which leads to irreversible destruction of joints and subsequently to significant morbidity, disability for patients, and costs for society.

Disclosure Statement: R. Knevel has nothing to disclose. Funding: METEOR (RP 2014-03), Niels Stensen Fellowship (R152568/P43317), Reumafonds (15-3-301); T.W.J. Huizinga: the Department of Rheumatology LUMC has received lecture fees/consultancy fees from Merck, UCB, Bristol-Myers Squibb, Biotest AG, Pfizer, GSK, Novartis, Roche, Sanofi-Aventis, Abbott, Crescendo Bioscience, Nycomed, Boeringher, Takeda, Zydus, Epirus, and Eli Lilly; F. Kurreeman has nothing to disclose. Funding: LUMC fellowship, Reumafonds en ZonMW DTL grant.
[a] Brigham and Women's Hospital, Division of Genetics, Raychaudhuri Lab, 77 Avenue Louis Pasteur, 2th Floor, Room 255, Boston, MA 02115, USA; [b] Harvard Medical School, 25 Shattuck Street, Boston, MA 02115, USA; [c] Leiden University Medical Center, Albinusdreef 2, 2333 ZA, Leiden, The Netherlands; [d] The Broad Institute, 415 Main Street, Cambridge, MA 02142, USA
* Corresponding author. Brigham and Women's Hospital, Division of Genetics, Raychaudhuri Lab, 77 Avenue Louis Pasteur, 2th Floor, Room 255, Boston, MA 02115.
E-mail address: rknevel@bwh.harvard.edu

Current treatment options are such that the decreased life expectancy as well as the severe joint destruction can substantially be reduced. Still, a high degree of variability in disease outcome and treatment response is observed among the group of RA patients. A problem in the treatment and diagnosis of RA is that the underlying abnormality is incompletely understood and patients are diagnosed with RA if they fulfill a subset of a list of criteria. Typically, treatment is targeted against inflammatory processes in general.

Therefore, an important aim in RA research is to improve the knowledge of the abnormality. The current understanding of RA is that it follows a multiple hit model that includes different preclinical phases, eventually crossing a threshold leading to the manifestation of clinical symptoms and ultimately joint damage. Likely, genetic predisposition combined with environmental factors influence the transition from one disease stage to another. The importance of genetics in understanding RA is underlined by the observation that RA heritability is ~40% to 65% for seropositive RA and ~20% for seronegative RA.[1,2] A family history of RA confers a 3- to 5-fold increased risk of developing RA.[1] These findings have fueled genetic studies and improved the understanding of RA.

After decades of genetic research in RA, the question arises whether this information has changed the clinical care. In this review, the authors aim to give the reader an overview of the major findings and issues in the field of RA genomics from a clinical perspective.

GENETICS OF RHEUMATOID ARTHRITIS SUSCEPTIBILITY

Most genetic studies explored RA susceptibility by comparing the prevalence of genetic variants between cases and controls. These studies have led to a large number of discoveries, especially after the introduction of genome-wide association studies. Still, the major genetic risk region, the HLA region, was discovered decades ago (see Vincent van Drongelen and Joseph Holoshitz's article, "HLA-Disease Associations in Rheumatoid Arthritis," in this issue).

Human Leukocyte Antigen in Rheumatoid Arthritis Susceptibility

HLA is a region of greater than 200 genes that encodes the major histocompatibility complex (MHC), which plays a crucial role in immune regulation. MHC molecules are located on the surface of many immune cells (such as macrophages, B cells, and especially dendritic cells), where they recognize pathogens and present them to T cells.

The fact that this genetic region is highly variable, spans a large region with many immune genes, and is characterized by strong linkage disequilibrium makes it a challenging region to study. The increasing insight into the region and methods to study this region has led to a repeatedly changing nomenclature and improved the precision of its association with RA. The dominant RA association within the HLA region is with the HLA-DRB1 locus. Until recently, the major association of this gene with RA was considered to be the HLA-Shared Epitope (HLA-SE), a 5-position amino acid motif at position 70 to 74 at the HLA-DRB1 gene encoding the amino acid sequences QKRAA, QRRAA, or RRRAA.[3]

Recent studies were able to study the region more precisely by the availability of highly dense genome-wide association studies (GWAS) and the development of imputation methods to more precisely define the highly polymorphic HLA region from single nucleotide polymorphism (SNP) data. These studies showed that the most significant associations within the HLA region are a combination of amino acid residues encoded at positions 11, 13, 71, and 74 (odds ratios [OR] range between 0.59 and 4.44), HLA-B position 9 [OR 2.12], and HLA-DPB1 position 9 [OR 1.40] for autoantibody-positive patients.[4] Similar risk associations have been found in the less well-studied anticitrullinated protein antibody (ACPA)-negative RA subsets, except for HLA-DRB1 position 11 for which an opposite risk effect is described for ACPA-negative individuals.[5] Although most of the HLA studies have been identified in European populations, the risk associated with the amino acid–based HLA model has been found in Asians and African Americans as well.[6,7]

HLA is not only associated with increased risk, HLA-DRB*13, which encompasses position 70 to 74 of the 5-amino acid sequence DERAA, appears to protect against the development of RA (OR 0.54 for DERAA and 0.24 for *13:01) as does HLA-A position 77 (OR 0.85) both in ACPA-positive patients.[5,8,9] In total, these HLA associations account for 13% of the variance in the genetic risk for RA.[4,10]

Much is known about the function of the HLA genes. HLA-DRB1 and HLA-DPB1 encode the MHC class II molecules that present peptide antigens to CD4+ T cells. HLA-B encodes the MHC class I protein that functions to present antigen to CD8+ T cells. These findings underlines the notion that (self) peptide binding plays an important role in RA pathogenesis.[10] An interesting theory is that HLA-DRB1 plays a critical role in the binding of ACPAs, which implies that HLA is important before the onset of inflammation.[10,11] Combined with studies on ACPA development, the current notion is that HLA does not play a role in the development of ACPAs itself but to the expansion of the ACPA response, which then leads to RA[12] (see Vincent van Drongelen and Joseph Holoshitz's article, "HLA-Disease Associations in Rheumatoid Arthritis," in this issue).

Non–Human Leukocyte Antigen Genetic Variants in Rheumatoid Arthritis Susceptibility

As the HLA region explains only part of the heritability of RA, many studies have focused on the non-HLA regions. These studies have used SNPs (either common >1% or rare <1%) and studied their association with RA. Studies in more than 100,000 individuals led to the discovery of 101 non-HLA genetic variants covering 98 genes.[10] The study of Okada and colleagues included both ACPA-positive and ACPA-negative RA patients from either European or Asian descent. Still, it is likely that most of the risk factors are confined to ACPA-positive RA, because many of the risk variants have been described in ACPA-positive RA, whereas ACPA-negative GWAS in both the Europeans and the Asians did not find any association that reached genome-wide significance ($P<5 \times 10^{-8}$) (**Fig. 1A**, **Table 1**).[13,14] Very recently, the largest ACPA-negative RA association study was published, using Immunochip (a selection of 186 Immune-related genes) as genotyping platform. This study found 2 variants associated with ACPA-negative RA that were not associated with ACPA-positive RA: one in the intergenic domain between the prolactin and the neurensin 1 (OR = 1.13) gene and the other in intronic region in nuclear factor I/A (OR = 0.85).[15] Although these findings did not reach genome-wide significance, they were independently replicated in a second cohort (OR 0.87, $P = 3.8 \times 10^{-3}$).

The translation of these genetic associations into a better understanding of RA abnormality is a challenging task for several reasons:

1. Because of strong linkage disequilibrium the discovered genetic variants are not necessarily the causal variants;
2. Most discovered variants are located in regions (introns) of which the function is still unknown;
3. The ultimate method to prove the function of a certain genetic variant is to alter the variant and study the consequences. This practice is impossible (or unethical) in

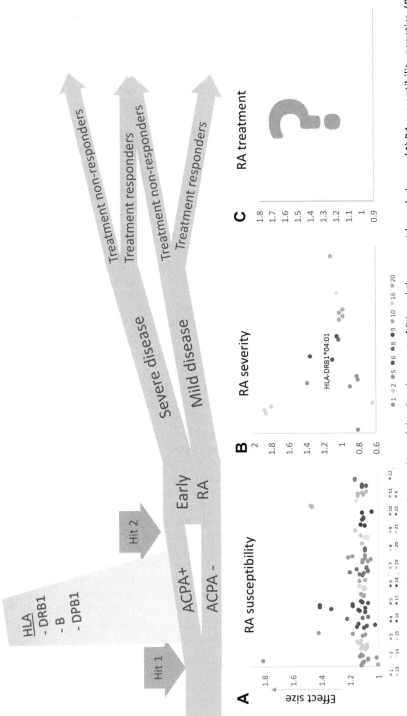

Fig. 1. A schematic depiction of the current understanding of the development of RA and the current knowledge on (A) RA susceptibility genetics, (B) severity genetics, and (C) treatment genetics.

Table 1
Genetic (non–human leukocyte antigen) variants associated with rheumatoid arthritis susceptibility

SNP	Gene	Chr	A1/A2	OR	95% Confidence Interval		P Value
chr1:2523811	TNFRSF14-MMEL1	1	G/A	1.12	1.09	1.16	2.20E−10
rs227163	TNFRSF9	1	C/T	1	0.97	1.03	.94
rs2301888	PADI4	1	G/A	1.11	1.06	1.15	5.50E−09
rs28411352	MTF1-INPP5B	1	T/C	1.11	1.07	1.16	5.20E−09
rs12140275	LOC339442	1	A/T	1.1	1.06	1.14	3.60E−07
rs2476601	PTPN22	1	A/G	1.81	1.73	1.9	1.60E−149
rs2228145	IL6R	1	A/C	1.07	1.04	1.11	4.50E−06
rs2317230	FCRL3	1	T/G	1.07	1.04	1.1	1.00E−05
rs4656942	LY9-CD244	1	G/A	1.01	0.98	1.05	.48
rs72717009	FCGR2A	1	T/C	1.13	1.08	1.19	1.10E−06
rs2105325	LOC100506023	1	C/A	1.11	1.08	1.15	1.00E−08
rs17668708	PTPRC	1	C/T	1.12	1.06	1.18	1.70E−05
rs10175798	LBH	2	A/G	1.09	1.06	1.13	1.30E−07
rs34695944	REL	2	C/T	1.12	1.09	1.16	4.40E−14
rs13385025	B3GNT2	2	A/G	1.08	1.02	1.15	.01
rs1858037	SPRED2	2	T/A	1.11	1.08	1.14	5.90E−10
rs9653442	AFF3	2	C/T	1.11	1.08	1.15	3.60E−12
rs6732565	ACOXL	2	A/G	1.08	1.04	1.13	8.80E−05
rs11889341	STAT4	2	T/C	1.13	1.09	1.17	6.50E−12
rs6715284	CFLAR-CASP8	2	G/C	1.14	1.08	1.2	2.90E−07
rs3087243	CTLA4	2	G/A	1.15	1.11	1.19	9.20E−20
rs1980422	CD28	2	C/T	1.12	1.09	1.16	6.00E−11
rs4452313	PLCL2	3	T/A	1.11	1.08	1.15	2.70E−10
rs3806624	EOMES	3	G/A	1.09	1.05	1.12	6.10E−08
rs73081554	DNASE1L3-ABHD6-PXK	3	T/C	1.18	1.11	1.25	4.70E−08
rs9826828	IL20RB	3	A/G	1.42	1.25	1.62	9.20E−08
rs13142500	CLNK	4	C/T	1.1	1.05	1.15	2.40E−06
rs11933540	C4orf52	4	C/T	1.15	1.11	1.19	9.20E−17
rs2664035	TEC	4	A/G	1.08	1.04	1.11	2.50E−06
rs10028001	ANXA3	4	T/A	1.02	0.98	1.06	.27
rs45475795	IL2-IL21	4	G/A	1.14	1.08	1.2	4.40E−06
rs7731626	ANKRD55	5	G/A	1.22	1.16	1.27	7.90E−23
rs2561477	C5orf30	5	G/A	1.11	1.08	1.15	5.20E−10
rs657075	IL3-CSF2	5	A/G	1.07	1.01	1.12	.011
rs9378815	IRF4	6	C/G	1.09	1.05	1.12	1.60E−07
chr6:14103212	CD83	6	T/C	1.13	1.04	1.23	.0046
rs2234067	ETV7	6	C/A	1.14	1.09	1.19	4.10E−08
rs2233424	NFKBIE	6	T/C	1.33	1.2	1.47	3.30E−08
rs9372120	ATG5	6	G/T	1.09	1.04	1.12	1.20E−05

(continued on next page)

Table 1
(continued)

SNP	Gene	Chr	A1/A2	OR	95% Confidence Interval		P Value
rs17264332	TNFAIP3	6	G/A	1.41	1.3	1.52	1.40E−17
rs17264332	TNFAIP3	6	G/A	1.18	1.14	1.22	7.10E−19
rs7752903	TNFAIP3	6	G/T	1.41	1.3	1.52	1.40E−17
rs7752903	TNFAIP3	6	G/T	1.18	1.14	1.22	7.10E−19
rs9373594	PPIL4	6	T/C	1.07	1.01	1.13	.012
rs2451258	TAGAP	6	T/C	1.11	1.07	1.14	6.60E−10
rs1571878	CCR6	6	C/T	1.12	1.1	1.16	4.90E−15
rs67250450	JAZF1	7	T/C	1.1	1.05	1.14	1.90E−06
rs4272	CDK6	7	G/A	1.1	1.06	1.15	3.40E−07
chr7:128580042	IRF5	7	G/A	1.12	1.09	1.15	4.20E−12
rs2736337	BLK	8	C/T	1.1	1.06	1.14	1.60E−07
rs998731	TPD52	8	T/C	1.09	1.05	1.12	1.30E−07
rs678347	GRHL2	8	G/A	1.1	1.05	1.14	1.40E−07
rs1516971	PVT1	8	T/C	1.13	1.08	1.18	5.30E−07
rs11574914	CCL19-CCL21	9	A/G	1.13	1.09	1.16	1.50E−13
rs10985070	TRAF1-C5	9	C/A	1.09	1.05	1.12	1.70E−08
rs706778	IL2RA	10	T/C	1.11	1.08	1.15	7.10E−12
rs947474	PRKCQ	10	A/G	1.13	1.08	1.17	2.80E−09
rs3824660	GATA3	10	C/T	1.1	1.06	1.14	3.60E−09
rs12413578	10p14	10	C/T	1.2	1.12	1.3	3.30E−07
rs793108	ZNF438	10	T/C	1.07	1.04	1.1	8.20E−06
rs2671692	WDFY4	10	A/G	1.07	1.03	1.1	6.60E−05
rs71508903	ARID5B	10	T/C	1.15	1.11	1.2	3.80E−13
rs6479800	RTKN2	10	C/G	1.08	1.03	1.12	.0022
rs726288	SFTPD	10	T/C	1.08	0.95	1.22	.24
rs331463	TRAF6-RAG1/2	11	T/A	1.11	1.06	1.15	5.70E−06
rs508970	CD5	11	A/G	1.07	1.04	1.11	4.40E−06
rs968567	FADS1-FADS2-FADS3	11	C/T	1.11	1.06	1.15	7.40E−07
rs11605042	ARAP1	11	G/A	1.05	1.01	1.09	.014
rs4409785	CEP57	11	C/T	1.09	1.05	1.14	1.20E−05
chr11:107967350	ATM	11	A/G	1.21	1.12	1.3	4.50E−07
rs10790268	CXCR5	11	G/A	1.18	1.12	1.22	3.30E−15
rs73013527	ETS1	11	C/T	1.09	1.05	1.12	2.00E−06
rs773125	CDK2	12	A/G	1.09	1.06	1.12	8.50E−08
rs1633360	CDK4	12	T/C	1.09	1.05	1.12	9.10E−08
rs10774624	SH2B3-PTPN11	12	G/A	1.09	1.05	1.12	2.40E−07
rs9603616	COG6	13	C/T	1.11	1.08	1.15	8.40E−11
rs3783782	PRKCH	14	A/G	1.07	0.9	1.27	.45
rs1950897	RAD51 B	14	T/C	1.09	1.06	1.13	2.50E−07
rs2582532	PLD4-AHNAK2	14	C/T	1.07	0.83	1.39	.59

(continued on next page)

Table 1
(continued)

SNP	Gene	Chr	A1/A2	OR	95% Confidence Interval		P Value
rs8032939	RASGRP1	15	C/T	1.12	1.09	1.16	2.40E−12
rs8026898	LOC145837	15	A/G	1.16	1.12	1.19	2.40E−17
rs4780401	TXNDC11	16	T/G	1.09	1.05	1.12	5.00E−07
rs13330176	IRF8	16	A/T	1.12	1.08	1.17	9.00E−09
rs72634030	C1QBP	17	A/C	1.11	1.05	1.18	.00047
rs1877030	MED1	17	C/T	1.1	1.05	1.15	1.50E−05
chr17:38031857	IKZF3-CSF3	17	G/T	1.1	1.06	1.14	2.00E−09
rs8083786	PTPN2	18	G/A	1.11	1.08	1.16	1.20E−07
rs2469434	CD226	18	C/T	1.04	1.01	1.08	.012
rs34536443	TYK2	19	G/C	1.46	1.33	1.6	4.60E−16
chr19:10771941	ILF3	19	C/T	1.47	1.3	1.67	8.70E−10
rs4239702	CD40	20	C/T	1.15	1.1	1.18	4.20E−14
rs73194058	IFNGR2	21	C/A	1.14	1.09	1.19	7.10E−08
rs8133843	RUNX1-LOC100506403	21	A/G	1.1	1.06	1.14	6.00E−09
chr21:35928240	RCAN1	21	C/T	1.14	1.09	1.19	2.90E−07
rs1893592	UBASH3A	21	A/C	1.11	1.07	1.15	9.80E−09
rs2236668	ICOSLG-AIRE	21	C/T	1.08	1.04	1.11	1.20E−05
rs11089637	UBE2L3-YDJC	22	C/T	1.11	1.06	1.16	5.60E−07
rs3218251	IL2RB	22	A/T	1.08	1.04	1.11	2.00E−05
rs909685	SYNGR1	22	A/T	1.11	1.08	1.15	3.10E−10
chrX:78464616	P2RY10	X	A/C	1.16	0.78	1.75	.46
rs5987194	IRAK1	X	C/G	1.16	1.11	1.22	2.80E−12

This list reports the findings of Okada et al on the European population. The selection of the list is a result of an analysis on European and Asian ACPA-positive RA patients.

Data from Okada Y, Kim K, Han B, et al. Risk for ACPA-positive rheumatoid arthritis is driven by shared HLA amino acid polymorphisms in Asian and European populations. Hum Mol Genet 2014;23(25):6916–26.

humans, and the current RA mouse models provide only a suggestion of what really happens in humans.

4. Finally, the interactions between genes and environment increase the difficulty in finding the exact mechanism. The presence of gene-environment interaction in RA has clearly been demonstrated by the increased risk of ACPA-positive RA for HLA-SE–positive people who smoke,[16] more precisely for subjects positive for HLA–DRB1 4-amino-acid haplotypes.[17]

At this moment, the significantly strongest, widest replicated, and functionally best understood SNPs are with *PTPN22* (OR = 1.8, 1p13), *PADI4* (OR = 1.11, 1p36), *CTLA4* (OR = 1.15, 2q33), *STAT4* (OR = 1.13, 2q32), and *TRAF1-C5* (OR = 1.08, 9q3) (ORs are for the European population). The reduced expression of *PTPN22* associated with the risk allele diminishes its inhibitory effect on T- and B-cell activation, leading to increased T-cell, dendritic-cell, and B-cell activation.[18] Possibly, *PTPN22* interacts with *PADI4*, which is involved in regulating the citrullination process by which ACPA might ultimately be formed.[19] The stability of the gene is linked to the *PADI4* risk allele, and the PTPN22 risk allele disrupts the interaction of *PTPN22* with PADI4, which leads to hypercitrullination in peripheral blood mononuclear cells.[20] Also, *CTLA4* and *STAT4* are known to influence T cells. *STAT4* enhances the maturation of T-helper cells and acts as a transcription factor. The possible association of prolactin with ACPA-negative RA still has to be further validated, but this finding is particularly interesting because parity and breastfeeding are associated with RA susceptibility.

Most of the functional studies have been performed in mouse models, and the proof that these concepts work in a similar manner in humans remains the subject of further study. When considering that it is not necessarily individual SNPs that generate risk, but rather a series of events, the 100 non-HLA loci reveal 3 pathways that may inform us about the disease process: JAK-STAT signaling, NF-kB, and T-cell receptor signaling.[21] Interestingly, drugs targeting these pathways already exist and have in part been (partially) tested in clinical trials or are currently under use in the clinic.

At a statistical level, the non-HLA genetic risk variants together explain 5% of the variance of RA susceptibility. There are several possible explanations for why so many genetic risk factors explain such a small proportion of the disease heritability:

a. Not all heritable factors are studied: DNA modulation factors (the so-called epigenetics) influence the heritability of the disease but are not necessary captured by studying SNPs.
b. Gene-gene interactions are not taken into account.
c. Gene-environment interactions are not taken into account.

These latter explanations could mean that some of the genetic risk variants are only relevant in the presence of other risk factors, whereby the effect sizes are underestimated or even missed if studied in the total RA population.

Constructing Clinically Applicable Models for Rheumatoid Arthritis Susceptibility

Thus far, the effect size of the associations of the identified genetic variants is not large enough to be useful in clinical settings. Even HLA testing in people at risk or patients with arthritis has little additional value to available clinical measures. For HLA specifically, this is due to the strong association of HLA-DRB1 with ACPA positivity, the fact that ACPA is present before onset of disease, and the widely available ACPA tests (often measured with anti-cyclic citrullinated peptide 2 kits), which make ACPA of more clinical value than specific HLA genes or amino acid chains.

To improve the clinical value of genetic testing, the logical next step is to study the predictive value of the combination of genetic risk factors. Therefore, genetic risk scores (GRS; the total number of risk alleles carried weighted by their odds ratio in the population) have been developed. One model, combining HLA risk alleles with 34 non-HLA SNPs, has an area under the receiver operating characteristic curve (AUC) of 0.56 to 0.70 in predicting RA as outcome.[22] When this model is combined with environmental factors such as smoking, alcohol intake, parity (in case of women), body mass index (BMI), and family history of RA, the model improved to an AUC of 0.70 to 0.83, which outperformed the models of only nongenetic risk factors. Translated into ORs, the combination of a positive family history, greater than 10 pack-years, BMI greater than 25, and a high GRS (>75th percentile) has an OR of 20.89 to develop ACPA-positive RA, whereas without the GRS, this OR is 9.4. The ORs are not as high for ACPA-negative RA or for patients without family history of RA. Intriguingly, it appears that the value of the current available GRSs is confined to subgroups and not to the whole RA population. This confinement could be the result of the focus of genetic studies on ACPA-positive disease. Another explanation is that RA, as it is now known, is not the optimal phenotype to study.

Rheumatoid Arthritis Heterogeneity

A problem of genetic studies in RA is that RA defines a very heterogeneous patient group. This heterogeneity is the direct result of the lack of knowledge of RA abnormality, and as a consequence of that, the fact that classification criteria are imperfect. There is substantial scientific support that the RA population consists of subsets. The most compelling indications are that:

a. Known risk factors are present in only a limited number of patients;
b. The variance in the phenotypical features of the disease is large;
c. Different patients respond to different therapeutic interventions;
d. The heritability estimate of RA is much larger than can be explained by the genetic risk variants currently identified (see discussion of missing heritability in Vincent A. Laufer and colleagues' article, "Integrative Approaches to Understanding the Pathogenic Role of Genetic Variation in Rheumatic Diseases," in this issue).

By using ACPA to optimize heterogeneity, genetic studies have demonstrated a clearly distinct association at the HLA locus for ACPA-negative and ACPA-positive RA patients.[5] The same study demonstrated that the shared genetic structure between the ACPA subsets might be attributable to phenotypical misclassifications, underlining the problem of clinical heterogeneity. Although ACPA positivity is strongly associated with a more severe form of RA, the presence of ACPA on its own appears not to be the optimal (or sole) distinctive feature, because it only explains 23% of the variance of RA severity.[23]

Subsequently, interrogation of the genome with RA disease characteristics is attractive because this can highlight subgroups within RA for which the underlying pathologic mechanisms might differ as well as improve the understanding of processes that are fundamental to RA progression.

GENETIC INFLUENCES ON RHEUMATOID ARTHRITIS SEVERITY

The genetic influences on RA severity are less extensively studied than RA susceptibility. The most widely studied RA severity measure is joint destruction as assessed by radiographs. This outcome has the advantage that it is a reflection of the cumulative burden of inflammation over time, and it can be studied reliably using quantitative measures, such as the modified Sharp score (Sharp van der Heijde score [SHS]) and the Larsen score.[24,25] Furthermore, the heritability of joint destruction is estimated at 45% to 58%.[26] For the purpose of this review, the associations that have been replicated or remained significant in a meta-analysis of cohorts are discussed.

Human Leukocyte Antigen and Rheumatoid Arthritis Joint Destruction

HLA, and particularly HLA-DRB1, is associated with RA severity, although the association is much weaker than for RA susceptibility. HLA-SE is associated with joint destruction in many cohorts. HLA-SE explains 4% of the variance in joint destruction over SHS over 6 years.[23] Possibly, this risk is explained by the ACPA positivity among the HLA-SE–positive patients, as within an ACPA-positive subset of the same study HLA-SE explained less than 0.01% of the total variation.[23] However, studying the HLA-DRB1 amino acids at position 11, 71, and 74 showed an OR of 1.75 for the presence of joint destruction after 5 years in patients with Valine at position 11. This association was independent of ACPA status if a quantitative measure for joint destruction (Larsen) was used.[15]

Notably, this amino acid position was also associated with mortality (hazard ratio 1.16),[15] severity of inflammation, arthritis, and disability in inflammatory polyarthritis.[27]

Non–Human Leukocyte Antigen Genetic Variants in Rheumatoid Arthritis Joint Destruction

The challenges of individual SNP studies are magnified in severity studies by the absence of large cohorts with sensitive data. Most of the findings are the results of candidate gene studies, and if GWAS or Immunochip-wide studies were used, they lack independent replication because of the limited availability of large replication cohorts. There are some variants that either had independent replication or were significant in meta-analysis (see **Fig. 1**B; **Table 2**).

As most of the findings are the result of candidate gene studies, the possible underlying mechanisms are generally bone related or concern perpetuation of inflammation.[23] Several severity studies succeeded in translating the genetic associations into a next step of understanding by adding expression quantitative trait loci (eQTL) or serum protein levels to the analyses (see Vincent A. Laufer and colleagues' article, "Integrative Approaches to Understanding the Pathogenic Role of Genetic Variation in Rheumatic Diseases," in this issue). However, to the authors' knowledge, none of these findings were confirmed by additional studies (see **Table 2** for an overview).

Together, most of the genetic severity factors explained 12% to 18% of the variance in radiologic progression.[23]

Constructing Clinically Applicable Models for Rheumatoid Arthritis Severity

Once a patient has been diagnosed with RA, risk for severe disease is attractive because more intensive treatment strategies could be used. At this moment, clinical models for RA severity are not yet accurate. In particular, patients who developed progressive disease are misclassified in these models.[23,28,29] Adding genetic severity risk markers to a risk model with traditional risk factors (age, gender, symptom duration at first visit, localization initial joint symptoms, 66-swollen joint count, BMI, ACPA-positivity, immunoglobulin M rheumatoid factor positivity, and erythrocyte sedimentation rate) improved the correct classification of RA patients from 54% to 62%. Still, the 38% incorrectly classified patients underscore the limited value for its use in clinical practice for now.

DISCUSSION AND FUTURE PERSPECTIVES

Knowledge on the role of genetics in RA has improved substantially. This improvement is mainly due to the improved genotyping methods, enabling us to densely genotype large regions of the genome and is further facilitated by the large number of patients included in current cohorts. These studies have improved the insights in the functional pathways that are involved, such as CD4$^+$ T cells, JAK-STAT, and B cells, and pointed out a large number of genetic variants that associated with RA susceptibility. Some of those variants are also associated with RA severity, although the severity phenotype has its own risk alleles as well. Intriguingly, these genetic association studies have pointed out treatment targets of which some have already proven to be effective in clinical practice. These findings demonstrates the value of studying the genome in relation to complex diseases such RA. Still, there are many discovered association that have not yet resulted in new insights into RA biology or treatment (**Fig. 1**C). The translation from a genetic association to an understanding of the biology is more complicated than anticipated decades ago.

Therefore, it is important to improve the understanding of a gene's function so every single step can be traced between the observed genetic variance to the clinical phenotypes. It is hoped that recent technical developments such as eQTL analyses to test the association of genetic variation on RNA expression,[30] technical developments such as the ability to measure many markers on a single cell CyTOF,[31] understanding of epigenetics, and plenty of additional valuable genomic research will allow further

Table 2
Genetic variants that are associated with rheumatoid arthritis severity (as defined by joint destruction)

Chr	Genetic Variant	Gene	MAF	Minor Allele	ACPA	Ethnicity	Beta	Description Beta	Validation[a]	Severity Measure
[c] 2	rs7607479[37]	SPAG16	0.33	C	+	C	0.81	SHS/y phase I	A.	SHS
[c] 4	rs7667746[26,38]	IL-15	0.33		Mixed	C	1.86	SHS/y phase I	B.	SHS and Larsen
[c] 4	rs7665842[38]	IL-15	0.4	G	Mixed	C	1.88	SHS/y phase I	B.	SHS and Larsen
[c] 4	rs4371699[38]	IL-15	0.19	A	Mixed	C	1.80	SHS/y phase I	B.	SHS and Larsen
[c] 4	rs6821171[38]	IL-15	0.29	C	Mixed	C	0.64	SHS/y phase I	B.	SHS and Larsen
[c] 5	rs26232[39]	C5orf30	0.29	T	Mixed	C	0.90	Incidence rate ratio (time not completely clear)	A.	SHS and Larsen
5	rs7445819[40]	CAPSL	0.11	T	Mixed	C (MA & EA)	1.39	SHS/y phase I	A.	SHS hands
5	rs10043548[40]	LOC100132524/RAI14	0.28	T	Mixed	C (MA & EA)	0.81	SHS/y phase I	A.	SHS hands
5	rs10058554[40]	LOC100132524/RAI14	0.27	T	Mixed	C (MA & EA)	0.82	SHS/y phase I	A.	SHS hands
6	DRB1*04:01[41]	HLA_DRB1		P vs A[b]	Mixed	C	1.10	Larsen/y?	A.	SHS hands
[c] 6	rs981042[40]	CDKAL1	0.07	T	Mixed	C (MA & EA)	1.35	SHS/y phase I	A.	SHS hands
[c] 8	rs1485305[42]	OPG	0.44	T	Mixed	C	1.03	Phase I SHS/y	B.	SHS and Larsen
[c] 9	rs2900180[43]	C5-traf1	36	A	—	C	1.05	Phase I SHS/y	A.	SHS
[c] 10	rs1896368[44]	DKK-1	0.47	G	Mixed	C	1.02	SHS/y phase I	B.	SHS and Larsen
[c] 10	rs1896367[44]	DKK-1	0.41	A	Mixed	C	0.98	SHS/y phase I	B.	SHS and Larsen
[c] 10	rs1528873[44]	DKK-1	0.47	A	Mixed	C	1.02	SHS/y phase I	B.	SHS and Larsen
[c] 10	rs2104286[45]	IL2RA	0.24	C	Mixed	C	0.98	SHS/y phase I	A.	SHS
[c] 14	rs8192916[45]	GRZB	0.42	A	Mixed	C	1.05	SHS/y phase I	B.	SHS and Larsen
[c] 14	rs451066[46]	RAD51ZFP36L1	0.2	A	Mixed	C	N/A	SHS/y phase I	A.	SHS
[c] 16	rs1119132[47]	IL-4R	0.13	A	Mixed	C	1.02	SHS/y phase I	B.	SHS and Larsen
[c] 20	rs4810485[48]	CD40	0.24	T	+	C	1.12	SHS/y phase I	A.	SHS
[c] 20	rs11908352[46]	MMP-9	0.21	A	Mixed	C	N/A	SHS/y phase I	A.	SHS

Abbreviations: C, Caucasian; EA, European American; MA, Mexican American; N/A, not available.

[a] Validated through (A) independent replication, (B) meta-analysis.
[b] Present versus absent.
[c] SNPs included in the explained variance calculation of van Steenbergen et al ARD 2015.[23]

understanding.[32] It is hoped that the better understanding of DNA function will translate into better understanding of clinical phenotypes.

The persistence of this knowledge gap is largely explained by the small effect sizes of individual variants that are often located in introns, regions that in general are considered nonfunctional. These small effect sizes are probably the result of a combination of issues:

1. The known risk variants are a proxy of the causal variant(s).
2. Not one, but a combination of genetic risk variants creates a risk profile.
3. The studied phenotype (which concerns RA itself as well as RA severity and RA treatment response) is not well defined whereby the studied groups are too heterogeneous.

To remove this obstacle and improve the understanding of RA, ingenious methods are needed that are able to deal with many factors and high dimensional data (see Vincent A. Laufer and colleagues' article, "Integrative Approaches to Understanding the Pathogenic Role of Genetic Variation in Rheumatic Diseases," in this issue). This is where, it is hoped, the relatively young and growing field of bioinformatic research adds value to disentangling complex combination of events and information. For example, several computational methods to tackle the situation mentioned above have been developed:

- Prioritization methods; to enable identification of possible causal variants based on the discovered risk variants.[33,34]
- Gene interaction testing models.[35]
- Methods to discern genetic heterogeneity.[36]

In addition to the data management and interpretation methods, the clinical field keeps improving the definition of all different phenotypic aspect of (pre-) clinical RA.

Challenges lie in many different fields of expertise (genetics, biology, bioinformatics, pharmacology, clinical medicine, and so forth). As knowledge and methodologies improve in each of these areas, combining them will result in an exponential increase in the understanding of RA.

With regard to clinical application of genetic testing for RA patients, we have to wait for the models to be improved. However, considering the currently fairly high accuracy of the genetic prediction models and the rapid increase in genetic understanding, soon the applicability of such models will likely be restricted by the absence of appropriate intervention methods than by a lack of accuracy.

REFERENCES

1. Jiang X, Frisell T, Askling J, et al. To what extent is the familial risk of rheumatoid arthritis explained by established rheumatoid arthritis risk factors? Arthritis Rheumatol 2015;67(2):352–62.
2. McInnes IB, Schett G. The pathogenesis of rheumatoid arthritis. N Engl J Med 2011;365(23):2205–19.
3. Gregersen PK, Silver J, Winchester RJ. The shared epitope hypothesis. An approach to understanding the molecular genetics of susceptibility to rheumatoid arthritis. Arthritis Rheum 1987;30(11):9.
4. Raychaudhuri S, Sandor C, Stahl EA, et al. Five amino acids in three HLA proteins explain most of the association between MHC and seropositive rheumatoid arthritis. Nat Genet 2012;44(3):291–6.
5. Han B, Diogo D, Eyre S, et al. Fine mapping seronegative and seropositive rheumatoid arthritis to shared and distinct HLA alleles by adjusting for the effects of heterogeneity. Am J Hum Genet 2014;94(4):522–32.

6. Okada Y, Kim K, Han B, et al. Risk for ACPA-positive rheumatoid arthritis is driven by shared HLA amino acid polymorphisms in Asian and European populations. Hum Mol Genet 2014;23(25):6916–26.

7. Reynolds RJ, Ahmed AF, Danila MI, et al. HLA-DRB1-associated rheumatoid arthritis risk at multiple levels in African Americans: hierarchical classification systems, amino acid positions, and residues. Arthritis Rheumatol 2014;66(12): 3274–82.

8. Oka SF H, Kawasaki A, Shimada K, et al. Protective effect of the HLA-DRB1*13:02 allele in Japanese rheumatoid arthritis patients. PLoS one 2014;9(6):e99453.

9. van der Woude D, Lie BA, Lundstrom E, et al. Protection against anti-citrullinated protein antibody-positive rheumatoid arthritis is predominantly associated with HLA-DRB1*1301: a meta-analysis of HLA-DRB1 associations with anti-citrullinated protein antibody-positive and anti-citrullinated protein antibody-negative rheumatoid arthritis in four European populations. Arthritis Rheum 2010;62(5):1236–45.

10. Okada Y, Wu D, Trynka G, et al. Genetics of rheumatoid arthritis contributes to biology and drug discovery. Nature 2014;506(7488):376–81.

11. Viatte S, Plant D, Han B, et al. Association of HLA-DRB1 haplotypes with rheumatoid arthritis severity, mortality, and treatment response. JAMA 2015;313(16): 1645–56.

12. van der Woude D, Catrina AI. HLA and anti-citrullinated protein antibodies: building blocks in RA. Best Pract Res Clin Rheumatol 2015;29(6):692–705.

13. Bossini-Castillo L, de Kovel C, Kallberg H, et al. A genome-wide association study of rheumatoid arthritis without antibodies against citrullinated peptides. Ann Rheum Dis 2015;74(3):e15.

14. Terao C, Ohmura K, Kochi Y, et al. Anti-citrullinated peptide/protein antibody (ACPA)-negative RA shares a large proportion of susceptibility loci with ACPA-positive RA: a meta-analysis of genome-wide association study in a Japanese population. Arthritis Res Ther 2015;17:104.

15. Viatte S, Massey J, Bowes J, et al. Replication of associations of genetic loci outside the HLA region with susceptibility to anti-cyclic citrullinated peptide-negative rheumatoid arthritis. Arthritis Rheumatol 2016;68(7):1603–13.

16. Jiang X, Kallberg H, Chen Z, et al. An Immunochip-based interaction study of contrasting interaction effects with smoking in ACPA-positive versus ACPA-negative rheumatoid arthritis. Rheumatology (Oxford) 2016;55(1):149–55.

17. Kim K, Jiang X, Cui J, et al. Interactions between amino acid-defined major histocompatibility complex class II variants and smoking in seropositive rheumatoid arthritis. Arthritis Rheumatol 2015;67(10):2611–23.

18. Rieck M, Arechiga A, Onengut-Gumuscu S, et al. Genetic variation in PTPN22 corresponds to altered function of T and B lymphocytes. J Immunol 2007; 179(7):4704–10.

19. Suzuki A1 YR, Chang X, Tokuhiro S, et al. Functional haplotypes of PADI4, encoding citrullinating enzyme peptidylarginine deiminase 4, are associated with rheumatoid arthritis. Nat Genet 2003;34(4):8.

20. Chang HH, Dwivedi N, Nicholas AP, et al. The W620 polymorphism in PTPN22 disrupts its interaction with peptidylarginine deiminase type 4 and enhances citrullination and NETosis. Arthritis Rheumatol 2015;67(9): 2323–34.

21. Messemaker TC, Huizinga TW, Kurreeman F. Immunogenetics of rheumatoid arthritis: understanding functional implications. J Autoimmun 2015;64:74–81.

22. Sparks JA, Chen CY, Jiang X, et al. Improved performance of epidemiologic and genetic risk models for rheumatoid arthritis serologic phenotypes using family history. Ann Rheum Dis 2015;74(8):1522–9.
23. van Steenbergen HW, Tsonaka R, Huizinga TW, et al. Predicting the severity of joint damage in rheumatoid arthritis; the contribution of genetic factors. Ann Rheum Dis 2015;74(5):876–82.
24. Boini S, Guillemin F. Radiographic scoring methods as outcome measures in rheumatoid arthritis: properties and advantages. Ann Rheum Dis 2001;60:11.
25. van der Helm-van Mil AH, Knevel R, van der Heijde D, et al. How to avoid phenotypic misclassification in using joint destruction as an outcome measure for rheumatoid arthritis? Rheumatology (Oxford, England) 2010;49(8):1429–35.
26. Knevel R, Grondal G, Huizinga TW, et al. Genetic predisposition of the severity of joint destruction in rheumatoid arthritis: a population-based study. Ann Rheum Dis 2012;71(5):707–9.
27. Ling SF, Viatte S, Lunt M, et al. HLA-DRB1 amino acid positions 11/13, 71, and 74 are associated with inflammation level, disease activity, and the health assessment questionnaire score in patients with inflammatory polyarthritis. Arthritis Rheumatol 2016;68(11):2618–28.
28. Visser K, Goekoop-Ruiterman YP, de Vries-Bouwstra JK, et al. A matrix risk model for the prediction of rapid radiographic progression in patients with rheumatoid arthritis receiving different dynamic treatment strategies: post hoc analyses from the BeSt study. Ann Rheum Dis 2010;69(7):1333–7.
29. Lillegraven S, Paynter N, Prince FH, et al. Performance of matrix-based risk models for rapid radiographic progression in a cohort of patients with established rheumatoid arthritis. Arthritis Care Res (Hoboken) 2013;65(4):526–33.
30. Westra HJ, Arends D, Esko T, et al. Cell specific eQTL analysis without sorting cells. PLoS Genet 2015;11(5):e1005223.
31. Cheung RK, Utz PJ. Screening: CyTOF-the next generation of cell detection. Nat Rev Rheumatol 2011;7(9):502–3.
32. Trynka G, Sandor C, Han B, et al. Chromatin marks identify critical cell types for fine mapping complex trait variants. Nat Genet 2013;45(2):124–30.
33. Farh KK, Marson A, Zhu J, et al. Genetic and epigenetic fine mapping of causal autoimmune disease variants. Nature 2015;518(7539):337–43.
34. Trynka G, Westra HJ, Slowikowski K, et al. Disentangling the effects of colocalizing genomic annotations to functionally prioritize non-coding variants within complex-trait loci. Am J Hum Genet 2015;97(1):139–52.
35. Li J, Huang D, Guo M, et al. A gene-based information gain method for detecting gene-gene interactions in case-control studies. Eur J Hum Genet 2015;23(11):1566–72.
36. Han B, Pouget JG, Slowikowski K, et al. A method to decipher pleiotropy by detecting underlying heterogeneity driven by hidden subgroups applied to autoimmune and neuropsychiatric diseases. Nat Genet 2016;48(7):803–10.
37. Knevel R, Klein K, Somers K, et al. Identification of a genetic variant for joint damage progression in autoantibody-positive rheumatoid arthritis. Ann Rheum Dis 2014;73(11):2038–46.
38. Knevel R, Krabben A, Brouwer E, et al. Genetic variants in IL15 associate with progression of joint destruction in rheumatoid arthritis: a multicohort study. Ann Rheum Dis 2012;71(10):1651–7.
39. Teare MD, Knevel R, Morgan MD, et al. Allele-dose association of the C5orf30 rs26232 variant with joint damage in rheumatoid arthritis. Arthritis Rheum 2013;65(10):2555–61.

40. Arya R, Del Rincon I, Farook VS, et al. Genetic variants influencing joint damage in Mexican Americans and European Americans with rheumatoid arthritis. Genet Epidemiol 2015;39(8):678–88.

41. Scott IC, Rijsdijk F, Walker J, et al. Do genetic susceptibility variants associate with disease severity in early active rheumatoid arthritis? J Rheumatol 2015; 42(7):1131–40.

42. Knevel R, de Rooy DP, Saxne T, et al. A genetic variant in osteoprotegerin is associated with progression of joint destruction in rheumatoid arthritis. Arthritis Res Ther 2014;16(3):R108.

43. van Steenbergen HW, Rodriguez-Rodriguez L, Berglin E, et al. A genetic study on C5-TRAF1 and progression of joint damage in rheumatoid arthritis. Arthritis Res Ther 2015;17:1.

44. de Rooy DP, Yeremenko NG, Wilson AG, et al. Genetic studies on components of the Wnt signalling pathway and the severity of joint destruction in rheumatoid arthritis. Ann Rheum Dis 2013;72(5):769–75.

45. Knevel R, de Rooy DP, Zhernakova A, et al. Association of variants in IL2RA with progression of joint destruction in rheumatoid arthritis. Arthritis Rheum 2013; 65(7):1684–93.

46. de Rooy DP, Zhernakova A, Tsonaka R, et al. A genetic variant in the region of MMP-9 is associated with serum levels and progression of joint damage in rheumatoid arthritis. Ann Rheum Dis 2014;73(6):1163–9.

47. Krabben A, Wilson AG, de Rooy DP, et al. Association of genetic variants in the IL4 and IL4R genes with the severity of joint damage in rheumatoid arthritis: a study in seven cohorts. Arthritis Rheum 2013;65(12):3051–7.

48. van der Linden MP, Feitsma AL, le Cessie S, et al. Association of a single-nucleotide polymorphism in CD40 with the rate of joint destruction in rheumatoid arthritis. Arthritis Rheum 2009;60(8):2242–7.

Human Leukocyte Antigen–Disease Associations in Rheumatoid Arthritis

Vincent van Drongelen, PhD, Joseph Holoshitz, MD*

KEYWORDS

- HLA • Rheumatoid arthritis • Autoimmunity • Shared epitope

KEY POINTS

- Certain human leukocyte antigen (HLA) alleles have been found to be associated with immune mediated or autoimmune diseases, but the underlying mechanisms are largely unknown.
- Rheumatoid arthritis (RA) strongly associates with *HLA-DRB1* alleles that encode a sequence motif called shared epitope (SE), and there is variability in the strength of RA-SE association among ethnic and racial populations.
- The SE shows interaction with environmental factors (tobacco exposure) and together significantly amplify the disease risk.
- In contrast to RA risk-conferring SE-coding alleles, there are several other *DRB1* alleles that protect against the disease.
- Genome-wide association studies discovered many non-HLA RA risk loci, but their aggregate contribution to RA risk is outweighed by that of the SE.

Disclosure: The authors have nothing to disclose.
Funding Sources: Dr J. Holoshitz has been supported by the Eleanor and Larry Jackier Research Award from the UM–Israel Partnership for Research program and by grants from The National Institute of Environmental Health Sciences (R21 ES024428), The National Institute of General Medical Sciences (R01 GM088560), The National Institute of Dental and Craniofacial Research (R21 DE023845), and The National Institute of Arthritis and Musculoskeletal and Skin Diseases (R01 AR059085). The content is solely the responsibility of the authors and does not necessarily represent the official views of the National Institutes of Health.

Department of Internal Medicine, University of Michigan, 1150 West Medical Center Drive, Ann Arbor, MI 48109, USA
* Corresponding author. University of Michigan, 5520D MSRB1, SPC 5680, 1150 West Medical Center Drive, Ann Arbor, MI 48109-5680.
E-mail address: jholo@umich.edu

Rheum Dis Clin N Am 43 (2017) 363–376
http://dx.doi.org/10.1016/j.rdc.2017.04.003
0889-857X/17/© 2017 Elsevier Inc. All rights reserved.

rheumatic.theclinics.com

INTRODUCTION

Rheumatoid arthritis (RA) is a common inflammatory disease in which both genetic and environmental factors play a role in disease development. Based on twin studies, the heritability of the disease was estimated at around 60%.[1] Among all the genetic risk factors found to date, the human leukocyte antigen (HLA) locus is the most significant one. A particularly strong association between RA and *HLA-DRB1* alleles that encode an HLA-DRβ chain containing a 5 amino acid sequence motif called the shared epitope (SE) has long been documented.[2] Here the authors review salient immunogenetic, clinical, and mechanistic features of RA association with the HLA locus, focusing primarily on the SE.

Human Leukocyte Antigen Genes and Their Products

The immune system is composed of various cells that work together to protect the host against invading pathogens without harming its own tissues. Therefore, the host has to recognize which antigens are self and which are foreign. To discriminate between such self- and foreign antigens, the major histocompatibility complex (MHC) antigens, known in humans as HLA, have evolved. MHC molecules have the ability to recognize and present foreign antigens to the immune system but at the same time disregard self-antigens. This ability to discriminate between self and foreign is established through a process called "MHC restriction."[3] During the development of T cells in the thymus, T cells that react to self-antigens are eliminated, whereas those that respond to foreign antigens that are presented by a self-HLA molecule are preserved. This selection results in CD4[+] and CD8[+] T cells that only respond to foreign antigens that are presented by self-HLA molecules. Despite their ability to selectively recognize and respond to foreign antigens, many HLA alleles have been found to confer susceptibility to various diseases, most of which involve dysregulated immunity or autoimmunity.

The HLA locus is located on the short arm of chromosome 6 and covers a 7.6-Mb region that contains more than 250 highly polymorphic genes.[4] The region is organized in 3 subregions: class I, class II, and class III, which all have different functions. Both class I and II regions encode for glycoproteins that are expressed as cell surface receptors, whereas the class III region contains genes that encode for a variety of secreted immune system proteins, including complement factors and cytokines.

The class I region encodes for 3 main subsets of HLA molecules: HLA-A, HLA-B, and HLA-C. Class I HLA molecules are composed of an HLA-coded heavy α-chain and an invariant light chain, beta-2 microglobulin, which is essential for functional expression of the HLA molecule at the cell surface. The α-chain is folded to form a peptide-binding cleft that is closed and can accommodate short antigenic peptides, typically 8 to 10 amino acids long. These class I molecules are expressed on all nucleated cells and specialize in presentation of intracellular antigens, including viral antigens, to cytotoxic (CD8[+]) T cells. Genes in the class II region encode for HLA-DR, HLA-DP, and HLA-DQ molecules as well as a few other related proteins. Class II HLA molecules are composed of an α-chain and a β-chain, both coded by the HLA class II region. Unlike the class I molecules, the peptide-binding cleft of class II molecules are open, which allows the accommodation of larger peptides of 15 to 20 amino acids long. Class II molecules are initially expressed on the cell surface of immune cells, in particular antigen-presenting cells, such as macrophages or dendritic cells, as well as B cells and activated T cells. These molecules present antigens from outside the cell to (CD4[+]) T cells, which in turn stimulate B cells to produce antibodies toward that specific antigen, resulting in an antigen-specific immune response. After activation of the immune system, the HLA class II molecules can be expressed on other cells.

Human Leukocyte Antigen–Associated Diseases

The HLA locus is a highly polymorphic region. Its high gene density, presence of clusters of genes with related functions, enormous polymorphism, and a strong linkage disequilibrium (LD) between alleles, renders it difficult to unravel the comprehensive HLA functions. During the last several decades, various conditions, such as infectious diseases,[5] cancer,[6] or autoimmune diseases,[7] have been found to be more prevalent in individuals who carry certain HLA alleles. Most HLA-associated diseases can be classified as autoimmune or immune-mediated disease and have been observed with merely HLA class I alleles (eg, ankylosing spondylitis [AS])[8] or merely class II alleles (eg, seropositive RA).[9] Additionally, some autoimmune diseases have been found to be influenced by both HLA class I and class II genes (eg, diabetes mellitus type I).[10] In addition to HLA alleles that predispose to disease, there are also several HLA alleles that are protective against disease.

How certain HLA alleles predispose to or protect against (autoimmune) diseases and what the underlying molecular mechanisms are is currently unclear. The hypotheses that have been proposed over the years commonly implicate atypical presentation of self-antigens,[11,12] an immune response to altered self-antigens[13] or cross-reactivity with foreign or self-antigens.[14,15] These hypotheses may seem plausible based on HLA function and their role in the immune response. However, despite their plausibility, the mechanistic and epidemiologic evidence that is currently available is difficult to reconcile with presentation of specific antigens being the underlying mechanism for HLA-disease association.

Several examples of HLA alleles are associated with more than one disease with completely different target tissues and pathogeneses, which defies the notion that antigen presentation should be specific for both the antigen and the presenting HLA molecule. Examples of such HLA alleles are *HLA-DRB1*04:01*, which is associated with both RA and type 1 diabetes,[16] and *HLA-DQB1*03:02*, which is associated with both type 1 diabetes and celiac disease.[17,18] In addition, there are certain HLA alleles that predispose to one disease but protect against another; for example, *HLA-DRB1*04:02* has been found to confer susceptibility to pemphigus vulgaris (PV) but at the same time protect against RA (discussed later).

Furthermore, the most significant HLA-disease association to date has been found for a brain disorder (narcolepsy), which is not known to involve antigen presentation.[19] Also, certain HLA molecules have been found to have functions unrelated to antigen presentation, including cognition,[20] olfaction, and the activation of innate immune signaling (reviewed in Ref.[21]).

In addition, some disease-associated alleles have been shown to demonstrate cross-species susceptibility; for example, *HLA-DRB1*04:01* associates with human RA and also confers susceptibility to inflammatory arthritis in mice.[22]

Moreover, despite extensive efforts to identify target antigens in autoimmune diseases, they have only been identified for a very small number of diseases. Also, presence of T-cell clonality, a phenomenon that can be expected in case of the presence of a specific antigen, has not been convincingly demonstrated in HLA-associated diseases.

Lastly, RA disease severity has been shown to correlate with HLA allele dose, that is, two allele copies confer greater susceptibility, severity, and penetrance compared with one copy (discussed later). Such allele-dose impact on RA disease severity cannot be explained by antigen presentation–based hypotheses.

HUMAN LEUKOCYTE ANTIGEN-RHEUMATOID ARTHRITIS ASSOCIATIONS
The Shared Epitope

RA association with HLA has been known since 1969,[23] and the associations with specific DR4 allotypes were identified in the late 1970s.[24,25] The term *shared epitope*[2] was coined in the late 1980s following the discovery that most patients with RA share a 5 amino acid sequence motif (ie, QKRAA, QRRAA, or RRRAA) in residues 70 to 74 of the DRβ chain, coded by several distinct *DRB1* alleles in individuals expressing DR4 and non-DR4 allotypes. Recent genomic imputation analyses suggest that in addition to residues 70 to 74 in the α helical rim of DRβ chain, the classically defined SE, residues 11 and/or 13, located in the floor of the HLA-DR groove, are also associated with RA susceptibility,[26,27] suggesting that presentation of peptide antigens may play a role in RA cause. However, this imputation-based hypothesis awaits experimental validation; the relevance of these statistical data to RA cause has recently been questioned.[28] Additionally, despite several decades of research, the identity of putative arthritis-causing peptides remains elusive. The findings of a recent study raise further doubts on the notion of specific antigen presentation by SE-expressing RA-associated DR molecules because a comparative analysis identified only negligible overlaps in the repertoires of peptides eluted from different SE-expressing HLA-DR molecules.[29] The epidemiologic and clinical aspects of RA genetics, including the SE, have been reviewed elsewhere.[30,31]

The SE not only confers a higher risk for RA but also increases the likelihood of developing earlier disease onset, more severe bone erosions,[9,32–34] and anticitrulli-nated protein antibodies (ACPA).[35] SE-RA association and disease severity are gene-dose dependent. For example, in individuals carrying one SE-coding allele, the odds ratio (OR) of developing joint damage compared with SE-negative individuals is 2.38. With 2 SE-coding alleles, the OR increases to 3.92.[36] Furthermore, there is additional evidence of an allele-dose effect, in which early disease onset, severity of bone destruction, and higher disease concordance among monozygotic twins all correlate with the number of SE-coding *HLA-DRB1* alleles.[9,33,34]

It is worth mentioning that not only inherited genes confer SE-RA association. Non-inherited maternal HLA antigens (NIMA) carrying SE motifs have been shown to confer RA risk in SE-negative individuals,[37] especially in younger-onset RA in women.[38] Thus, minute amounts of maternal SE acquired during the fetal period is sufficient to determine RA susceptibility. This mechanism may account for some of the SE-negative subset of RA.

Ethnic and Racial Factors That Affect Shared Epitope–Rheumatoid Arthritis Association

Considerable ethnic and racial stratification exists within the SE-positive RA subset in terms of association with specific SE-coding *DRB1* alleles (reviewed in[39]). For example, in European patients with RA, *DRB1*04:01*, *04:04*, *01:01*, and *10:01* are the predominant SE-coding alleles, whereas in East Asians, the most common SE-coding allele is *DRB1*04:05*. In Pima, Tlingit, Yakima, and Chippewa Native American individuals, an SE-coding allele *DRB1*14:02* has been found to be a significant genetic risk factor for severe RA.[40,41]

RA is generally less common among Africans compared with populations of European descent,[42,43] and the frequency of SE-coding alleles in African American patients with RA is approximately one-third of that reported in European patients with RA.[44] Nonetheless, SE-coding *DRB1* alleles are almost twice as common in African American patients with RA compared with healthy control subjects.[44] This finding indicates that the SE is a significant risk factor in African Americans, albeit to a lesser extent than in Caucasians. Importantly, the prevalence of SE-coding alleles in African Americans correlates positively with the extent of estimated European ancestry, regardless of RA status, suggesting that genetic admixture between European and African American populations is responsible for introducing RA risk in the latter population.[44]

Shared Epitope and Anticitrullinated Protein Antibodies

ACPA (or anticyclic citrullinated peptide [anti-CCP]) is a useful disease marker in RA. These antibodies associate with severe, erosive disease[45,46] and relevant to this review, they are strongly associated with SE-coding *DRB1* alleles.[35,47] Among different patients with SE-positive RA, those carrying the *DRB1*04* group of alleles display higher ACPA titers compared with those carrying *DRB1*01* alleles.[48] An early study on patients with RA in the Netherlands[49] demonstrated an OR of 3.3 for anti-CCP positivity in patients with RA with a single SE-coding allele (*DRB1*01, *04, *10*). The OR in patients with RA with 2 SE-coding alleles was 13.3, suggesting an SE gene-dose effect on anti-CCP positivity. In anti-CCP–negative European patients with RA, on the other hand, a significant RA association (OR = 1.84) with the DR3 allotype was reported.[50] In Japanese individuals, who rarely carry the *DRB1*03:01* allele, a significant association with DR14 and DR8 was found.[51] Thus, the ACPA-positive and -negative subsets of RA associate with different *HLA-DRB1* alleles and should be, therefore, considered immunogenetically distinct diseases.

The strong association between SE-coding alleles and ACPA suggest a cause-effect relationship, although the precise underlying mechanism remains unknown. A common hypothesis states that the SE represents an obligatory amino acid sequence in the HLA-DR antigen presentation pocket that is critical and necessary for antigen-specific presentation of citrullinated antigen-derived peptides to citrullinated protein-specific helper T cells, which help B cells to produce ACPA. According to this scenario, ACPA react against tissue citrullinated proteins, which results in autoimmunity.[52,53] Although this hypothesis is plausible, it is difficult to reconcile with the findings that ACPA can be detected in patients with RA years before disease onset.[54,55] Furthermore, ACPA in RA sera display promiscuous specificity against multiple citrullinated proteins, which do not share sequence homology, such as vimentin,[56] a-enolase,[57] collagen type II,[58] or fibrin,[59] among other candidate self-proteins. Such promiscuity is inconsistent with the HLA-restricted antigen-presentation concept.

In addition to the antigen specificity paradox discussed earlier, the hypotheses that postulate an effector role for ACPA in disease pathogenesis seem to dismiss a sizable body of literature implicating presence of polymorphisms in the peptidyl arginine deiminase 4 (*PADI4*) gene in certain populations[60,61] and evidence for enzyme dysregulation and overabundance of citrullinated proteins in RA.[62–64] These data suggest that citrullinated proteins, independent of ACPA, are at least partially accountable for RA pathogenesis. Although definitive explanations of this paradox are absent, it is worth mentioning that the HLA Cusp Theory[65,66] has previously proposed that, in addition to antigen presentation, HLA-DR molecules may perform other, non–antigen-presentation allele-specific functions, through the third allelic hypervariable region of the DRβ chain, as depicted graphically in **Fig. 1**. The authors' group has demonstrated that the SE acts as a signal transduction ligand that leads to immune dysregulation and osteoclast activation, independent of its putative antigen-presentation role.[67–74] It remains to be seen if a non–antigen-presentation mechanism, such as SE ligand-activated signaling, could shed light on the SE-ACPA association paradox.

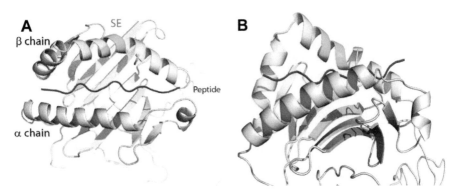

Fig. 1. The SE ligand. Crystal structure of HLA-DR4 (*DRB1*04:01*) molecule in top (*A*) and side (*B*) views. The DRα chain is colored in gray; the DRβ chain is shown in yellow, and the groove peptide is shown in red. The SE (residues 70–74) is shown in cyan.

Shared epitope–environment interaction

Approximately two-thirds of RA risk is attributed to genetic factors, of which the SE is the most significant one. The remaining one-third of disease susceptibility is attributed to nongenetic mechanisms that are most likely triggered by environmental factors. Over the years, ample evidence has been gathered to support the role of environmental factors in disease onset. For example, the disease is historically thought to have gained higher prevalence in the Old World concomitant with the Industrial Revolution; prevalence of the disease is higher in urban populations; the disease incidence varies by birth cohort; and most importantly, conclusive evidence has been established for an association between RA and exposure to cigarette smoke.[75] Several studies have identified interactions between the SE and tobacco exposure.[76–78] For example, a Swedish group reported a strong interaction between SE and smoking in RA risk, particularly in SE homozygous individuals.[77] Similar conclusions have been reached by a Danish study,[78] and a very large US survey has demonstrated strong interaction between heavy smoking and SE in RA.[76] In African Americans, the contribution of cigarette smoking to RA was found to be limited to those with more than 10 years of exposure, particularly among patients carrying SE-coding *DRB1* alleles.[79] Thus, there is compelling evidence for interaction between SE and tobacco exposure in the cause of RA in diverse populations.

The mechanistic basis of SE-smoking interaction in RA cause and pathogenesis is unknown. A popular model for the cause of RA suggests that the association between smoking and RA is due to the ability of the former to enhance SE-dependent immune reaction to citrullinated proteins, which, in turn, trigger disease.[80] According to this model, smoking increases the abundance of citrullinated proteins in the lung, which in SE-positive individuals may provide an antigenic stimulus for ACPA generation. More recently, another group has reported that SE-smoking interaction does not shape the reactivity of the ACPA response, suggesting that smoking activates antigen-nonspecific citrullination.[81]

Bacterial infection has long been proposed as an environmental etiologic factor for RA.[82] Given that ACPA may be found years before disease onset in RA, it has been speculated that before RA, extra-articular infections may be the culprit. For example, recently, there has been a growing interest in the possible contribution of smoking-induced lung infection as an extra-articular source of disease-triggering infection. A recent study suggested that smoking-associated bronchiectasis might be an

RA-triggering cause due to enhanced production of ACPA in such individuals.[83] Periodontal disease (PD), another extra-articular chronically infected site, has been proposed as a culprit in RA because of the known association between the two diseases[84]; the fact that a well-studied PD-triggering bacterium, *Porphyromonas gingivalis*, expresses the bacterial PAD enzyme.[85] In the context of this review, however, it should be pointed out that PD has been shown to associate with SE-coding alleles independent of RA.[86,87] How this confounding factor affects the interpretation of studies focusing on the etiologic role of oral bacterial agents on RA cause is currently unclear.

Protective DRB1 Alleles

Although the QKRAA, QRRAA, or RRRAA sequences in position 70 to 74 of the DRβ chain have been shown to increase RA risk, alleles that code for D instead of Q or R in position 70,[88,89] particularly the 70-DERAA-74 sequence, which is coded by several alleles, including *DRB1*01:03, DRB1*13:01, DRB1*13:02,* or *DRB1*04:02,* exert a protective effect.[90,91] Interestingly, diametrically opposite of the pro-RA effect of SE-expressing NIMA,[37,38] DERAA-expressing NIMA have been shown to protect against the disease.[92]

The mechanism of this allele-based protection is unknown, although it was recently proposed that this association is due to cross-reactivity between citrullinated-vinculin and microbial proteins, due to presentation of the DERAA sequence by *DQB* alleles that are in LD with SE-coding *DRB1* alleles.[15] Nonetheless, besides the fact that this intriguing hypothesis awaits experimental validation, it also seems to contradict published data from the same group that indicate that DERAA-expressing alleles are protective against RA independent of an SE-coding *DRB1* allele[90] and the dominant protective effect of a DERAA-expressing transgene on the development of Collagen-Induced Arthritis (CIA) independent of any DQ molecules.[93] Moreover, this hypothesis does not explain why exposure of SE-positive haplotypes to the DERAA sequence, ubiquitously expressed by microbial proteins, cannot mount a similar immune protective effect in individuals without DERAA-coding alleles. Finally, DERAA-coding *DRB1* alleles have been shown to be protective against several other autoimmune diseases besides RA,[94,95] suggesting an antigen-nonspecific modulatory effect, rather than antigen presentation-based mechanism.

The 70-DERAA-74 sequence coded by *HLA-DRB1*0402,* as well as by several other alleles, exerts a dominant protective effect in RA[90,91]; presence of one DERAA-coding *HLA-DRB1* allele provides protection against RA even in the presence of predisposing SE-positive alleles.[90]

However, this allele has been shown to predispose to PV, a potentially lethal autoimmune disease that is characterized by blistering of the skin and the mucosal membranes. Although this disease is relatively rare, it is associated with considerable morbidity and mortality.[96] Little is currently known about the mechanistic basis of the association of *HLA-DRB1*04:02* with PV, but some have postulated that this allele binds and allows presentation of desmoglein 3, an identified autoantigen in PV. However, the evidence supporting this hypothesis is ambiguous. The dual role of *HLA-DRB1*04:02* in HLA-disease association, being protective in RA and at the same time being a genetic risk factor for PV, is currently not understood.

Non–Shared Epitope–coding Human Leukocyte Antigen Alleles in Rheumatoid Arthritis

As mentioned earlier, although ACPA-positive RA strongly associates with SE-coding *DRB1* alleles, the ACPA-negative subset has been shown to associate with other, non-SE-coding HLA alleles, such as *DRB1*03:01*, *DR14*, or *DR8*. In East Asians, associations of RA with a homozygous non–SE-coding allele *DRB1*09:01*[97] or a heterozygous combination of *DRB1*04:05/09:01* alleles[98] have been anecdotally reported. Although the prevalence and mechanistic basis of these associations remain to be better explored, it is clear that there is more to learn about the stringency of the SE motif as an RA genetic risk factor.

The *DR* and *DQ* loci are inherited in strong linkage disequilibrium. It is, therefore, not surprising that both loci are statistically found to associate with RA. RA-associated *DRB1* alleles have been particularly demonstrated in haplotypes with certain *DQ* loci. For example, the SE-coding *DRB1*04:01* has been found in haplotypes that include *DQA1*03-DQB1*03:01* or *DQA1*03-DQB1*03:02* alleles, the SE-coding *DRB1*04:04* has been shown to form haplotypes with *DQA1*03-DQB1*03:02*.[99] However, although extensive evidence exists to substantiate a direct role of the *DRB1* locus in RA, evidence to support such role for the *DQ* locus remains to be conclusively shown.

Associations with Non–Human Leukocyte Antigen Genes

With the advent of GWAS technologies over the past decade, the field has seen major expansion in the number of single nucleotide polymorphism (SNP) sites that identify RA susceptibility gene candidates. A large meta-analysis of multiple independent GWAS data sets,[100] covering more than 100,000 subjects of European or Asian ancestries, identified 101 RA risk loci corresponding to 98 biological candidate genes.

Among the SNPs identified, there are many that involve immune system genes and/or known targets of approved therapy.[100] For example, a missense variant of protein tyrosine phosphatase nonreceptor 22, coded by *PTPN22* that introduces an R620W substitution, is associated with RA as well as with many other autoimmune diseases in Caucasian patients.[101] This variant has been shown to affect immune responses relevant to autoimmunity.[102] Another important RA-associated polymorphism involves *PADI4*,[103] the gene that codes for the citrullinating enzyme PAD4. The risk variant is associated with increased *PADI4* transcription stability and has been shown to associate with RA primarily in Asians. An interesting SNP association has been reproducibly found in the tumor necrosis factor-a protein 3 (*TNFAIP3*) locus.[104] The variant leads to impaired A20, an enzyme that inhibits nuclear factor (NF)-κB activity. As a result, NF-κB signaling is enhanced; in mice with ablation of *Tnfaip3*, there is spontaneous inflammatory polyarthritis.[105] Additional information about GWAS-based RA association data is discussed elsewhere.[100,106–108]

Finally, it should be added that the contribution of the HLA locus to RA susceptibility is far higher than any of the known non-HLA loci, with the *DRB1*-associated risk alone being greater than the aggregate contribution of all known non-HLA risk loci. Additionally, even when the genetic contributions of the entire list of known HLA and non-HLA risk loci are compiled, there is still a large percentage of heritability that remains unaccounted for. The research challenges in the coming years will be to fill in the missing hereditability gaps, address the role of gene-environment and gene-gene interactions, and validate the functional roles of the SE and a myriad of GWAS-based RA risk loci.

REFERENCES

1. MacGregor AJ, Snieder H, Rigby AS, et al. Characterizing the quantitative genetic contribution to rheumatoid arthritis using data from twins. Arthritis Rheum 2000;43:30–7.

2. Gregersen PK, Silver J, Winchester RJ. The shared epitope hypothesis. An approach to understanding the molecular genetics of susceptibility to rheumatoid arthritis. Arthritis Rheum 1987;30:1205–13.

3. Zinkernagel RM, Doherty PC. The discovery of MHC restriction. Immunol Today 1997;18:14–7.

4. Trowsdale J, Knight JC. Major histocompatibility complex genomics and human disease. Annu Rev Genomics Hum Genet 2013;14:301–23.

5. Kaslow RA, Shaw S. The role of histocompatibility antigens (HLA) in infection. Epidemiol Rev 1981;3:90–114.

6. Gill TJ 3rd. Role of the major histocompatibility complex region in reproduction, cancer, and autoimmunity. Am J Reprod Immunol 1996;35:211–5.

7. Gough SC, Simmonds MJ. The HLA region and autoimmune disease: associations and mechanisms of action. Curr Genomics 2007;8:453–65.

8. Reveille JD. Major histocompatibility genes and ankylosing spondylitis. Best Pract Res Clin Rheumatol 2006;20:601–9.

9. Mattey DL, Hassell AB, Dawes PT, et al. Independent association of rheumatoid factor and the HLA-DRB1 shared epitope with radiographic outcome in rheumatoid arthritis. Arthritis Rheum 2001;44:1529–33.

10. Erlich H, Valdes AM, Noble J, et al. HLA DR-DQ haplotypes and genotypes and type 1 diabetes risk: analysis of the type 1 diabetes genetics consortium families. Diabetes 2008;57:1084–92.

11. Nepom GT, Kwok WW. Molecular basis for HLA-DQ associations with IDDM. Diabetes 1998;47:1177–84.

12. Ridgway WM, Fathman CG. The association of MHC with autoimmune diseases: understanding the pathogenesis of autoimmune diabetes. Clin Immunol Immunopathol 1998;86:3–10.

13. Yin L, Dai S, Clayton G, et al. Recognition of self and altered self by T cells in autoimmunity and allergy. Protein Cell 2013;4:8–16.

14. Oldstone MB. Molecular mimicry and immune-mediated diseases. FASEB J 1998;12:1255–65.

15. van Heemst J, Jansen DT, Polydorides S, et al. Cross-reactivity to vinculin and microbes provides a molecular basis for HLA-based protection against rheumatoid arthritis. Nat Commun 2015;6:6681.

16. Tait BD, Drummond BP, Varney MD, et al. HLA-DRB1*0401 is associated with susceptibility to insulin-dependent diabetes mellitus independently of the DQB1 locus. Eur J Immunogenet 1995;22:289–97.

17. Sabbah E, Savola K, Kulmala P, et al. Disease-associated autoantibodies and HLA- DQB1 genotypes in children with newly diagnosed insulin-dependent diabetes mellitus (IDDM). The childhood diabetes in Finland study group. Clin Exp Immunol 1999;116:78–83.

18. Setty M, Hormaza L, Guandalini S. Celiac disease: risk assessment, diagnosis, and monitoring. Mol Diagn Ther 2008;12:289–98.

19. Nishino S, Okuro M, Kotorii N, et al. Hypocretin/orexin and narcolepsy: new basic and clinical insights. Acta Physiol (Oxf) 2010;198:209–22.

20. Shepherd CE, Piguet O, Broe GA, et al. Histocompatibility antigens, aspirin use and cognitive performance in non-demented elderly subjects. J Neuroimmunol 2004;148:178–82.

21. Jonsson AH, Yokoyama WM. Natural killer cell tolerance licensing and other mechanisms. Adv Immunol 2009;101:27–79.

22. Taneja V, Behrens M, Mangalam A, et al. New humanized HLA-DR4-transgenic mice that mimic the sex bias of rheumatoid arthritis. Arthritis Rheum 2007;56: 69–78.

23. Astorga GP, Williams RC Jr. Altered reactivity in mixed lymphocyte culture of lymphocytes from patients with rheumatoid arthritis. Arthritis Rheum 1969;12: 547–54.

24. McMichael AJ, Sasazuki T, McDevitt HO, et al. Increased frequency of HLA-Cw3 and HLA-Dw4 in rheumatoid arthritis. Arthritis Rheum 1977;20:1037–42.

25. Stastny P. Association of the B-cell alloantigen DRw4 with rheumatoid arthritis. N Engl J Med 1978;298:869–71.

26. Kim K, Jiang X, Cui J, et al. Interactions between amino acid-defined major histocompatibility complex class II variants and smoking in seropositive rheumatoid arthritis. Arthritis Rheumatol 2015;67:2611–23.

27. Raychaudhuri S, Sandor C, Stahl EA, et al. Five amino acids in three HLA proteins explain most of the association between MHC and seropositive rheumatoid arthritis. Nat Genet 2012;44:291–6.

28. van Heemst J, Huizinga TJ, van der Woude D, et al. Fine-mapping the human leukocyte antigen locus in rheumatoid arthritis and other rheumatic diseases: identifying causal amino acid variants? Curr Opin Rheumatol 2015;27:256–61.

29. Scholz E, Mestre-Ferrer A, Daura X, et al. A comparative analysis of the peptide repertoires of HLA-DR molecules differentially associated with rheumatoid arthritis. Arthritis Rheumatol 2016;68:2412–21.

30. Furukawa H, Oka S, Shimada K, et al. Human leukocyte antigen polymorphisms and personalized medicine for rheumatoid arthritis. J Hum Genet 2015;60: 691–6.

31. Kurko J, Besenyei T, Laki J, et al. Genetics of rheumatoid arthritis - a comprehensive review. Clin Rev Allergy Immunol 2013;45:170–9.

32. Gonzalez-Gay MA, Garcia-Porrua C, Hajeer AH. Influence of human leukocyte antigen-DRB1 on the susceptibility and severity of rheumatoid arthritis. Semin Arthritis Rheum 2002;31:355–60.

33. Plant MJ, Jones PW, Saklatvala J, et al. Patterns of radiological progression in early rheumatoid arthritis: results of an 8 year prospective study. J Rheumatol 1998;25:417–26.

34. Weyand CM, Goronzy JJ. Disease mechanisms in rheumatoid arthritis: gene dosage effect of HLA-DR haplotypes. J Lab Clin Med 1994;124:335–8.

35. Huizinga TW, Amos CI, van der Helm-van Mil AH, et al. Refining the complex rheumatoid arthritis phenotype based on specificity of the HLA-DRB1 shared epitope for antibodies to citrullinated proteins. Arthritis Rheum 2005;52:3433–8.

36. Marotte H, Pallot-Prades B, Grange L, et al. The shared epitope is a marker of severity associated with selection for, but not with response to, infliximab in a large rheumatoid arthritis population. Ann Rheum Dis 2006;65:342–7.

37. van der Horst-Bruinsma IE, Hazes JM, Schreuder GM, et al. Influence of non-inherited maternal HLA-DR antigens on susceptibility to rheumatoid arthritis. Ann Rheum Dis 1998;57:672–5.

38. Guthrie KA, Tishkevich NR, Nelson JL. Non-inherited maternal human leukocyte antigen alleles in susceptibility to familial rheumatoid arthritis. Ann Rheum Dis 2009;68:107–9.

39. Plenge RM. Recent progress in rheumatoid arthritis genetics: one step towards improved patient care. Curr Opin Rheumatol 2009;21:262–71.

40. Ferucci ED, Templin DW, Lanier AP. Rheumatoid arthritis in American Indians and Alaska Natives: a review of the literature. Semin Arthritis Rheum 2005;34: 662–7.
41. Nelson JL, Boyer G, Templin D, et al. HLA antigens in Tlingit Indians with rheumatoid arthritis. Tissue Antigens 1992;40:57–63.
42. Brighton SW, de la Harpe AL, van Staden DJ, et al. The prevalence of rheumatoid arthritis in a rural African population. J Rheumatol 1988;15:405–8.
43. Silman AJ, Ollier W, Holligan S, et al. Absence of rheumatoid arthritis in a rural Nigerian population. J Rheumatol 1993;20:618–22.
44. Hughes LB, Morrison D, Kelley JM, et al. The HLA-DRB1 shared epitope is associated with susceptibility to rheumatoid arthritis in African Americans through European genetic admixture. Arthritis Rheum 2008;58:349–58.
45. Mustila A, Korpela M, Haapala AM, et al. Anti-citrullinated peptide antibodies and the progression of radiographic joint erosions in patients with early rheumatoid arthritis treated with FIN-RACo combination and single disease-modifying antirheumatic drug strategies. Clin Exp Rheumatol 2011;29:500–5.
46. van Venrooij WJ, van Beers JJ, Pruijn GJ. Anti-CCP antibodies: the past, the present and the future. Nat Rev Rheumatol 2011;7:391–8.
47. Lundstrom E, Kallberg H, Alfredsson L, et al. Gene-environment interaction between the DRB1 shared epitope and smoking in the risk of anti-citrullinated protein antibody-positive rheumatoid arthritis: all alleles are important. Arthritis Rheum 2009;60:1597–603.
48. Snir O, Widhe M, von Spee C, et al. Multiple antibody reactivities to citrullinated antigens in sera from patients with rheumatoid arthritis: association with HLA-DRB1 alleles. Ann Rheum Dis 2009;68:736–43.
49. van Gaalen FA, van Aken J, Huizinga TW, et al. Association between HLA class II genes and autoantibodies to cyclic citrullinated peptides (CCPs) influences the severity of rheumatoid arthritis. Arthritis Rheum 2004;50:2113–21.
50. Verpoort KN, van Gaalen FA, van der Helm-van Mil AH, et al. Association of HLA-DR3 with anti-cyclic citrullinated peptide antibody-negative rheumatoid arthritis. Arthritis Rheum 2005;52:3058–62.
51. Terao C, Ohmura K, Ikari K, et al. ACPA-negative RA consists of two genetically distinct subsets based on RF positivity in Japanese. PLoS One 2012;7:e40067.
52. Amara K, Steen J, Murray F, et al. Monoclonal IgG antibodies generated from joint-derived B cells of RA patients have a strong bias toward citrullinated autoantigen recognition. J Exp Med 2013;210:445–55.
53. Scally SW, Petersen J, Law SC, et al. A molecular basis for the association of the HLA-DRB1 locus, citrullination, and rheumatoid arthritis. J Exp Med 2013;210: 2569–82.
54. Nielen MM, van Schaardenburg D, Reesink HW, et al. Specific autoantibodies precede the symptoms of rheumatoid arthritis: a study of serial measurements in blood donors. Arthritis Rheum 2004;50:380–6.
55. Rantapaa-Dahlqvist S, de Jong BA, Berglin E, et al. Antibodies against cyclic citrullinated peptide and IgA rheumatoid factor predict the development of rheumatoid arthritis. Arthritis Rheum 2003;48:2741–9.
56. Vossenaar ER, Despres N, Lapointe E, et al. Rheumatoid arthritis specific anti-Sa antibodies target citrullinated vimentin. Arthritis Res Ther 2004;6:R142–50.
57. Kinloch A, Tatzer V, Wait R, et al. Identification of citrullinated alpha-enolase as a candidate autoantigen in rheumatoid arthritis. Arthritis Res Ther 2005;7: R1421–9.

58. Burkhardt H, Sehnert B, Bockermann R, et al. Humoral immune response to citrullinated collagen type II determinants in early rheumatoid arthritis. Eur J Immunol 2005;35:1643–52.

59. Masson-Bessiere C, Sebbag M, Girbal-Neuhauser E, et al. The major synovial targets of the rheumatoid arthritis-specific antifilaggrin autoantibodies are deiminated forms of the alpha- and beta-chains of fibrin. J Immunol 2001;166:4177–84.

60. Ikari K, Kuwahara M, Nakamura T, et al. Association between PADI4 and rheumatoid arthritis: a replication study. Arthritis Rheum 2005;52:3054–7.

61. Lee YH, Rho YH, Choi SJ, et al. PADI4 polymorphisms and rheumatoid arthritis susceptibility: a meta-analysis. Rheumatol Int 2007;27:827–33.

62. Andrade F, Darrah E, Gucek M, et al. Autocitrullination of human peptidyl arginine deiminase type 4 regulates protein citrullination during cell activation. Arthritis Rheum 2010;62:1630–40.

63. Giles JT, Fert-Bober J, Park JK, et al. Myocardial citrullination in rheumatoid arthritis: a correlative histopathologic study. Arthritis Res Ther 2012;14:R39.

64. Suzuki A, Yamada R, Yamamoto K. Citrullination by peptidylarginine deiminase in rheumatoid arthritis. Ann N Y Acad Sci 2007;1108:323–39.

65. de Almeida DE, Holoshitz J. MHC molecules in health and disease: at the cusp of a paradigm shift. Self Nonself 2011;2:43–8.

66. Holoshitz J. The quest for better understanding of HLA-disease association: scenes from a road less travelled by. Discov Med 2013;16:93–101.

67. De Almeida DE, Ling S, Pi X, et al. Immune dysregulation by the rheumatoid arthritis shared epitope. J Immunol 2010;185:1927–34.

68. Fu J, Ling S, Liu Y, et al. A small shared epitope-mimetic compound potently accelerates osteoclast-mediated bone damage in autoimmune arthritis. J Immunol 2013;191:2096–103.

69. Holoshitz J, Ling S. Nitric oxide signaling triggered by the rheumatoid arthritis shared epitope: a new paradigm for MHC disease association? Ann N Y Acad Sci 2007;1110:73–83.

70. Holoshitz J, Liu Y, Fu J, et al. An HLA-DRB1-coded signal transduction ligand facilitates inflammatory arthritis: a new mechanism of autoimmunity. J Immunol 2013;190:48–57.

71. Ling S, Lai A, Borschukova O, et al. Activation of nitric oxide signaling by the rheumatoid arthritis shared epitope. Arthritis Rheum 2006;54:3423–32.

72. Ling S, Li Z, Borschukova O, et al. The rheumatoid arthritis shared epitope increases cellular susceptibility to oxidative stress by antagonizing an adenosine-mediated anti-oxidative pathway. Arthritis Res Ther 2007;9:R5.

73. Ling S, Pi X, Holoshitz J. The rheumatoid arthritis shared epitope triggers innate immune signaling via cell surface calreticulin. J Immunol 2007;179:6359–67.

74. Naveh S, Tal-Gan Y, Ling S, et al. Developing potent backbone cyclic peptides bearing the shared epitope sequence as rheumatoid arthritis drug-leads. Bioorg Med Chem Lett 2012;22:493–6.

75. Klareskog L, Padyukov L, Lorentzen J, et al. Mechanisms of disease: genetic susceptibility and environmental triggers in the development of rheumatoid arthritis. Nat Clin Pract Rheumatol 2006;2:425–33.

76. Karlson EW, Chang SC, Cui J, et al. Gene-environment interaction between HLA-DRB1 shared epitope and heavy cigarette smoking in predicting incident rheumatoid arthritis. Ann Rheum Dis 2010;69:54–60.

77. Padyukov L, Silva C, Stolt P, et al. A gene-environment interaction between smoking and shared epitope genes in HLA-DR provides a high risk of seropositive rheumatoid arthritis. Arthritis Rheum 2004;50:3085–92.

78. Pedersen M, Jacobsen S, Garred P, et al. Strong combined gene-environment effects in anti-cyclic citrullinated peptide-positive rheumatoid arthritis: a nationwide case-control study in Denmark. Arthritis Rheum 2007;56:1446–53.

79. Mikuls TR, Sayles H, Yu F, et al. Associations of cigarette smoking with rheumatoid arthritis in African Americans. Arthritis Rheum 2010;62:3560–8.

80. Klareskog L, Stolt P, Lundberg K, et al. A new model for an etiology of rheumatoid arthritis: smoking may trigger HLA-DR (shared epitope)-restricted immune reactions to autoantigens modified by citrullination. Arthritis Rheum 2006;54: 38–46.

81. Willemze A, van der Woude D, Ghidey W, et al. The interaction between HLA shared epitope alleles and smoking and its contribution to autoimmunity against several citrullinated antigens. Arthritis Rheum 2011;63:1823–32.

82. Carty SM, Snowden N, Silman AJ. Should infection still be considered as the most likely triggering factor for rheumatoid arthritis? Ann Rheum Dis 2004; 63(Suppl 2):ii46–9.

83. Quirke AM, Perry E, Cartwright A, et al. Bronchiectasis is a model for chronic bacterial infection inducing autoimmunity in rheumatoid arthritis. Arthritis Rheumatol 2015;67:2335–42.

84. Detert J, Pischon N, Burmester GR, et al. The association between rheumatoid arthritis and periodontal disease. Arthritis Res Ther 2010;12:218.

85. McGraw WT, Potempa J, Farley D, et al. Purification, characterization, and sequence analysis of a potential virulence factor from Porphyromonas gingivalis, peptidylarginine deiminase. Infect Immun 1999;67:3248–56.

86. Bonfil JJ, Dillier FL, Mercier P, et al. A "case control" study on the role of HLA DR4 in severe periodontitis and rapidly progressive periodontitis. Identification of types and subtypes using molecular biology (PCR.SSO). J Clin Periodontol 1999;26:77–84.

87. Marotte H, Farge P, Gaudin P, et al. The association between periodontal disease and joint destruction in rheumatoid arthritis extends the link between the HLA-DR shared epitope and severity of bone destruction. Ann Rheum Dis 2006;65:905–9.

88. Mackie SL, Taylor JC, Martin SG, et al. A spectrum of susceptibility to rheumatoid arthritis within HLA-DRB1: stratification by autoantibody status in a large UK population. Genes Immun 2012;13:120–8.

89. Shadick NA, Heller JE, Weinblatt ME, et al. Opposing effects of the D70 mutation and the shared epitope in HLA-DR4 on disease activity and certain disease phenotypes in rheumatoid arthritis. Ann Rheum Dis 2007;66:1497–502.

90. van der Helm-van Mil AH, Huizinga TW, Schreuder GM, et al. An independent role of protective HLA class II alleles in rheumatoid arthritis severity and susceptibility. Arthritis Rheum 2005;52:2637–44.

91. van der Woude D, Lie BA, Lundstrom E, et al. Protection against anti-citrullinated protein antibody-positive rheumatoid arthritis is predominantly associated with HLA- DRB1*1301: a meta-analysis of HLA-DRB1 associations with anti-citrullinated protein antibody-positive and anti-citrullinated protein antibody-negative rheumatoid arthritis in four European populations. Arthritis Rheum 2010;62:1236–45.

92. Feitsma AL, van der Helm-van Mil AH, Huizinga TW, et al. Protection against rheumatoid arthritis by HLA: nature and nurture. Ann Rheum Dis 2008; 67(Suppl 3):iii61–3.

93. Taneja V, Taneja N, Behrens M, et al. HLA-DRB1*0402 (DW10) transgene protects collagen-induced arthritis-susceptible H2Aq and DRB1*0401 (DW4) transgenic mice from arthritis. J Immunol 2003;171:4431–8.

94. Bettencourt A, Carvalho C, Leal B, et al. The protective role of HLA-DRB1(*)13 in autoimmune diseases. J Immunol Res 2015;2015:948723.

95. Cruz-Tapias P, Perez-Fernandez OM, Rojas-Villarraga A, et al. Shared HLA class II in six autoimmune diseases in Latin America: a meta-analysis. Autoimmune Dis 2012;2012:569728.

96. Langan SM, Smeeth L, Hubbard R, et al. Bullous pemphigoid and pemphigus vulgaris–incidence and mortality in the UK: population based cohort study. BMJ 2008;337:a180.

97. Wakitani S, Imoto K, Murata N, et al. The homozygote of HLA- DRB1*0901, not its heterozygote, is associated with rheumatoid arthritis in Japanese. Scand J Rheumatol 1998;27:381–2.

98. Lee HS, Lee KW, Song GG, et al. Increased susceptibility to rheumatoid arthritis in Koreans heterozygous for HLA-DRB1*0405 and *0901. Arthritis Rheum 2004; 50:3468–75.

99. Zanelli E, Breedveld FC, de Vries RR. HLA class II association with rheumatoid arthritis: facts and interpretations. Hum Immunol 2000;61:1254–61.

100. Okada Y, Wu D, Trynka G, et al. Genetics of rheumatoid arthritis contributes to biology and drug discovery. Nature 2014;506:376–81.

101. Zheng J, Ibrahim S, Petersen F, et al. Meta-analysis reveals an association of PTPN22 C1858T with autoimmune diseases, which depends on the localization of the affected tissue. Genes Immun 2012;13:641–52.

102. Zheng J, Petersen F, Yu X. The role of PTPN22 in autoimmunity: learning from mice. Autoimmun Rev 2014;13:266–71.

103. Suzuki A, Yamada R, Chang X, et al. Functional haplotypes of PADI4, encoding citrullinating enzyme peptidylarginine deiminase 4, are associated with rheumatoid arthritis. Nat Genet 2003;34:395–402.

104. Thomson W, Barton A, Ke X, et al. Rheumatoid arthritis association at 6q23. Nat Genet 2007;39:1431–3.

105. Matmati M, Jacques P, Maelfait J, et al. A20 (TNFAIP3) deficiency in myeloid cells triggers erosive polyarthritis resembling rheumatoid arthritis. Nat Genet 2011;43:908–12.

106. Amagai M, Tsunoda K, Suzuki H, et al. Use of autoantigen-knockout mice in developing an active autoimmune disease model for pemphigus. J Clin Invest 2000;105:625–31.

107. Diogo D, Okada Y, Plenge RM. Genome-wide association studies to advance our understanding of critical cell types and pathways in rheumatoid arthritis: recent findings and challenges. Curr Opin Rheumatol 2014;26:85–92.

108. Kochi Y, Suzuki A, Yamamoto K. Genetic basis of rheumatoid arthritis: a current review. Biochem Biophys Res Commun 2014;452:254–62.

Precision Medicine in Rheumatoid Arthritis

James Bluett, MBBS, PhD[a],*, Anne Barton, FRCP, PhD[a,b]

KEYWORDS

- Methotrexate • Anti-TNF • Anti-TNF response • Genetic • Genomic
- Rheumatoid arthritis • Pharmacogenomics

KEY POINTS

- Treatment of rheumatoid arthritis (RA) has improved in recent years but response is not universal.
- Clinical predictors of response alone are not sufficiently predictive to aid treatment decisions.
- Understanding the pharmacogenomics of RA would allow more personalized health care.

INTRODUCTION

Rheumatoid arthritis (RA) is a heterogenous disease and can range from a mild, self-limiting arthritis to rapidly progressive joint damage. Treatment is based on controlling inflammation, and early effective therapy reduces disability, joint damage, and mortality.[1] A range of treatment options are available but none are universally effective, so treatment selection is based on a "trial-and-error" approach, trying different therapies until a drug that induces low disease activity or remission is identified.[2] Time on multiple ineffective medications affects the patient's quality of life, may lead to irreversible joint damage,[3] exposes the patient to potential adverse events, and is a waste of health care resources. Therefore, considerable research effort has been applied to identifying predictors of drug response to allow more rational prescribing of the drug most likely to be effective in individual patients, an approach known as precision (or stratified) medicine.

Methotrexate (MTX) is the first-line therapy for RA,[2] whereas biologic therapies target specific molecular pathways, including the tumor necrosis factor (TNF),

Disclosure Statement: The authors have nothing to disclose.
[a] Division of Musculoskeletal and Dermal Sciences, Arthritis Research UK Centre for Genetics and Genomics, Centre for Musculoskeletal Research, Manchester Academic Health Science Centre, The University of Manchester, Room 2.607, Stopford Building, Oxford Road, Manchester M13 9PT, UK; [b] NIHR Manchester Biomedical Research Centre, Central Manchester University Hospitals NHS Foundation Trust, Manchester Academic Health Science Centre, Manchester M139WU, UK
* Corresponding author.
E-mail address: james.bluett@manchester.ac.uk

interleukin-6, B-cell and T-cell costimulation pathways. The biologic drugs are typically reserved for those with an inadequate response to nonbiologic disease-modifying antirheumatic drugs,[2] but there is currently no guidance on which biologic agent to use first.[4] Each drug has a significant failure rate; for example, TNF inhibitors (TNFi) are ineffective in up to 30% patients,[5] yet remain the most commonly prescribed first-line biologic. As most research has investigated biomarkers predictive of response to MTX and TNFi biologics, the current review limits the focus to these drug classes.

Treatment response is likely to be multifactorial and influenced by clinical, psychological, and biological factors. For example, robust clinical predictors of TNFi response include disease severity, smoking status, concomitant MTX, and patient disability, but account for a small proportion ($r^2 = 0.17$) of the variance in response and so, alone, are not useful in informing therapy selection decisions.[6] There is, therefore, a need for accurate predictors (biomarkers) of response to RA therapies to enable precision medicine, defined by National Academy of Sciences as the use of genomic, epigenomic, exposure, and other data to define individual patterns of disease, potentially leading to better individual treatment.[7]

The use of genomic variants as predictors of response has several theoretic advantages. Genetic variants are stable and will not change because of the environment, unlike epigenetics or expression profiling. Genetic variants that are associated with response are likely to be involved in key molecular pathways and can therefore provide insight into the mechanisms of nonresponse. Whole-genome genotyping is now economically viable, and the assays are standardized, enabling their use in the clinical setting. Indeed, genetic biomarkers are already being used to personalize health care. In cystic fibrosis, for example, ivacaftor, a drug that targets the CFTR molecule, is recommended in the 4% of patients with the G551D mutation[8] whereas in rheumatology, screening for the enzyme TPMT, responsible for the metabolism of 6-mercaptopurine and related compounds, is recommended to identify the 13% of the population with reduced activity and who are at increased risk of toxicity to azathioprine.[9] There are currently more than 200 examples of US Food and Drug Administration–approved drugs that contain information on genomic biomarkers that may be used to inform treatment decisions.[10] Although many of these are not commonly used in clinical practice, TPMT screening is frequently in the United Kingdom.

STUDIES INVESTIGATING GENOMIC PREDICTORS OF METHOTREXATE

Given that MTX remains the treatment of choice for patients with newly diagnosed RA, several studies have investigated genes involved in the key molecular pathways affecting MTX absorption, metabolism, or its target enzymes as predictive biomarkers of response (**Fig. 1**).

The most consistent evidence for association is for the solute carrier family 19 member 1 (SLC19A1) gene, one of several transport carriers that allow MTX to enter cells. Studies have reported that the rs1051266 variant associates with intracellular MTX-polyglutamate levels and a recent meta-analysis of 12 studies (n = 2049) reported an association with MTX treatment response (odds ratio [OR] = 1.49 of AA genotype, $P = .001$).[11,12] Methylene tetrahydrofolate reductase is another key enzyme in the MTX pathway and has also been extensively investigated with several studies reporting associations with efficacy and toxicity. However, a meta-analysis including 17 previous studies revealed no association with either outcome,[13] and this finding has been replicated in 2 subsequent meta-analyses.[14,15] MTX is thought to exert an

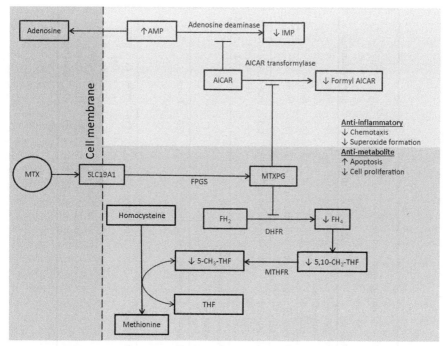

Fig. 1. The MTX metabolic pathway. 5-CH$_3$-THF, 5-methyltetrahydrofolate; 5,10-CH$_2$-THF, 5,10-methyltetrahydrofolate; AMP, adenosine monophosphate; DHFR, dihydrofolate reductase; FH$_2$, dihydrofolate; FH$_4$, tetrahydrofolate; FPGS, folylpolyglutamate synthetase; IMP, inosine monophosphate; MTHRF, methylene tetrahydrofolate reductase; MTXPG, methotrexate polyglutamate; SLC19A1, solute carrier family 19 member 1; THF, tetrahydrofolate.

anti-inflammatory effect through inhibiting aminoimidazole carboxamido tibo nucleotide (AICAR) transformylase (ATIC) leading to an increase in AICAR levels and the anti-inflammatory agent adenosine.[16] Several studies have associated the (ATIC 347 C > G single nucleotide polymorphism [SNP] rs2372536) with toxicity,[17–19] but this finding has not been consistently replicated.[20–22]

As well as investigating MTX pathway genes, the major RA susceptibility gene, HLA-DRB1, has also been studied. As the gene is associated with more severe disease,[23] it was hypothesized that carriers of the risk allele would be less likely to respond to MTX monotherapy. In a study of 309 patients from an early inflammatory polyarthritis inception cohort, the presence of the HLA-DRB1 allele was associated with MTX monotherapy inefficacy at 2 years (OR = 3.04, P = .02), but this finding requires replication in other data sets.[24]

STUDIES INVESTIGATING GENOMIC PREDICTORS OF RESPONSE TO TUMOR NECROSIS FACTOR INHIBITOR

Early candidate gene studies investigating the pharmacogenomics of TNFi therapy revealed inconsistent findings, none of which have been robustly replicated. This review focuses on genome-wide association studies (GWAS): candidate gene studies where findings have been replicated by at least one group and candidate gene studies performed in sample sizes exceeding 1500 individuals (**Table 1**).

Table 1
Summary of pharmacogenomic studies investigating response to tumor necrosis factor inhibitors reported to date

Study	N	Study Design	Platform	SNPs for Analysis	Results	Validation Study	n	SNPs Validated
Liu et al,[25] 2008	89	GWAS	Illumina Beadstation and Hap300 chips	283,348	16 SNPs of suggestive association	Suarez-Gestal et al,[26] 2010	151	None
						Krintel et al,[27] 2012	196	None
Plant et al,[28] 2011	566	GWAS	Affymetrix GeneChip 500K	459,446	7 SNPs of suggestive association	Krintel et al,[27] 2012	196	None
Krintel et al,[27] 2012	196	GWAS	Illumina HumanHap550K duo array	561,466	10 SNPs of suggestive association	Acosta et al,[29] 2013	315	$PDEA3A\text{-}SLC01C1$ (OR = 2.63, $P = 1.74 \times 10^{-5}$)
Mirkov et al,[30] 2013	882	GWAS	HumanHap550-Duo/Human660W-Quad BeadChips	2,557,253	No SNP of suggestive association			
Cui et al,[31] 2013	2706	GWAS	Various	>2,000,000	1 SNP of suggestive association in etanercept-treated cohort	Cui et al,[31] 2013	139	None
Cui et al,[32] 2010	1283	Candidate gene study	Various	31	1 SNP of suggestive association	Plant et al,[33] 2012	1115	$PTPRC$ ($\beta = 0.19$, $P = .04$)
						Ferreiro-Iglesias et al,[34] 2016	755	$PTPRC$ ($\beta = 0.33$, $P = .006$)
						Pappas et al,[35] 2013	233	Not validated
						Zervou et al,[36] 2013	183	Not validated

WHOLE-GENOME STUDIES

To date, 5 GWAS have been undertaken with the first including just 89 patients.[25] Sixteen SNPs showed suggestive association ($P<5 \times 10^{-5}$), but none exceeded genome-wide significance thresholds and none have been replicated in subsequent, larger studies.[26]

A second GWAS undertaken by Plant and colleagues[28] in 2011 included a 3-stage design with an initial GWAS investigating change in Disease Activity Score on 28 joints (DAS-28) over 6 months (n = 566); variants with $P<10^{-3}$ were subsequently genotyped in an independent cohort with a subsequent meta-analysis. In stage 3, variants whereby the signal was strengthened were investigated in a third independent cohort, and finally, a second meta-analysis of the data was performed. The results demonstrated 7 loci associated with response, but 3 SNPs showed an opposite effect in the meta-analysis compared with the first stage and no SNP reached genome-wide significance ($P<5 \times 10^{-8}$). Neither the Liu[25] or Plant[28] and colleagues results have been replicated subsequently.

In 2012, Krintel and colleagues[27] performed a GWAS of 196 Danish RA patients treated with TNFi, most of whom were treated with infliximab, and performed a subsequent meta-analysis with the Liu and colleagues and Plant and colleagues datasets. Response was defined as the change in DAS-28 over 14 weeks. Suggestive association was detected at the PDE3A-SLCO1C1 locus, where a C > T polymorphism at rs3794271 was associated with reduced efficacy according to the European League Against Rheumatism (EULAR) criteria (OR = 3.2, $P = 3.5 \times 10^{-6}$).[37] A Spanish study by Acosta-Colman and colleagues[29] tested the same variant in 315 RA patients and replicated the association (OR = 2.63, $P = 1.74 \times 10^{-5}$). The variant was associated with response to infliximab and etanercept but not adalimumab. A subsequent meta-analysis strengthened the association (OR = 2.91, $P = 3.34 \times 10^{-10}$). The PDE3A gene encodes a phosphodiesterase, inhibition of which suppresses TNF production in lipopolysaccharide-stimulated monocytes.[38] The association was not reported in previous GWA studies, but the variant was not tested by the Plant and colleagues study. However, a subsequent study in a UK population found no evidence for association.[39]

A multistage GWAS in 2013 recruited 882 Dutch patients and 2 further validation cohorts (n = 954 and 867, respectively)[30] through international collaboration. Response was defined as 3-month change in DAS-28, a shorter time period than previous studies, but no variants were associated even at suggestive association thresholds ($P<5 \times 10^{-5}$).

In 2013, Cui and colleagues[31] performed the largest GWAS to date. Following international collaboration, 2706 RA patients from 13 different cohorts treated with etanercept, infliximab, or adalimumab were investigated. Response was defined as the change in DAS-28 at 3 to 12 months. No association reaching genome-wide significance was detected. A subset analysis revealed SNP rs6427528 nearing genome-wide significance ($P = 8 \times 10^{-8}$) in the etanercept-treated group. rs6427528 is thought to disrupt transcription binding site motifs of CD84 and is associated with higher CD84 expression in peripheral blood mononuclear cells. CD84 is involved in T-cell activation and maturation[40] and acts as a costimulatory molecule for interferon-γ secretion.[41] Despite the strong initial association, the SNP failed to replicate in Portuguese and Japanese cohorts (n = 290).

Recently, a rigorous community-based assessment of the utility of SNP data for predicting anti-TNF treatment efficacy in RA patients was performed in the context of a DREAM Challenge (http://www.synapse.org/RA_Challenge).[42] This approach enabled the comparative evaluation of treatment response predictions developed by 73 research groups using the most comprehensive available data on TNFi response and genome-wide data. Unfortunately, no significant genetic contribution to prediction accuracy was observed.

PROTEIN TYROSINE PHOSPHATASE RECEPTOR TYPE C, HUMAN LEUKOCYTE ANTIGEN-DRB1, AND RESPONSE TO TUMOR NECROSIS FACTOR INHIBITOR

In 2010, Cui and colleagues[32] hypothesized that genetic factors associated with RA susceptibility and severity may also be important in predicting treatment response. The investigators investigated Caucasian individuals (n = 1283) receiving infliximab, etanercept, or adalimumab. Response was defined according to the EULAR criteria at 3 to 12 months posttreatment. An association within the *PTPRC* gene was reported (rs10919563; OR = 0.55, $P = 10^{-5}$) with the strongest effect in the seropositive cohort. Subgroup analysis revealed *PTPRC* was associated with infliximab and etanercept response but not adalimumab. PTPRC is a transmembrane receptor-like molecule that regulates T- and B-cell antigen receptor signaling[43] and is a mediator of TNF secretion from monocytes.[44] The *PTPRC* association has been replicated by 2 independent studies,[33,34] but 2 other studies failed to replicate the association,[35,36] possibly because of lack of power as the 2 negative studies had smaller sample sizes (see **Table 1**). The *PTPRC* variant accounted for only 0.5% of the variance in response to TNFi and will therefore not be clinically useful at the individual patient level.

The shared epitope HLA-DRB1 amino acid at positions 11, 71, and 74 confer the largest susceptibility risk of RA and are associated with disease progression.[45] In a candidate gene study investigating the association between loci within the *HLA DRB1* gene and EULAR response in 1846 RA patients treated with TNFi, a VKA haplotype at the 3 amino acid positions was also significantly associated with improved EULAR response (OR = 1.23, $P = .007$).[23] The work suggests that the same variants may be associated with susceptibility, severity, and treatment response but with a sequential reduction in effect size, meaning that larger sample sizes are required for treatment response studies.

DISCUSSION

Despite the large number of studies investigating the pharmacogenetics and genomics of RA, results to date have been disappointing and have not yielded a change in clinical practice. There are several possible reasons for this. It could be argued that there is no genetic heritability for treatment response in RA, and the results to date are false positives, but 2 studies have reported that there is detectable heritability.[46,47] These observations, therefore, begs the question of where the missing heritability is (see Vincent A. Laufer and colleagues' article, "Integrative Approaches to Understanding the Pathogenic Role of Genetic Variation in Rheumatic Diseases", in this issue), and there are several explanations for the failure to consistently detect genetic predictors of response.

First, most studies have investigated common variants, with limited power to detect the effect of rare variants on treatment response. Technology is advancing at a staggering pace, and with the reducing cost of whole genome sequencing, it is now economically viable to evaluate the effect of rare variants; however, a recent exon sequencing study of candidate genes found no evidence for association with TNFi response in ~1000 individuals.[48]

Second, RA is not a simple monogenic disease, but a polygenic disease whereby environmental and multiple genetic loci increase the individuals risk of developing disease. It is therefore likely that treatment response is in part due to the multiple effects of many genetic variants, each of small effect size. A recent study used simulations to show that successful application of common polygenic modeling approaches would require sample sizes greater than 1000 individuals for traits with less than 50% heritability,[49] yet few studies, to date, have included such numbers.

Third, response in RA is difficult to capture, and several composite scores are used in clinical practice. Many research studies also use these measures, including DAS-28, American College of Rheumatology, or EULAR response criteria, which include subjective measures of disease and are known to have a placebo effect.[50] Previous research has reported that the swollen joint count and erythrocyte sedimentation rate are response markers that are associated with the greatest genetic influence and that psychological factors correlate with the subjective visual analogue score.[47,51] Some investigators have used imaging to objectively assess disease activity (synovitis) and to re-weight the DAS-28[52] score to more accurately reflect that feature as biologic drugs target that aspect of disease, but routine MR imaging remains impractical in the clinical setting.

Fourth, adherence to therapy is a potential confounder of predictive studies that is rarely accounted for; it has been shown, for example, that up to 20% of RA patients self-report nonadherence to TNFi therapy when asked and that nonadherence is associated with poorer clinical outcome.[53] Thus, a patient who is genetically predisposed to respond to treatment may be classified as a nonresponder because they are not taking the drug but, to date, no study has adjusted for inadequate adherence to treatment.

Finally, RA may not be one disease, but different diseases, with different molecular mechanisms that present as a similar, if heterogeneous, phenotype. For example, it is known that there are significant clinical and genetic differences between anticyclic citrullinated peptide (CCP) -positive and anti-CCP-negative patients.[54] Including all patients who fulfill classification criteria for RA may cause admixture of RA subsets, reducing the power of a study to detect genetic association. Furthermore, although response to TNFi therapies is broadly similar, there are differences illustrated by the fact that patients may experience inefficacy with one but subsequently respond to another.[55] Differences in the mechanism of action are recognized; for example, infliximab and adalimumab are licensed for Crohn disease, whereas etanercept is ineffective,[56] is associated with a lower risk of development of tuberculosis,[57] and appears to be the least immunogenic, with a reported incidence of 1% to 18% of antidrug antibodies without an effect on response.[58] Despite this, most studies investigate response by grouping together all TNFis, potentially reducing the power to detect association in subgroups.

THE FUTURE

Pharmacogenetic and genomic studies have the potential to enable precision medicine by providing biomarkers to target the right drug to the right patients. Current guidelines offer little advice as to which biologic therapy to offer patients first, but stratifying patients according to increased probability of response to a particular drug would be of major benefit.[4] However, studies to date have illustrated that it is unlikely that a single genetic variant will be highly and confidently predictive of an individual's response to drug treatment in RA. Progress in this area will require larger sample sizes with well-described patient cohorts to allow for adjustment of confounding clinical factors such as nonadherence, antidrug antibodies, disease severity, and smoking status. These study design changes would facilitate adequately powered studies to evaluate the effect of genetic variants on different TNFi therapies and gene-gene interactions. Alternative measures of response that are able to objectively characterize true responders are also required.

Patients are currently treated in a trial-and-error approach until an effective therapy is identified, but each cycle of trying a drug destined to be ineffective increases the probability of adverse events, cost to the state, patient dissatisfaction, and the development of disability. It is therefore vital that further research is conducted to develop precision medicine approaches, moving medicine into the twenty-first century.

REFERENCES

1. Scire CA, Lunt M, Marshall T, et al. Early remission is associated with improved survival in patients with inflammatory polyarthritis: results from the Norfolk Arthritis Register. Ann Rheum Dis 2014;73(9):1677–82.
2. Smolen JS, Landewe R, Breedveld FC, et al. EULAR recommendations for the management of rheumatoid arthritis with synthetic and biological disease-modifying antirheumatic drugs: 2013 update. Ann Rheum Dis 2014;73(3):492–509.
3. Finckh A, Liang MH, van Herckenrode CM, et al. Long-term impact of early treatment on radiographic progression in rheumatoid arthritis: a meta-analysis. Arthritis Rheum 2006;55(6):864–72.
4. National Institute for Health and Care Excellence. TA375: adalimumab, etanercept, infliximab, certolizumab pegol, golimumab, tocilizumab and abatacept for rheumatoid arthritis not previously treated with DMARDs or after conventional DMARDs only have failed. 2016. Available at: https://www.nice.org.uk/guidance/ta375. Accessed August 9, 2016.
5. Gibbons LJ, Hyrich KL. Biologic therapy for rheumatoid arthritis: clinical efficacy and predictors of response. BioDrugs 2009;23(2):111–24.
6. Hyrich KL, Watson KD, Silman AJ, et al. Predictors of response to anti-TNF-alpha therapy among patients with rheumatoid arthritis: results from the British Society for Rheumatology Biologics register. Rheumatology (Oxford) 2006;45(12): 1558–65.
7. National Academy of Sciences. Toward precision medicine: building a knowledge network for biomedical research and a new taxonomy of disease. Washington, DC: National Academy of Sciences; 2011.
8. North of England Specialised Commissioning Group. Clinical commissioning policy: ivacaftor for cystic fibrosis. 2013. Available at: https://www.england.nhs.uk/wp-content/uploads/2013/04/a01-p-b.pdf. Accessed August 9, 2016.
9. Reuther LO, Vainer B, Sonne J, et al. Thiopurine methyltransferase (TPMT) genotype distribution in azathioprine-tolerant and -intolerant patients with various disorders. The impact of TPMT genotyping in predicting toxicity. Eur J Clin Pharmacol 2004;59(11):797–801.
10. US Food and Drug Administration. Table of pharmacogenomic biomarkers in drug labeling. 2016. Available at: http://www.fda.gov/drugs/scienceresearch/researchareas/pharmacogenetics/ucm083378.htm. Accessed August 9, 2016.
11. Li X, Hu M, Li W, et al. The association between reduced folate carrier-1 gene 80G/A polymorphism and methotrexate efficacy or methotrexate related-toxicity in rheumatoid arthritis: a meta-analysis. Int Immunopharmacol 2016;38:8–15.
12. Dervieux T, Kremer J, Lein DO, et al. Contribution of common polymorphisms in reduced folate carrier and gamma-glutamylhydrolase to methotrexate polyglutamate levels in patients with rheumatoid arthritis. Pharmacogenetics 2004;14(11):733–9.
13. Owen SA, Lunt M, Bowes J, et al. MTHFR gene polymorphisms and outcome of methotrexate treatment in patients with rheumatoid arthritis: analysis of key polymorphisms and meta-analysis of C677T and A1298C polymorphisms. Pharmacogenomics J 2013;13(2):137–47.

14. Spyridopoulou KP, Dimou NL, Hamodrakas SJ, et al. Methylene tetrahydrofolate reductase gene polymorphisms and their association with methotrexate toxicity: a meta-analysis. Pharmacogenet Genomics 2012;22(2):117–33.

15. Lee YH, Song GG. Associations between the C677T and A1298C polymorphisms of MTHFR and the efficacy and toxicity of methotrexate in rheumatoid arthritis: a meta-analysis. Clin Drug Investig 2010;30(2):101–8.

16. Cronstein BN, Naime D, Ostad E. The antiinflammatory mechanism of methotrexate. Increased adenosine release at inflamed sites diminishes leukocyte accumulation in an in vivo model of inflammation. J Clin Invest 1993;92(6): 2675–82.

17. Dervieux T, Greenstein N, Kremer J. Pharmacogenomic and metabolic biomarkers in the folate pathway and their association with methotrexate effects during dosage escalation in rheumatoid arthritis. Arthritis Rheum 2006;54(10): 3095–103.

18. Weisman MH, Furst DE, Park GS, et al. Risk genotypes in folate-dependent enzymes and their association with methotrexate-related side effects in rheumatoid arthritis. Arthritis Rheum 2006;54(2):607–12.

19. Grabar PB, Rojko S, Logar D, et al. Genetic determinants of methotrexate treatment in rheumatoid arthritis patients: a study of polymorphisms in the adenosine pathway. Ann Rheum Dis 2010;69(5):931–2.

20. Takatori R, Takahashi KA, Tokunaga D, et al. ABCB1 C3435T polymorphism influences methotrexate sensitivity in rheumatoid arthritis patients. Clin Exp Rheumatol 2006;24(5):546–54.

21. Stamp LK, Chapman PT, O'Donnell JL, et al. Polymorphisms within the folate pathway predict folate concentrations but are not associated with disease activity in rheumatoid arthritis patients on methotrexate. Pharmacogenet Genomics 2010; 20(6):367–76.

22. Owen SA, Hider SL, Martin P, et al. Genetic polymorphisms in key methotrexate pathway genes are associated with response to treatment in rheumatoid arthritis patients. Pharmacogenomics J 2013;13(3):227–34.

23. Viatte S, Plant D, Han B, et al. Association of HLA-DRB1 haplotypes with rheumatoid arthritis severity, mortality, and treatment response. JAMA 2015;313(16): 1645–56.

24. Hider SL, Silman AJ, Thomson W, et al. Can clinical factors at presentation be used to predict outcome of treatment with methotrexate in patients with early inflammatory polyarthritis? Ann Rheum Dis 2009;68(1):57–62.

25. Liu C, Batliwalla F, Li W, et al. Genome-wide association scan identifies candidate polymorphisms associated with differential response to anti-TNF treatment in rheumatoid arthritis. Mol Med 2008;14(9–10):575–81.

26. Suarez-Gestal M, Perez-Pampin E, Calaza M, et al. Lack of replication of genetic predictors for the rheumatoid arthritis response to anti-TNF treatments: a prospective case-only study. Arthritis Res Ther 2010;12(2):R72.

27. Krintel SB, Palermo G, Johansen JS, et al. Investigation of single nucleotide polymorphisms and biological pathways associated with response to TNFalpha inhibitors in patients with rheumatoid arthritis. Pharmacogenet Genomics 2012;22(8): 577–89.

28. Plant D, Bowes J, Potter C, et al. Genome-wide association study of genetic predictors of anti-tumor necrosis factor treatment efficacy in rheumatoid arthritis identifies associations with polymorphisms at seven loci. Arthritis Rheum 2011; 63(3):645–53.

29. Acosta-Colman I, Palau N, Tornero J, et al. GWAS replication study confirms the association of PDE3A-SLCO1C1 with anti-TNF therapy response in rheumatoid arthritis. Pharmacogenomics 2013;14(7):727–34.

30. Umicevic Mirkov M, Cui J, Vermeulen SH, et al. Genome-wide association analysis of anti-TNF drug response in patients with rheumatoid arthritis. Ann Rheum Dis 2013;72(8):1375–81.

31. Cui J, Stahl EA, Saevarsdottir S, et al. Genome-wide association study and gene expression analysis identifies CD84 as a predictor of response to etanercept therapy in rheumatoid arthritis. PLoS Genet 2013;9(3):e1003394.

32. Cui J, Saevarsdottir S, Thomson B, et al. Rheumatoid arthritis risk allele PTPRC is also associated with response to anti-tumor necrosis factor alpha therapy. Arthritis Rheum 2010;62(7):1849–61.

33. Plant D, Prajapati R, Hyrich KL, et al. Replication of association of the PTPRC gene with response to anti-tumor necrosis factor therapy in a large UK cohort. Arthritis Rheum 2012;64(3):665–70.

34. Ferreiro-Iglesias A, Montes A, Perez-Pampin E, et al. Replication of PTPRC as genetic biomarker of response to TNF inhibitors in patients with rheumatoid arthritis. Pharmacogenomics J 2016;16(2):137–40.

35. Pappas DA, Oh C, Plenge RM, et al. Association of rheumatoid arthritis risk alleles with response to anti-TNF biologics: results from the CORRONA registry and meta-analysis. Inflammation 2013;36(2):279–84.

36. Zervou MI, Myrthianou E, Flouri I, et al. Lack of association of variants previously associated with anti-TNF medication response in rheumatoid arthritis patients: results from a homogeneous Greek population. PLoS One 2013;8(9):e74375.

37. van Gestel AM, Prevoo ML, van 't Hof MA, et al. Development and validation of the European League Against Rheumatism response criteria for rheumatoid arthritis. Comparison with the preliminary American College of Rheumatology and the World Health Organization/International league against rheumatism criteria. Arthritis Rheum 1996;39(1):34–40.

38. Prabhakar U, Lipshutz D, Bartus JO, et al. Characterization of cAMP-dependent inhibition of LPS-induced TNF alpha production by rolipram, a specific phosphodiesterase IV (PDE IV) inhibitor. Int J Immunopharmacol 1994;16(10):805–16.

39. Smith SL, Plant D, Lee XH, et al. Previously reported PDE3A-SLCO1C1 genetic variant does not correlate with anti-TNF response in a large UK rheumatoid arthritis cohort. Pharmacogenomics 2016;17(7):715–20.

40. Tangye SG, Nichols KE, Hare NJ, et al. Functional requirements for interactions between CD84 and Src homology 2 domain-containing proteins and their contribution to human T cell activation. J Immunol 2003;171(5):2485–95.

41. Martin M, Romero X, de la Fuente MA, et al. CD84 functions as a homophilic adhesion molecule and enhances IFN-gamma secretion: adhesion is mediated by Ig-like domain 1. J Immunol 2001;167(7):3668–76.

42. Sieberts SK, Zhu F, Garcia-Garcia J, et al. Crowdsourced assessment of common genetic contribution to predicting anti-TNF treatment response in rheumatoid arthritis. Nat Commun 2016;7:12460.

43. Hermiston ML, Xu Z, Weiss A. CD45: a critical regulator of signaling thresholds in immune cells. Annu Rev Immunol 2003;21:107–37.

44. Hayes AL, Smith C, Foxwell BM, et al. CD45-induced tumor necrosis factor alpha production in monocytes is phosphatidylinositol 3-kinase-dependent and nuclear factor-kappaB-independent. J Biol Chem 1999;274(47):33455–61.

45. Plant D, Thomson W, Lunt M, et al. The role of rheumatoid arthritis genetic susceptibility markers in the prediction of erosive disease in patients with early

inflammatory polyarthritis: results from the Norfolk arthritis register. Rheumatology (Oxford, England) 2011;50(1):78–84.

46. Umicevic Mirkov M, Janss L, Vermeulen SH, et al. Estimation of heritability of different outcomes for genetic studies of TNFi response in patients with rheumatoid arthritis. Ann Rheum Dis 2015;74(12):2183–7.

47. Plant D, Bowes J, Orozco G, et al. Estimating heritability of response to treatment with anti-TNF biologic agents using linear mixed models. Ann Rheum Dis 2013; 71(Suppl 3):474–5.

48. Cui J, Diogo D, Stahl EA, et al. The role of rare protein-coding variants to anti-TNF treatment response in rheumatoid arthritis. Arthritis Rheumatol 2017;69(4): 735–41.

49. Marshall SL, Guennel T, Kohler J, et al. Estimating heritability in pharmacogenetic studies. Pharmacogenomics 2013;14(4):369–77.

50. Strand V, Cohen S, Crawford B, et al. Patient-reported outcomes better discriminate active treatment from placebo in randomized controlled trials in rheumatoid arthritis. Rheumatology (Oxford, England) 2004;43(5):640–7.

51. Cordingley L, Prajapati R, Plant D, et al. Impact of psychological factors on subjective disease activity assessments in patients with severe rheumatoid arthritis. Arthritis Care Res 2014;66(6):861–8.

52. Baker JF, Conaghan PG, Smolen JS, et al. Development and validation of modified disease activity scores in rheumatoid arthritis: superior correlation with magnetic resonance imaging-detected synovitis and radiographic progression. Arthritis Rheumatol 2014;66(4):794–802.

53. Bluett J, Morgan C, Thurston L, et al. Impact of inadequate adherence on response to subcutaneously administered anti-tumour necrosis factor drugs: results from the Biologics in Rheumatoid Arthritis Genetics and Genomics Study Syndicate cohort. Rheumatology (Oxford, England) 2015;54(3):494–9.

54. van der Helm-van Mil AH, Verpoort KN, Breedveld FC, et al. Antibodies to citrullinated proteins and differences in clinical progression of rheumatoid arthritis. Arthritis Res Ther 2005;7(5):R949–58.

55. Soliman MM, Hyrich KL, Lunt M, et al. Rituximab or a second anti-tumor necrosis factor therapy for rheumatoid arthritis patients who have failed their first anti-tumor necrosis factor therapy? Comparative analysis from the British Society for rheumatology biologics register. Arthritis Care Res 2012;64(8):1108–15.

56. Sandborn WJ, Hanauer SB, Katz S, et al. Etanercept for active Crohn's disease: a randomized, double-blind, placebo-controlled trial. Gastroenterology 2001; 121(5):1088–94.

57. Dixon WG, Hyrich KL, Watson KD, et al. Drug-specific risk of tuberculosis in patients with rheumatoid arthritis treated with anti-TNF therapy: results from the British Society for Rheumatology Biologics Register (BSRBR). Ann Rheum Dis 2010;69(3):522–8.

58. Emi Aikawa N, de Carvalho JF, Artur Almeida Silva C, et al. Immunogenicity of Anti-TNF-alpha agents in autoimmune diseases. Clin Rev Allergy Immunol 2010;38(2–3):82–9.

Genomic Influences on Hyperuricemia and Gout

Tony Merriman, PhD

KEYWORDS

- Genome-wide association studies • Gout • Hyperuricemia • ABCG2 • SLC2A9
- Urate • Uric acid

KEY POINTS

- Genome-wide association studies have identified nearly 30 loci associated with urate concentrations, dominated by loci containing renal and gut uric acid excretion regulators.
- The SLC2A9 gene, that encodes a renal uric acid reuptake transporter, has a major effect on urate concentrations and the risk of gout, and exhibits non-additive interactions with sex and dietary exposures.
- The ABCG2 gene, that encodes a gut and renal uric acid secretory transporter, also has a major effect. The causal 141K variant results in ABCG2 internalization with the defect able to be rescued by small molecules.
- To date only small genome-wide association studies have been done in gout meaning that little is known about the genetic control of progression from hyperuricemia to gout.

INTRODUCTION

Gout is an inflammatory arthritis caused by an extremely painful but self-limiting innate immune response to monosodium urate (MSU) crystals deposited in synovial fluid.[1] Without effective management, in some individuals, gout can become chronic, with the development of tophi (organized lumps of urate and immune cells[2]) and permanent bony erosion and disability. Gout is also comorbid with other metabolic-based conditions, such as heart and kidney disease and type 2 diabetes,[3] with the causal relationships that are of much clinical interest, remaining unclear. An elevated concentration of serum urate (hyperuricemia) is necessary, but not sufficient, for the development of gout with host-specific and environmental factors required for the progression from hyperuricemia to gout. Approximately 30 genetic loci, including SLC2A9 and ABCG2 that have major effects, influence serum urate concentrations[4] with less understood about the genetic control of the formation of MSU crystals and the subsequent inflammatory response. Urate-lowering therapy, in particular use of the

Department of Biochemistry, University of Otago, 710 Cumberland Street, Dunedin 9054, New Zealand
E-mail address: tony.merriman@otago.ac.nz

Rheum Dis Clin N Am 43 (2017) 389–399
http://dx.doi.org/10.1016/j.rdc.2017.04.004
0889-857X/17/© 2017 Elsevier Inc. All rights reserved.

rheumatic.theclinics.com

xanthine oxidase inhibitor allopurinol, is a cornerstone of gout management, but for a variety of reasons it is often not effective.[1]

Hyperuricemia and gout are more prevalent in men than women, with the prevalence of both increasing with age and particularly in women after menopause.[5] The prevalence of gout is typically 3% to 4% in people of European ancestry, up to 1% in populations of Asian ancestry, and 6% to 8% in Taiwanese Aboriginals and Polynesian people (Maori and Pacific Islanders) living in New Zealand.[5] The increased prevalence of gout in the latter populations has a strong contribution from the inherent hyperuricemia in these groups.[6,7] Serum urate levels are a balance of overproduction and renal and gut underexcretion,[8] with renal excretion particularly important. The renal fractional excretion of uric acid is reduced in hyperuricemia compared with normouricemia, in men compared with women, and in Pacific Islanders and New Zealand Maori compared with Europeans.[9,10] Regarding overproduction, urate is the end product of purine metabolism, with the liver a major site of production. For example, the liver produces urate as a by-product of fructose and alcohol-induced purine nucleotide degradation.

Monogenic disorders of purine metabolism including hypoxanthine-guanine phosphoribosyltransferase deficiency (Lesch-Nyhan syndrome) and 5-phosporibosyl-1-pyrophosphate synthetase superactivity generate rare pediatric syndromes of hyperuricemia, early-onset gout, and kidney stones. Familial juvenile hyperuricemic nephropathy is a disorder of renal uric acid underexcretion caused by mutations in uromodulin leading to hyperuricemia, early-onset gout, and chronic kidney disease. These rare disorders provide insights into purine metabolism and renal uric acid excretion mechanisms but account for an extremely small proportion of hyperuricemia and gout in the general population. Genome-wide association studies (GWAS) for common genetic variants contributing to the polygenic component of hyperuricemia and gout in the general population exhibit very little to no overlap (with the possible exception of a locus containing the *PRPSAP1* gene) with monogenic disorders. This review, therefore, focuses on insights into the common genetic variants contributing to the development of gout, in particular on recent and other pertinent findings regarding the 2 major urate and gout loci, *SLC2A9* and *ABCG2*.

GENOME-WIDE ASSOCIATION STUDIES IN URATE

In the context of medically important metabolites, urate is very tractable to research on etiology. It is easily measured and levels typically do not fluctuate over short periods; this allows good quality of phenotyping for studies of genetic and environmental risk factors. Approximately 90% of variance in renal uric acid handling and approximately 60% of variance in serum urate concentrations are explained by inherited genetic variants.[11,12] The largest GWAS to date was carried out in people of European ancestry.[4] A total of 110,347 individuals were genotyped at 2.45 million single nucleotide polymorphism (SNP) markers. Of these markers, 2201 were associated with serum urate concentrations at an experiment-wide level of significance ($P < 5 \times 10^{-8}$) that accounts for the multiple testing inherent in a GWAS. These markers were spread over 28 distinct regions of the genome; each region can be considered a locus containing one or more genetic variants with a causal role in determining serum urate concentrations. Predictably, most of these loci are also associated with the risk of gout in multiple ancestral groups.[4,13,14] Within the 28 loci, renal and gut uric acid excretion genes are prominent, some with a very strong effect, particularly *SLC2A9* and *ABCG2*. The urate-raising allele at *SLC2A9* associates with an average 0.37 mg/dL increase in serum urate, the urate-raising allele at *ABCG2* with an average 0.22 mg/dL increase.

The amount of variance in serum urate concentrations explained by *SLC2A9* (GLUT9) is 2% to 3% and *ABCG2* is approximately 1%, both very strong effects in the context of complex phenotype loci. In comparison, the established and strongest effect weight locus (*FTO/IRX3*) in Europeans explains approximately 0.3% of variance in body mass index.[15] Other loci with renal and gut uric acid transporters or auxiliary molecules identified are *SLC17A1-A3* (NPT1, NPT3, NPT4), *SLC22A12* (URAT1), *SLC22A11* (OAT4), and *PDZK1*. Smaller GWAS for serum urate concentrations have been performed in people of East Asian, African, and Pacific ancestry.[16–19] The East Asian study included 51,327 participants and approximately 2.4 million SNPs with 4 loci identified, all overlapping with those discovered in the European study (*SLC2A9*, *ABCG2*, *SLC22A12*, and *MAF*). Two African American GWAS, both published in 2011, included 5820[19] and 1017[16] participants, so were inadequately powered to detect loci of moderate to weak effect. *SLC2A9* was detected in both studies. The larger study[19] also detected *SLC22A12* and a novel locus containing the *SLC2A12* and *SGK1* genes that encode the GLUT12 transporter and serine/threonine protein kinase serum/glucocorticoid-regulated kinase 1, respectively. Finally, the study by Kenny and colleagues[18] had 2906 participants from the Micronesian island of Kosrae. The only locus detected at a genome-wide level of significance was *SLC22A12* (URAT1). Interestingly, the signal at *SLC22A12* was a considerable distance (500 kb) upstream of *SLC22A12*, suggesting it may represent a novel locus.

SLC2A9

Hundreds of single nucleotide variants are associated with urate concentrations and the risk of gout over a several hundred kilobase region on chromosome 4 encompassing the *SLC2A9* gene.[4] *SLC2A9* confers an extremely strong single genetic effect in the context of complex phenotypes, reminiscent of the human leukocyte antigen (HLA) locus in autoimmune disease. Like the HLA locus in autoimmunity, dissection of the complex genetic architecture at *SLC2A9* and identification of causal genetic variant(s) is challenging, with relatively little progress yet at *SLC2A9*. Circumstantial evidence suggests that the major *SLC2A9* genetic effect is associated with isoform expression, whereby the urate-raising causal genetic variant increases the expression of an SLC2A9 isoform (SLC2A9-S) that has a 28-residue portion missing from the N-terminus.[20,21] This isoform is expressed on the apical (urine) side of the collecting duct, where it presumably increases reuptake of secreted uric acid, whereas the full-length version (SLC2A9-L) is expressed on the basolateral side where it is the major basolateral uric acid exit route into the circulation.[22] There are multiple independent causal genetic effects at *SLC2A9*.[23] Aside from mutations that cause type 2 hereditary renal hypouricemia,[24–26] the precise common genetic variants that causally control serum urate concentrations are yet to be pinpointed.

ABCG2

The ATP binding cassette G2 (ABCG2) protein is one of a superfamily of 48 human ABC transporters that transport a wide array of substrates. A GWAS first identified the missense *rs2231142* (Q141K) variant to be associated with serum urate concentration in Europeans, with the 141K allele associated with increased urate concentration.[27] This genome-wide significant level of association has been consistently replicated in other GWAS in people of European and East Asian ancestry[4,17] but not in people of African American ancestry.[16,19] However, there is nominal evidence for association of the Q141K variant with serum urate concentration in African American individuals, with the 141K allele also associated with increased urate[27] and the risk of gout.[28] ABCG2 transports uric acid, with the 141K variant reducing by approximately 50% the ability to secrete uric acid and highly likely to be the lead causal variant at ABCG2.[28]

There is evidence for a second genetically and statistically independent effect at the ABCG2 locus, marked by SNP rs2622629 (**Table 1**).[29] This second effect is of clinical relevance, as the rs2622629-correlated SNPs (ie, those SNPs in linkage disequilibrium) include rs10011796 (r^2 = 0.84 in Europeans); rs10011796 is also implicated in gout and in allopurinol response (see **Table 1**).[30] The molecular mechanism whereby rs2622629 (or tightly correlated variants) influence serum urate levels is not known, but this variant maps within a DNaseI hypersensitivity cluster of approximately 150 bp (www.genome.ucsc.edu) identified by the Encode project (www.encodeproject.org), consistent with the effect being mediated through control of gene expression and/or mRNA editing.

Aside from Q141K, the only other common (>1%) missense variant in ABCG2 is V12M (rs2231137), situated in the intracellular portion of ABCG2. This variant is genetically independent of both Q141K (r^2 = 0.002 in Europeans) and rs2622629 (r^2 = 0.009 in Europeans). This variant is associated with serum urate and gout and can be considered a third independent effect on gout in ABCG2, after Q141K and rs10011796/rs2622629. The GWAS by Köttgen and colleagues[4] in serum urate in European individuals reported an increase in serum urate of 0.077 mg/dL and the GWAS by Okada and colleagues[17] in East Asian individuals reported an increase of 0.108 mg/dL per copy of the 12V allele. In gout, the major 12V allele consistently confers risk in 3 separate samples drawn from East Asian populations: Taiwanese Aborigines (odds ratio [OR] = 1.36),[31] Han Chinese in Taiwan (OR = 1.33),[31] and Han Chinese in Shanghai (OR = 1.82).[32] Any impact of this variant on the uric acid transport activity of ABCG2 is currently unknown.

Expression of most uric acid transporters is relatively high in the kidney or, for SLC22A12/URAT1, restricted to the kidney. However, expression of ABCG2 is also relatively high in the gut.[33] Recent work in a well-defined Japanese gout sample set has demonstrated the role of ABCG2 uric acid excretion in both the gut and kidney. It was possible to create grades of ABCG2 dysfunction based on Q141 K and Q126X genotype combinations, with individuals positive for the dysfunctional variants 126X and 141K having the highest serum urate concentrations and highest

Table 1
Major genetic variation in ABCG2 and impact on phenotype

Variant	Population Prevalence (EUR/EAS/SAS/AFR)	Urate	Gout	Allopurinol Response
V12M (rs2231137)	12M: 0.06/0.33/0.15/0.06	Decreases[4,17]	Decreased risk[31,32]	—
Q126X (rs72552713)	126X: 0.00/0.01/0.00/0.00	—	Increased risk[32,34]	—
Q141K (rs2231142)	141K: 0.09/0.29/0.10/0.01	Increases[4,17]	Increased risk[4,34,67]	Resistance[30,68]
rs10011796	T: 0.39/0.63/0.48/0.27	Increases[4]	Increased risk[69]	Resistance[30] Same[68]

Abbreviations: AFR, African; EAS, East Asian; EUR, European; SAS, South Asian.
The dashes indicate that no data are available.
Phenotype and prevalence information is given to the minor (alternative) allele. All phenotypes are compared with wild type.

risk for gout, and those homozygous for 141Q and 126Q having the lowest serum urate concentrations and lowest risk for gout.[34] The presence of the 141K (and 126X) alleles reduces excretion through the gut and adds to the circulating urate, overloading the kidney excretion system, resulting in increased urinary uric acid levels.

Restoring ABCG2 expression and function in people with detrimental genetic polymorphisms may be an important next step to limit urate levels and inflammatory responses. Recently, it has been shown that histone deacetylase (HDAC) inhibitors and colchicine can restore the function of the 141K ABCG2 variant by restoring trafficking and dimer expression. HDAC inhibitors and colchicine may impede targeting of 141K ABCG2 to the aggresome (an aggregation of misfolded proteins formed when the protein degradation system of a cell is overloaded) and promote relocalization on the cell surface.[35,36] Colchicine is an anti-inflammatory agent that acts by inhibiting microtubule polymerization via binding to tubulin. This suggests that HDAC inhibitors, as is the case with colchicine, inhibit trafficking of ABCG2 to the aggresome along microtubules. These results should encourage further research into the use of HDAC inhibitors and small molecules to restore defective ABCG2 function in patients with the 141K polymorphism.

OTHER URATE LOCI

Uric acid transporters at the SLC2A9, ABCG2, SLC22A11, SLC22A12, and SLC17A1 loci are extremely strong candidates for causal genes. At other urate loci reported by Köttgen and colleagues,[4] candidate genes were identified using Gene Relationships Across Implicated Loci (GRAIL),[37] a bioinformatic approach that looks for commonalities among associated SNPs, the literature, and published GWAS. This approach, however, does require prior published knowledge and is therefore limited in its ability to discover novel pathogenic mechanisms. Thus, without further evidence, the GRAIL-identified genes cannot be assumed as causal. Extensive linkage disequilibrium (inter-marker correlation) results in association signals extending for some distance across many loci with the possibility of long-range regulatory interactions, showing that causal genes can be located outside the region of association (eg, the FTO-IRX3 locus in weight control[38]). This means that multiple candidate genes can exist within a risk locus. Despite this, various lines of evidence strongly support PDZK1 and INHBB as the causal genes at their respective loci.[23] PDKZ1 is an accessory molecule that binds to the extreme C-terminus of all apical and secretory uric acid transporters, except ABCG2, and assists in the specific positioning of the transporters in the plasma membrane.[39] The INHBB gene encodes for the inhibin beta subunit B and combines with INHBA to form activin A. How activin A regulates serum urate concentrations is not known.

NONADDITIVE GENE-ENVIRONMENT (GxE) AND GENE-GENE (GxG) INTERACTIONS

Despite the etiologic variants at SLC2A9 not yet being identified, the urate-associated variants at this and other loci can be used as markers of the biological effect of SLC2A9 on urate concentrations. New insights have come from identification of nonadditive gene-environmental ('GxE') and gene-gene ('GxG') interactions,[40–45] and from use of the genetic variants as "instrumental variables" in Mendelian randomization studies to test for a causal effect of urate in other metabolic diseases comorbid with hyperuricemia and gout.[46]

A nonadditive (epistatic) GxG interaction between genetic variants in the genes encoding the NLRP3 inflammasome subunit CARD8 and interleukin (IL)-1β[47] is consistent with an etiology in which greater inflammasome activity from reduced CARD8 expression, combined with higher levels of pre–IL-1β expression, leads to increased production of mature IL-1β and an amplified immune response. There are also GxG interactions within the *SLC2A9* locus.[48] These interactions are enriched in enhancer elements that could regulate expression of *SLC2A9* and the neighboring *WDR1* gene.

There is a nonadditive interaction between sugar-sweetened beverage consumption and the *SLC2A9* gene in serum urate control and the risk of gout.[41] The rationale for this analysis was that *SLC2A9* encodes GLUT9, a uric acid and simple sugar transporter, and that ingestion of sugar-sweetened beverages is associated increased urate concentrations and with incident and prevalent gout.[41,49,50] It was found that exposure to sugar-sweetened beverages caused the normally urate-lowering allele at *SLC2A9* to flip into urate-raising behavior.[41] The biological mechanism underlying this genetic epidemiologic observation is not understood.

A nonadditive interaction between alcohol exposure and the *GCKR* and *LRP2* genes on the risk of gout was recently reported.[44,50] All urate-associated loci identified by GWAS[4] were tested, with *GCKR* showing experiment-wide evidence for nonadditive interaction. Given that no uric acid transporters showed evidence for nonadditive interactions,[50] this argues against current thinking that alcohol influences renal excretion of uric acid. Closer examination of ORs in the various genotype and alcohol exposure groups was informative. At *GCKR*, any alcohol exposure overcame ("swamped") the risk conferred by the genetic variant at *GCKR*: in people not exposed to alcohol the genetic risk was strong, whereas no genetic risk was observed in those exposed to any alcohol. The *GCKR* gene codes for the glucokinase regulatory protein that is involved in the hepatic glycolytic processing of sugar and alcohol, which generates urate as a consequence of ATP depletion.[51] It can be surmised that the glycolytic processing of alcohol overrides the genetic discrimination of genetic variation at *GCKR*. In the case of *LRP2* genetic associations with urate concentrations and the risk of gout have been reported in Polynesian and Asian populations.[44,52] In the Polynesian study, the nonadditive interaction of the *rs2544390* variant of *LRP2* with alcohol consumption in the risk of gout[44] was driven by alcohol consumption overriding the effect of the protective genotype.

In the previous examples, evidence for nonadditive interaction was detected by including an interaction term in the logistic and linear regression analyses. The basis of the interactions was subsequently characterized by evaluating risk in stratified groups. An alternative approach is to test for association of genotype with *variance* in phenotype, rather than the standard phenotypic average. A genotype-specific influence on variance is indicative of a second factor interacting with genotype. This could be an intrinsic (eg, age, sex, a second unlinked locus) or an extrinsic environmental exposure. The variance approach is a powerful way to first detect evidence for nonadditive interaction (particularly on a genome-wide basis[53]) and can be followed up with testing for nonadditive interaction with specific intrinsic and extrinsic exposures. This approach was used to analyze *SLC2A9*[45] with the urate-raising allele found to be associated with increased variance in serum urate levels in people of European ancestry. Subsequent testing revealed that this effect was far stronger in premenopausal women with a greater increase in urate concentration associated with the urate-increasing allele in women. This finding has generated the hypothesis that female hormones, and/or other factors that they influence or are associated with (such as iron levels, temperature, testosterone), interact with the *SLC2A9* genotype in women to determine urate concentration. The association of *SLC2A9* with greater variance in urate among premenopausal women may reflect the cyclical changes resulting from menstruation. Interestingly, there is epidemiologic evidence for association of increasing ferritin concentrations with increased urate concentrations,[54] warranting further testing of a possible causal role for iron metabolism in urate control.

MENDELIAN RANDOMIZATION AS A GENETIC EPIDEMIOLOGICAL TOOL TO DISENTANGLE CAUSAL RELATIONSHIPS

The burden of the major comorbidities of gout (eg, heart disease, kidney disease, type 2 diabetes) is considerable. The shared pathophysiology for type 2 diabetes, chronic kidney disease, heart disease, and gout has been highlighted by GWAS, with an ever-increasing list of shared predisposing loci (https://www.ebi.ac.uk/gwas/). However, the direction of causal relationships remains undefined. Understanding the molecular basis of the relationship between gout and shared metabolic comorbidities is important to improve the management of gout in the presence of these comorbidities (and vice versa).

Alleles of genetic variants are randomly inherited at conception; Mendelian randomization uses these variants as "instrumental variables" to test whether a risk factor is causal for a disease outcome. As proof of principle, association with gout of genetic variants associated with urate concentrations by GWAS[4,13] proves that hyperuricemia is causal of gout. For example, using Mendelian randomization, a possible causal effect of urate on renal function can be evaluated by testing the effect of a urate-associated genetic variant (eg, in *SLC2A9*) on renal function by comparing renal function between people inheriting the urate-increasing and urate-decreasing alleles. Because these alleles are inherited at conception, people with either allele are equally exposed to confounders. Importantly, an instrumental variable for Mendelian randomization needs to satisfy some basic assumptions, including lack of association with other metabolic conditions comorbid with hyperuricemia and gout. Thus, *SLC2A9* is an ideal instrumental variable, as it does not associate with such conditions,[55] in contrast to *GCKR*, for example, which associates with multiple metabolic conditions.[4,56,57]

Current results from Mendelian randomization studies (reviewed in Ref.[46]), in contrast to observational studies, do not support a causal role for serum urate levels in phenotypes associated with hyperuricemia, such as reduced renal function, ischemic heart disease, type 2 diabetes, hypertension, hypertriglyceridemia, and obesity. In fact, the reverse studies, using as instrumental variables genetic variants associated with the various metabolic conditions, show that increased body mass index and increased triglyceride concentrations are causal of increased serum urate levels.[58–62] As yet, no Mendelian randomization studies have been done focusing on the possible causal role of the intermittent chronic inflammation of gout with the comorbid metabolic conditions. This would require the use of genetic variants associated with gouty inflammation but not serum urate concentrations.

GENOME-WIDE ASSOCIATION STUDIES IN GOUT

As discussed previously, GWAS for urate concentrations have provided important insights into the control of urate and the risk of gout. Given that only a subset of hyperuricemic people progress to gout, there must, like the control of urate concentrations, also be genetic factors and environmental exposures controlling the progression to gout, that is, the deposition of monosodium urate crystals and subsequent innate immune response. However, only 4 small GWAS have been published in gout, as opposed to the control of urate concentration. The first was done in 956 Icelandic individuals with gout resulting in 2 low-frequency variants being detected: one at the *PDZK1* locus and the second a population-specific missense variant in the *ALDH16A1* gene.[63] Sulem and colleagues[63] postulated that the *ALDH16A1* effect plays a role in purine metabolism. The second GWAS was on 2115 cases of European ancestry nested within the serum urate GWAS done by Köttgen and colleagues,[4] with only *SLC2A9* and *ABCG2* detected at a genome-wide level of significance. In 2015, 2 GWAS were reported in Han Chinese and Japanese sample sets. The former studied 1255 male individuals with gout and, in addition to *ABCG2*, discovered associations at *BCAS3, RFX3,* and *KCNQ1*.[64] All these loci were also significantly associated with gout when asymptomatic hyperuricemic controls were used, an important test that indicates that the loci control the progression from hyperuricemia to gout, and not the progression to hyperuricemia. Interestingly, *KCNQ1* is an established type 2 diabetes susceptibility locus.[65] In addition to *ABCG2, SLC2A9,* and *GCKR,* the Japanese GWAS, using 945 male cases, reported associations at the *MYL2-CUX2* and *CNIH-2* loci.[66] However, it is unclear whether these loci control progression to hyperuricemia or the progression from hyperuricemia to gout. Certainly, considerably larger GWAS in gout are required.

REFERENCES

1. Dalbeth N, Merriman TR, Stamp LK. Gout. Lancet 2016;388(10055):2039–52.
2. Dalbeth N, Pool B, Gamble GD, et al. Cellular characterization of the gouty tophus: a quantitative analysis. Arthritis Rheum 2010;62:1549–56.
3. Choi HK, Atkinson K, Karlson EW, et al. Obesity, weight change, hypertension, diuretic use, and risk of gout in men: the health professionals follow-up study. Arch Intern Med 2005;165:742–8.
4. Köttgen A, Albrecht E, Teumer A, et al. Genome-wide association analyses identify 18 new loci associated with serum urate concentrations. Nat Genet 2013;45: 145–54.
5. Kuo CF, Grainge MJ, Zhang W, et al. Global epidemiology of gout: prevalence, incidence and risk factors. Nat Rev Rheumatol 2015;11:649–62.
6. Buckley H. Epidemiology of gout: perspectives from the past. Curr Rheum Rev 2011;7:106–13.
7. Merriman TR. Population heterogeneity in the genetic control of serum urate. Semin Nephrol 2011;31:420–5.
8. Ichida K, Matsuo H, Takada T, et al. Decreased extra-renal urate excretion is a common cause of hyperuricemia. Nat Comm 2012;3:764.
9. Gibson T, Waterworth R, Hatfield P, et al. Hyperuricaemia, gout and kidney function in New Zealand Maori men. Br J Rheumatol 1984;23:276–82.
10. Simmonds HA, McBride MB, Hatfield PJ, et al. Polynesian women are also at risk for hyperuricaemia and gout because of a genetic defect in renal urate handling. Br J Rheumatol 1994;33:932–7.
11. Krishnan E, Lessov-Schlaggar CN, Krasnow RE, et al. Nature versus nurture in gout: a twin study. Am J Med 2012;125:499–504.
12. Emmerson BT, Nagel SL, Duffy DL, et al. Genetic control of the renal clearance of urate: a study of twins. Ann Rheum Dis 1992;51:375–7.
13. Phipps-Green AJ, Merriman ME, Topless R, et al. Twenty-eight loci that influence serum urate levels: analysis of association with gout. Ann Rheum Dis 2016;75: 124–30.
14. Urano W, Taniguchi A, Inoue E, et al. Effect of genetic polymorphisms on development of gout. J Rheumatol 2013;40:1374–8.
15. Speliotes EK, Willer CJ, Berndt SI, et al. Association analyses of 249,796 individuals reveal 18 new loci associated with body mass index. Nat Genet 2010;42: 937–48.

16. Charles BA, Shriner D, Doumatey A, et al. A genome-wide association study of serum uric acid in African Americans. BMC Med Genomics 2011;4:17.

17. Okada Y, Sim X, Go MJ, et al. Meta-analysis identifies multiple loci associated with kidney function-related traits in east Asian populations. Nat Genet 2012; 44:904–9.

18. Kenny EE, Kim M, Gusev A, et al. Increased power of mixed models facilitates association mapping of 10 loci for metabolic traits in an isolated population. Hum Mol Genet 2011;20:827–39.

19. Tin A, Woodward OM, Kao WHL, et al. Genome-wide association study for serum urate concentrations and gout among African Americans identifies genomic risk loci and a novel URAT1 loss-of-function allele. Hum Mol Genet 2011;20:4056–68.

20. Döring A, Gieger C, Mehta D, et al. SLC2A9 influences uric acid concentrations with pronounced sex-specific effects. Nat Genet 2008;40:430–6.

21. Vitart V, Rudan I, Hayward C, et al. SLC2A9 is a newly identified urate transporter influencing serum urate concentration, urate excretion and gout. Nat Genet 2008; 40:437–42.

22. Kimura T, Takahashi M, Yan K, et al. Expression of SLC2A9 isoforms in the kidney and their localization in polarized epithelial cells. PLoS One 2014;9:e84996.

23. Merriman TR. An update on the genetic architecture of hyperuricemia and gout. Arthritis Res Ther 2015;17:98.

24. Androvitsanea A, Stylianou K, Maragkaki E, et al. Vanishing urate, acute kidney injury episodes and a homozygous SLC2A9 mutation. Int Urol Nephrol 2015;47: 1035–6.

25. Stiburkova B, Ichida K, Sebesta I. Novel homozygous insertion in SLC2A9 gene caused renal hypouricemia. Mol Genet Metab 2011;102:430–5.

26. Windpessl M, Ritelli M, Wallner M, et al. A novel homozygous SLC2A9 mutation associated with renal-induced hypouricemia. Am J Nephrol 2016;43:245–50.

27. Dehghan A, Kottgen A, Yang Q, et al. Association of three genetic loci with uric acid concentration and risk of gout: a genome-wide association study. Lancet 2008;372:1953–61.

28. Woodward OM, Kottgen A, Coresh J, et al. Identification of a urate transporter, ABCG2, with a common functional polymorphism causing gout. Proc Natl Acad Sci U S A 2009;106:10338–42.

29. Stahl E, Choi H, Cadzow M, et al. Conditional analysis of 30 serum urate loci identifies 25 additional independent effects. Arthritis Rheumatol 2014;66:S1294.

30. Wen C, Yee S, Liang X, et al. Genome-wide association study identifies ABCG2 (BCRP) as an allopurinol transporter and a determinant of drug response. Clin Pharmacol Ther 2015;97:518–25.

31. Tu HP, Ko AMS, Chiang SL, et al. Joint effects of alcohol consumption and ABCG2 Q141K on chronic tophaceous gout risk. J Rheumatol 2014;41:749–58.

32. Zhou D, Liu Y, Zhang X, et al. Functional polymorphisms of the ABCG2 gene are associated with gout disease in the Chinese Han male population. Int J Mol Sci 2014;15:9149–59.

33. Huls M, Brown CD, Windass AS, et al. The breast cancer resistance protein transporter ABCG2 is expressed in the human kidney proximal tubule apical membrane. Kidney Int 2008;73:220–5.

34. Matsuo H, Takada T, Ichida K, et al. Common defects of ABCG2, a high-capacity urate exporter, cause gout: a function-based genetic analysis in a Japanese population. Sci Transl Med 2009;1:5ra11.

35. Woodward OM, Tukaye DN, Cui J, et al. Gout-causing Q141K mutation in ABCG2 leads to instability of the nucleotide-binding domain and can be corrected with small molecules. Proc Natl Acad Sci U S A 2013;110:5223–8.

36. Basseville A, Tamaki A, Ierano C, et al. Histone deacetylase inhibitors influence chemotherapy transport by modulating expression and trafficking of a common polymorphic variant of the ABCG2 efflux transporter. Cancer Res 2012;72: 3642–51.

37. Raychaudhuri S, Plenge RM, Rossin EJ, et al. Identifying relationships among genomic disease regions: predicting genes at pathogenic SNP associations and rare deletions. PLos Genet 2009;5(6):e1000534.

38. Smemo S, Tena JJ, Kim KH, et al. Obesity-associated variants within FTO form long-range functional connections with IRX3. Nature 2014;507:371–5.

39. Mandal AK, Mount DB. The molecular physiology of uric acid homeostasis. Annu Rev Physiol 2015;77:323–45.

40. Bao Y, Curhan G, Merriman T, et al. Lack of gene–diuretic interactions on the risk of incident gout: the Nurses' Health Study and Health Professionals Follow-Up Study. Ann Rheum Dis 2015;74:1394–8.

41. Batt C, Phipps-Green AJ, Black MA, et al. Sugar-sweetened beverage consumption: a risk factor for prevalent gout with SLC2A9 genotype-specific effects on serum urate and risk of gout. Ann Rheum Dis 2014;73:2101–6.

42. Hamajima N, Naito M, Okada R, et al. Significant interaction between LRP2 rs2544390 in intron 1 and alcohol drinking for serum uric acid levels among a Japanese population. Gene 2012;503:131–6.

43. McAdams-DeMarco MA, Maynard JW, Baer AN, et al. A urate gene-by-diuretic interaction and gout risk in participants with hypertension: results from the ARIC study. Ann Rheum Dis 2013;72:701–6.

44. Rasheed H, Phipps-Green A, Topless R, et al. Association of the lipoprotein receptor-related protein 2 gene with gout and non-additive interaction with alcohol consumption. Arthritis Res Ther 2013;15:R177.

45. Topless RK, Flynn TJ, Cadzow M, et al. Association of SLC2A9 genotype with phenotypic variability of serum urate in pre-menopausal women. Front Genet 2015;6:313.

46. Robinson PC, Choi HK, Do R, et al. Insight into rheumatological cause and effect through the use of Mendelian randomization. Nat Rev Rheumatol 2016;12: 486–96.

47. McKinney C, Stamp LK, Dalbeth N, et al. Multiplicative interaction of functional inflammasome genetic variants in determining the risk of gout. Arthritis Res Ther 2015;17:288.

48. Wei WH, Guo Y, Kindt AS, et al. Abundant local interactions in the 4p16. 1 region suggest functional mechanisms underlying SLC2A9 associations with human serum uric acid. Hum Mol Genet 2014;23:5061–8.

49. Choi JW, Ford ES, Gao X, et al. Sugar-sweetened soft drinks, diet soft drinks, and serum uric acid level: the Third National Health and Nutrition Examination Survey. Arthritis Rheum 2008;59:109–16.

50. Rasheed H, Stamp LK, Dalbeth N, et al. Non-additive interaction of the GCKR and A1CF loci with alcohol consumption to influence the risk of gout. Arthritis Rheumatol 2016;68:S10.

51. Johnson RJ, Perez-Pozo SE, Sautin YY, et al. Hypothesis: could excessive fructose intake and uric acid cause type 2 diabetes? Endocr Rev 2009;30:96–116.

52. Kamatani Y, Matsuda K, Okada Y, et al. Genome-wide association study of hematological and biochemical traits in a Japanese population. Nat Genet 2010;42: 210–5.

53. Wei WH, Hemani G, Haley CS. Detecting epistasis in human complex traits. Nat Rev Genet 2014;15:722–33.

54. Ghio AJ, Ford ES, Kennedy TP, et al. The association between serum ferritin and uric acid in humans. Free Radic Res 2005;39:337–42.

55. Hughes K, Flynn T, de Zoysa J, et al. Mendelian randomization analysis associates increased serum urate, due to genetic variation in uric acid transporters, with improved renal function. Kidney Int 2014;85:344–51.

56. Köttgen A, Pattaro C, Boger CA, et al. New loci associated with kidney function and chronic kidney disease. Nat Genet 2010;42:376–84.

57. Orho-Melander M, Melander O, Guiducci C, et al. Common missense variant in the glucokinase regulatory protein gene is associated with increased plasma triglyceride and C-reactive protein but lower fasting glucose concentrations. Diabetes 2008;57:3112–21.

58. Burgess S, Daniel RM, Butterworth AS, et al. Network Mendelian randomization: using genetic variants as instrumental variables to investigate mediation in causal pathways. Int J Epidemiol 2015;44:484–95.

59. Lyngdoh T, Vuistiner P, Marques-Vidal P, et al. Serum uric acid and adiposity: deciphering causality using a bidirectional Mendelian randomization approach. PLoS One 2012;7:e39321.

60. Oikonen M, Wendelin-Saarenhovi M, Lyytikäinen LP, et al. Associations between serum uric acid and markers of subclinical atherosclerosis in young adults. The Cardiovascular Risk in Young Finns study. Atherosclerosis 2012;223:497–503.

61. Palmer TM, Nordestgaard BG, Benn M, et al. Association of plasma uric acid with ischaemic heart disease and blood pressure: mendelian randomisation analysis of two large cohorts. BMJ 2013;347:f4262.

62. Rasheed H, Hughes K, Flynn TJ, et al. Mendelian randomization provides no evidence for a causal role of serum urate in increasing serum triglyceride levels. Circ Cardiovasc Genet 2014;7:830–7.

63. Sulem P, Gudbjartsson DF, Walters GB, et al. Identification of low-frequency variants associated with gout and serum uric acid levels. Nat Genet 2011;43: 1127–30.

64. Li C, Li Z, Liu S, et al. Genome-wide association analysis identifies three new risk loci for gout arthritis in Han Chinese. Nat Comm 2015;6:7041.

65. Voight BF, Scott LJ, Steinthorsdottir V, et al. Twelve type 2 diabetes susceptibility loci identified through large-scale association analysis. Nat Genet 2010;42: 579–89.

66. Matsuo H, Yamamoto K, Nakaoka H, et al. Genome-wide association study of clinically defined gout identifies multiple risk loci and its association with clinical subtypes. Ann Rheum Dis 2015;75:652–9.

67. Phipps-Green AJ, Hollis-Moffatt J, Dalbeth N, et al. A strong role for the ABCG2 gene in susceptibility to gout in New Zealand Pacific Island and Caucasian, but not Maori, case and control sample sets. Hum Mol Genet 2010;19:4813–9.

68. Roberts R, Wallace M, Phipps-Green A, et al. ABCG2 loss-of-function polymorphism predicts poor response to allopurinol in patients with gout. Pharmacogenomics J 2017;17(2):201–3.

69. Merriman TR, Phipps-Green A, Boocock J, et al. Pleiotropic effect of ABCG2 in gout. Arthritis Rheumatol 2016;68:S10.

Genetics and the Causes of Ankylosing Spondylitis

Aimee Hanson[a], Matthew A. Brown, MBBS, MD, FRACP, FAHMS, FAA[b],*

KEYWORDS

- Axial spondyloarthritis • Ankylosing spondylitis • Genetics • Association • SNP
- Heritability

KEY POINTS

- Ankylosing spondylitis (AS) is a common, highly heritable inflammatory arthritis for which, thus far, 113 non-MHC genetic associations have been identified.
- Human leukocyte antigen (HLA)-B27 contributes approximately 20% of the heritability of AS, and nonmajor histocompatibility complex loci identified to date contribute another approximately 10%.
- The HLA associations of AS are complex and multiple non-B27 HLA alleles have been identified as being involved.
- Key pathways identified by AS genetic studies include the interleukin (IL)-23 and M1-aminopeptidase pathways, but multiple other pathways have been identified as increasing numbers of associations have been identified.
- Preliminary evidence suggesting involvement of killer immunoglobulin-like receptor (KIR) genes in AS pathogenesis needs replication in other cohorts.

INTRODUCTION

Genetic studies of ankylosing spondylitis (AS) have, over the past decade, provided major insights into the etiopathogenesis of the disease that have led to major therapeutic innovations. Some of these new treatments have already entered clinical practice, and others are in trials and undergoing development. It is well known that susceptibility to and severity of AS are largely genetically determined. Extensive progress has been made identifying susceptibility alleles in the disease, with

Disclosure Statement: A. Hanson has nothing to disclose. M.A. Brown has received research support, and acted as an advisor or as part of the speakers' bureau of Abbvie, Janssen, Novartis, Pfizer, and UCB.
[a] Translational Research Institute, Princess Alexandra Hospital, University of Queensland Diamantina Institute, Woolloongabba, Brisbane, Queensland, Australia; [b] Institute of Health and Biomedical Innovation, Translational Research Institute, Princess Alexandra Hospital, Queensland University of Technology, Woolloongabba, Brisbane, Queensland, Australia
* Corresponding author.
E-mail address: matt.brown@qut.edu.au

113 established loci identified, contributing roughly 10% of the heritability of AS, over and above the major effect of human leukocyte antigen (HLA)-B27, which determines approximately 20% of the genetic risk. Studies of the genetics of clinical manifestations of AS, such as the extent of bony ankylosis or presence of anterior uveitis, have been more challenging, though some genes have been found to influence uveitis risk beyond their effects on the risk of AS. This article seeks to present the current state of understanding of the genetic influences in AS, focusing on more recent advances and their contribution to understanding mechanisms of disease.

MAJOR HISTOCOMPATIBILITY COMPLEX AND ANKYLOSING SPONDYLITIS

Large scale case-control studies of HLA and other major histocompatibility complex (MHC) genes in AS have demonstrated that the genetic associations at this locus are far more complex than initially thought. Since the discovery of the association of HLA-B27 with AS, there have been many studies suggesting the presence of additional MHC-associated variants.[1–5] With the exception of the association of HLA-B60 with AS,[6,7] until recently, none of those have been convincingly replicated.

The MHC is under marked genetic selection pressure and HLA frequencies vary substantially between ethnic groups. The development of methods of HLA-typing using imputation from dense single nucleotide polymorphism (SNP) genotyping, together with the availability of large reference sets of subjects genotyped at both HLA loci and MHC SNPs, has enabled analysis of HLA and MHC associations in large case-control cohorts. Another methodologic advance in recent studies is principal components analysis; population stratification can be identified and controlled for, making the findings robust to differences in allele frequencies due to ethnic variation rather than disease affection status. Two such studies have now been published, 1 in subjects of European ancestry[8] and the other in Koreans.[9] Both show convincingly that there are additional HLA-B variants associated with AS, as well as other HLA class I and II variants (**Table 1**). Although these studies do not exclude the presence of other non-HLA MHC genetic associations, they do indicate that it is unlikely that variants of large effect exist within the MHC once the associations of HLA variants are accounted for.

Table 1
Association of HLA-B alleles with susceptibility to ankylosing spondylitis in European-descent subjects

Round	HLA-B Allele	Odds Ratio (95% CI)	P-Value
1	27:05	62.41	$<10^{-321}$
2	27:02	43.41	1.07×10^{-122}
3	07:02	0.82	5.04×10^{-6}
4	57:01	0.75	5.13×10^{-4}
5	51:01	1.33	2.14×10^{-3}
6	47:01	2.35	2.25×10^{-3}
7	40:02	1.59	4.65×10^{-3}
8	13:02	1.43	4.29×10^{-3}
9	40:01	1.22	4.93×10^{-3}

Findings are presented for consecutive conditional analyses, in which, for round 2 and onward, the test conditioned on the previous alleles.

The additional HLA-associations likely contribute to the known association of AS with other diseases. For example, *HLA-B51*, which is also a risk variant for AS, is the major risk allele for Behçet syndrome, a condition that can be complicated by sacroiliitis. *HLA-DRB1*0103* is AS-associated and is among the major risk alleles for Crohn disease, which frequently co-occurs with AS. *HLA-B7* has a major protective effect on AS and, interestingly, is used as a control allele in transgenic rats. In this model, excess copy numbers of *HLA-B27* induce a spondyloarthropathy, whereas rats with similar excess copy numbers of *HLA-B7* remain healthy.[10]

Using dense MHC SNP genotyping data, the amino-acid composition of the HLA alleles can be imputed and tested for association with disease, enabling the identification of the key amino-acids involved. This approach has been successfully used to extend the known amino-acids in the rheumatoid arthritis shared epitope, which provides a functional explanation for the association of HLA-DRB1 alleles with that disease.[11] In AS, in the populations studied, the identity of the amino-acid at position 97 in HLA-B was shown to determine the direction of association of the major HLA-B alleles with the disease (**Table 2**).[8] This does not mean that this amino acid alone is the sole HLA-B determinant of AS risk; rather it indicates that, in the context of the HLA-B alleles involved, this amino acid is a key determinant of disease risk.

AMINOPEPTIDASES AND ANKYLOSING SPONDYLITIS

A key recent discovery has been the demonstration that variants of the M1-aminopeptidase gene, *ERAP1*, are associated with AS,[12] and interact genetically with both the AS-associated HLA class I alleles HLA-B27 and HLA-B*4001.[8,13] Thus, *ERAP1* is only associated with AS in HLA-B27 positive cases, or HLA-B27-negative/HLA-B*4001 positive cases. The same *ERAP1* haplotypes interact with HLA-Cw6 in psoriasis,[14] and HLA-B51 in Behçet disease.[15] This locus is also strongly associated with the rare ocular uveitis birdshot retinopathy, which is strongly associated with HLA-A29, though in this disease the number of subjects studied is too small to

---

Table 2
Association analysis of single nucleotide polymorphisms and amino acids at position 97 of human leukocyte antigen-B

Amino Acid Residue	Multivariate Odds Ratio (95% CI)	P-Value	Classical *HLA-B* Allele
Asparagine (N)	16.51 (15.43–17.69)	$<1 \times 10^{-300}$	*27:02, *27:04, *27:05
Threonine (T)	1.12 (1.03–1.21)	4.50×10^{-3}	*13:02, *39:06, *40:06, *51:01, *51:08, *52:01, *55:01, *56:01
Arginine (R)	1.00 (Reference)	1	*15:01, *15:03, *15:10, *15:16, *15:17, *15:18, *18:01, *35:01, *35:02, *35:03, *35:08, *35:12, *37:01, *38:01, *38:02, *39:01, *39:10, *40:01, *41:01, *44:02, *44:03, *44:04, *44:05, *45:01, *47:01, *49:01, *50:01, *53:01, *58:01
Tryptophan (W)	1.00 (0.89–1.12)	.95	*14:01, *14:02
Serine (S)	0.86 (0.81–0.91)	4.81×10^{-8}	*07:02, *07:05, *08:01, *15:07, *27:07, *40:02, *41:02, *48:01
Valine (V)	0.68 (0.59–0.78)	1.41×10^{-8}	*57:01, *57:03

determine if the disease association is with *ERAP1*, the neighboring related gene *ERAP2*, or both.[16] The *ERAP2* association with AS is present in both HLA-B27-positive and HLA-B27-negative disease,[17] suggesting some subtle difference in its functional mechanism in causing AS. For example, ERAP2 may potentially affect peptide handling by other AS-associated HLA class I alleles for which ERAP1 peptide cleavage is less influential.

A recent paper has suggested that haplotypes of *ERAP1* variants are more strongly associated with disease and have greater functional effects than individual disease-associated variants.[18] However, the small sample size of this study (19 cases and 17 controls) is too few to distinguish haplotypic from single variant effects, and many of the haplotypic associations reported were not statistically significant.[19] The study also reports the opposite direction of association of the key AS *ERAP1* nonsynonymous SNP, rs30187, compared with all other studies, which included more than 1000 times more cases and controls, in multiple ethnic groups.[8,20–24] In the absence of further supportive evidence, this study should be considered hypothesis-generating.

Extensive studies of the functional mechanism of the associations of ERAP1 and ERAP2 variants and AS are underway. Both proteins are involved in peptide trimming in the endoplasmic reticulum (ER), changing particularly the length but also the amino acid composition of peptides available for HLA class I presentation.[25–28] Proposed mechanisms of association include

- Effects on the peptidome presented by HLA-B27 and thus leading either to presentation of arthritogenic peptides[29] or failure to present disease-protective peptides[30]
- Effects on HLA-B27 free heavy chain expression and killer immunoglobulin-like receptor (KIR) interactions, in turn influencing activation of interleukin (IL)-17 producing immune cells[31]
- Effects on HLA-B27 folding and ER accumulation leading to ER stress reactions.[32,33]

It is beyond the scope of this article to discuss these hypotheses and studies in detail. However, a common feature of each model is that variants that are disease-protective in AS exhibit reduced peptide cleavage function.[34–36] This and the fact that, apart from in Behçet disease, there is no convincing evidence in either humans or animal models that ERAP deficiency increases disease risk, has led to programs targeting these proteins as therapeutics for AS and related diseases.[37]

T CELLS AND ANKYLOSING SPONDYLITIS

How genetic variants predisposing to immune-mediated diseases are tied to altered immune system activity is a question of primary importance. Despite being among the first proposed mechanisms of disease development in AS, strongly supported by the robust ERAP1-HLA-B27 epistasis identified,[36] it has not been conclusively demonstrated that auto-reactive T cells recognize a B27-restricted peptide in AS patients to cause disease. T-cell receptors (TCRs) develop by the process of random recombination of numerous encoded gene segments to generate highly variable and cell-specific receptor chains. Unique cell surface TCRs on each T cell have the potential to engage different combinations and conformations of HLA bound peptides (**Fig. 1**). Clonally expanded T cells that have recognized an antagonistic antigen and proliferated to hone adaptive immune responses are a feature of many immune-mediated diseases and contribute to targeted inflammation.[38,39] Little evidence of such occurrence in AS patients has been published since the work of Mamedov

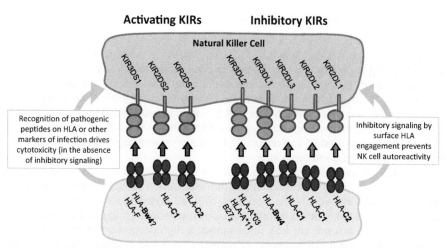

Fig. 1. KIR gene usage and interacting partners, and their effects on natural killer (NK) cell activation or inhibition.

and colleagues[40] in 2009, which characterized the T-cell populations of 2 patients and found stably expanded clones consistently representing between 5% and 50% of the profiled repertoire over several years. These T cells were found to be cytotoxic and proinflammatory in nature, predominantly CD8+/CD27-/CD28- (regarded as terminally differentiated effector or cytotoxic T cells), and expressed TCRs with homology to several previously reported clones in reactive arthritis,[41] rheumatoid arthritis,[42] and other AS subjects.[43] Earlier work demonstrated that a nonamer of the HLA-B*2705 molecule hypervariable region itself can be recognized by cytotoxic T lymphocytes in AS subjects.[44] Convergence of TCR sequences used by these nonamer-responsive T-cell populations found in the peripheral blood and synovial fluid of numerous AS subjects suggested a mechanism by which self-reactive T cells contribute to inflammation in a B27-dependent fashion. However other studies including in discordant twin pairs found no sharing of CD4+ or CD8+ peripheral T cell receptor Vβ repertoire.[45] TCR involvement in AS has also been looked at from the point of view of germline variable region genes, but neither linkage nor association of the TCRA or TCRB loci have been demonstrated with AS,[36,46] suggesting that these loci are not important in the familiality of the disease.

The future of immunogenetics studies in immune-mediated diseases with suspected autoreactive T-cell involvement will be in the high-resolution profiling of T-cell populations. Although yet to be conducted in an AS cohort, new immunosequencing techniques applied to a diversity of conditions, including juvenile idiopathic arthritis (JIA), has provided insight into the underlying nature of T-cell responses in disease.[47] The JIA study demonstrated a restricted TCRB repertoire in the peripheral blood and synovial fluid regulatory T cell (Treg) population of patients, with patient sharing of expanded clonotypes lacking in healthy children. Results suggested either appropriate but inefficient control of inflammatory processes by Tregs, which are typically an immensely diverse T-cell population, or perhaps pathogenicity of the expanded clones in disease. Clonal restriction of relevant T-cell populations in AS may very well be detected with the profiling of hundreds of thousands of TCRs in this fashion, providing support for the arthritogenic peptide model of disease.

PLEIOTROPY AND ANKYLOSING SPONDYLITIS

AS frequently co-occurs in individuals and families with psoriasis and inflammatory bowel disease, potentially because of shared genetic or environmental risk factors, or both. Using a genotyping chip targeting immunogenetically important loci,[48] the extensive role of genetic pleiotropy in these clinical associations has been demonstrated.[24] This cross-disease study showed extensive coheritability of AS with both ulcerative colitis and Crohn disease, as well as with psoriasis, albeit to a lesser extent. Using these data, the investigators identified an additional 17 genome-wide significant AS-associated loci, and 65 loci associated at genome-wide significance with combinations of diseases (pleiotropic loci).

The study further strengthened the evidence of the role of the IL-23 pathway in AS pathogenesis, building on the finding of the association of *IL23R* variants with the disease, which initiated the development of IL-23 pathway inhibitors for the disease.[12] Although the exact functional mechanisms underpinning most genetic associations with AS are not yet fully understood, a high proportion of AS-associated genes influence the IL-23 pathway. At some loci multiple disease-associated variants have been identified, often with differential associations with different diseases. For example, Ellinghaus and colleagues[24] identified 4 independent associations at *IL23R*, and additional variants have been identified as the primary variants associated with other immune-mediated diseases, such as Behçet syndrome, psoriatic arthritis, and Vogt-Koyanagi-Harada syndrome. This suggests that differences in transcriptional regulation, such as tissue specificity, or response to particular stimuli, underlie how these genes operate to cause clinically distinct diseases. Functional analysis of such variants will provide important information about the role of particular genes in disease, and inform therapeutic targeting of such genes. An excellent recent example of this has been the functional and immunogenetic dissection of the *RUNX3* locus, a potential therapeutic target for these diseases that is known to be associated with AS but also celiac disease, psoriasis,[49] and psoriatic arthritis.[50]

Other novel gene pathways identified in the cross-disease study include

- DNA methylation: DNA methyltransferase 3a and 3b (*DNMT3A*, *DNM3TB*) are de novo methyltransferases known to be involved in genomic imprinting and X-chromosome inactivation, to influence hematopoietic stem cell development, and activation of UBE2 ubiquitin ligases, a family of genes also known to be AS-associated. The known functions of these genes raise the hypothesis that they may be involved in the male gender bias in AS, which remains unexplained.
- Gut mucosal immunology: The AS-associated gene *FUT2* encodes a fucosyl transferase that determines the ability to secrete blood group antigens into body fluids. This has a major effect on the gut microbiome, providing further evidence that AS is a disease caused by interaction between an abnormal gut microbiome and the host immune system.[51]
- JAK (Janus kinase) signaling: JAK2 is the tyrosine kinase that signals from IL-23R, and is the only AS-associated *JAK*.[24] It was, therefore, predictable that agents such as tofacitinib, which primarily target other JAK proteins, would be only moderately effective in AS,[52] and suggests that more JAK2-specific inhibitors should undergo clinical trials.
- Toll-like receptor (TLR) signaling: The association of TLR4 with AS, which drives innate immune reactions, particularly to lipopolysaccharide (a key bacterial cell wall component), provides another non-HLA-B27–dependent pathway involved in causing the disease.[24]

These findings demonstrate that further hypothesis-free genetic studies are warranted in AS. Although many of the genes identified in recent studies lie in established pathways, new pathways are still being identified through new gene discoveries.

KILLER IMMUNOGLOBULIN-LIKE RECEPTORS

Another group of genes with suspected relevance in many immune-mediated diseases are the KIRs encoded within the lymphocyte receptor complex on chromosome 19. KIR disease associations have largely gone undetected by genetic studies because the biological consequences of receptor signaling on immune responses depends heavily on a multitude of factors that are highly variable in the population. The KIR locus is immensely polymorphic, encoding variable combinations of 17 different receptors that transduce either excitatory or inhibitory signals to natural killer (NK) and T cells on engagement with specific HLA class 1 or HLA-like ligands (**Fig. 2**). Given the large degree of allelic and expression variability that exists at each gene, and that the independent HLA background of an individual governs the compatibility of receptor-ligand engagements, KIR-mediated immune response are uniquely shaped in each individual[53] and thus difficult to study collectively. KIR associations with AS are varied. One disease model proposes that the ability of KIR3DL2 to recognize abnormal HLA-B27 cell surface homodimers is tied to pathogenicity[54]; others suggest that the balance of inhibitory and excitatory KIR receptors in AS patients is relevant in skewing inflammatory NK cell responses in disease.

Recent molecular studies have demonstrated that the KIR3DL2 receptor is upregulated on activated CD4+ T cells. It has been previously demonstrated that CD4+/KIR3DL2+ T cells are found in increased numbers in AS patients relative to healthy individuals.[31,55] The same research team found them to be expressed in the terminal

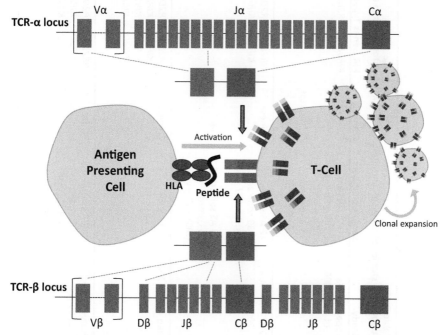

Fig. 2. TCR gene rearrangement pathway determining TCR usage by individual T cells.

Table 3
Association studies of killer-cell immunoglobulin-like receptor genes in ankylosing spondylitis

Study	Sample Numbers	Ethnicity	KIR Genes Typed	Main Findings
Lopez-Larrea et al,[60] 2006	71 AS subjects, 105 controls (HLA-B27 +ve)	Spanish	KIR3DL1, KIR3DS1	KIR3DL1 frequency decreased in subjects (Spanish P<.0001; Azorean P<.003)
	55 AS subjects, 75 controls (HLA-B27 +ve)	Portuguese		KIR3DS1 frequency increased in subjects (Spanish P<.0001; Azorean P<.003)
Diaz-Pena et al,[59] 2008	42 AS subjects, 30 controls (HLA-B27 +ve)	Chinese	KIR2DS1, KIR2DS2, KIR2DS3, KIR2DS5, KIR3DS1, KIR2DL1, KIR2DL2, KIR2DL3, KIR2DL5, KIR3DL1	KIR3DS1, KIR2DS5 and KIR2DL5 frequencies increased in subjects (Chinese P<.005, P<.001, P<.01 respectively; Thai P<.05, P<.05, P<.05 respectively)
	30 AS subjects, 16 controls (HLA-B27 +ve)	Thai		KIR3DL1/KIR3DL1 frequency decreased in subjects (Chinese P<.05; Thai P<.05) KIR3DL1/KIR3DS1 frequency increased in subjects (Chinese P<.005; Thai P<.05)
Jiao et al,[63] 2008	119 AS subjects, 128 controls	Chinese	KIR2DS1, KIR2DS2, KIR2DS3, KIR2DS4, KIR2DS5, KIR3DS1, KIR2DL1, KIR2DL2, KIR2DL3, KIR2DL4, KIR2DL5, KIR3DL1, KIR3DL2, KIR3DL3, KIR2DP1, KIR3DP1	KIR3DS1 and KIR2DL5 frequencies increased in subjects (P = .016 and P = .003 respectively) HLA-Cw02 frequency increased in subjects (P = 0) Genotype HLA-Cw02/KIR2DS1 frequency increased in subjects (P = .011)
Harvey et al,[58] 2009	200 AS subjects, 405 controls (KIR typing) 368 AS subjects, 366 controls (KIR3DL2 typing)	White	KIR2DS1, KIR2DS2, KIR2DS3, KIR2DS4, KIR2DS5, KIR3DS1, KIR2DL1, KIR2DL2, KIR2DL3, KIR2DL4, KIR2DL5, KIR3DL1, KIR3DL2, KIR3DL3	No significant difference between KIR gene or KIR3DL2 allele frequencies between subjects and controls

Study	Sample	Population	KIR genes	Findings
Jiao et al,[64] 2010	115 AS subjects, 119 controls (HLA-B27 +ve)	Chinese	KIR2DS1, KIR2DS2, KIR2DS3, KIR2DS4, KIR2DS5, KIR3DS1, KIR2DL1, KIR2DL2, KIR2DL3, KIR2DL4, KIR2DL5, KIR3DL1, KIR3DL2, KIR3DL3, KIR2DP1, KIR3DP1	KIR2DL1 and KIR2DL5 frequencies increased in subjects ($P = .012$ and $P = .009$ respectively) HLA-Cw08 frequency increased in subjects ($P = .001$)
Zvyagin et al,[61] 2010	83 AS subjects, 107 controls (HLA-B27 +ve)	Russian and white	KIR3DL1 (functional), KIR3DL1*004 (nonfunctional), KIR3DL1*005 (lowly expressed), KIR3DL1*007 (lowly expressed) KIR3DS1	KIR3DL1 frequency decreased in subjects ($P<.01$) KIR3DS1 frequency increased in subjects ($P<.01$) KIR3DL1/KIR3DL1 frequency decreased in subjects ($P = .005$) KIR3DL1/KIR3DS1 frequency increased in subjects ($P = .01$) KIR3DL1*F (functional alleles) frequency decreased in subjects ($P = .005$)
Mahmoudi et al,[65] 2016	200 AS subjects, 200 controls	Iranian	KIR2DS1, KIR2DS2, KIR2DS3, KIR2DS4, KIR2DS5, KIR3DS1, KIR2DL1, KIR2DL2, KIR2DL3, KIR2DL4 KIR2DL5, KIR3DL1, KIR3DL2, KIR3DL3 KIR2DP1, KIR3DP1	KIR2DL3 frequency increased is subjects ($P = .005$) KIR2DL5 frequency decreased in subjects ($P = .03$) HLA-C2 group and HLA-B27 frequency increased in subjects $KIR2DL1^+/HLA\text{-}CW^{Lys+}$, $KIR2DL2^-/HLA\text{-}CW^{asp80-}$, $KIR2DL3^+/HLA\text{-}CW^{asp80-}$, $KIR2DS1^+/HLA\text{-}CW^{Lys+}$, $KIR2DS2^-/HLA\text{-}CW^{asp80-}$ frequencies increased in subjects ($P = .0009$, $P = .01$, $P = .0008$, $P = .009$, $P = .002$ respectively) $KIR2DL1^+/HLA\text{-}CW^{Lys-}$, $KIR2DL2^+/HLA\text{-}CW^{asp80+}$, $KIR2DL3^-/HLA\text{-}CW^{asp80+}$, $KIR3DL1^+/HLA\text{-}Bw4^{Thr+}$, $KIR2DS1^-/HLA\text{-}CW^{Lys-}$, $KIR2DS1^+/HLA\text{-}CW^{Lys-}$, $KIR2DS2^+/HLA\text{-}CW^{asp80+}$ frequencies decreased in subjects ($P = .00008$, $P = .01$, $P = .002$, $P = .07$, $P = .02$, $P = .006$, $P = .004$, respectively)

ileum of early spondyloarthritis (SpA) subjects.[56] Engagement of KIR3DL2 with HLA-B27 homodimers or free heavy chains has been shown to provide a survival signal to these cell populations and to promote differentiation into T-helper 17 (Th17) cells, which secrete the proinflammatory cytokine IL-17 found at increased levels in AS patients.[31] The studies reporting these findings have been small, involved subjects with spondyloarthropathies other than AS, and have not been replicated.[57] Only KIR3DL2 and KIR3DL1 usage has been studied in AS to date. A study of KIR3DL2 genetic variation found no association with AS.[58] Given the potential significance of the studies of KIR3DL2 with AS, there is a clear need for independent replication of this finding and a more comprehensive survey of KIR usage should be performed.

Genetic studies looking to compare gene dosages of differing KIR receptors in AS cases and controls have revealed several other genes found more or less frequently in subjects, with potential ramifications for the control of NK cell immunity (**Table 3**). Of relevance are differences in the frequency of genes KIR3DS1 (increased in AS cohorts), and KIR3DL1 (decreased in AS cohorts),[59–61] given that the latter is an inhibitory receptor known to recognize HLA-Bw4 subgroups, including HLA-B27. Highly homologous KIR3DS1 encodes a lymphocyte-activating receptor and has been postulated to also respond to HLA-B27 ligands. KIR3DS1 co-occurrence with HLA-Bw4 is associated with slowed progression to AIDS in human immunodeficiency virus (HIV) individuals, evidence of its immune-activating potential.[62] Profiling the patterns of KIR and HLA inheritance in large disease cohorts is likely to be very informative in characterizing the involvement of KIR-expressing lymphocytes in AS.

SUMMARY

Genetic studies have identified multiple different pathways involved in AS and, as more genes are being identified, more pathways are being uncovered. These findings are helping solve the mystery about how HLA-B27 is involved in AS and in identifying new potential therapeutic targets. Although much more will be learned from further hypothesis-free studies in AS genomics, the research now needs to transition increasingly to functional genomics studies to determine the mechanisms underpinning these associations and to turn the genetic discoveries into new treatments as they have already with regard to IL-23 pathway inhibition in AS.

REFERENCES

1. Brown MA, Kennedy LG, Darke C, et al. The effect of HLA-DR genes on susceptibility to and severity of ankylosing spondylitis. Arthritis Rheum 1998;41(3): 460–5.
2. Milicic A, Lindheimer F, Laval S, et al. Interethnic studies of TNF polymorphisms confirm the likely presence of a second MHC susceptibility locus in ankylosing spondylitis. Genes Immun 2000;1(7):418–22.
3. Jaakkola E, Herzberg I, Laiho K, et al. Finnish HLA studies confirm the increased risk conferred by HLA-B27 homozygosity in ankylosing spondylitis. Ann Rheum Dis 2006;65(6):775–80.
4. Said-Nahal R, Miceli-Richard C, Gautreau C, et al. The role of HLA genes in familial spondyloarthropathy: a comprehensive study of 70 multiplex families. Ann Rheum Dis 2002;61(3):201–6.
5. Sims AM, Barnardo M, Herzberg I, et al. Non-B27 MHC associations of ankylosing spondylitis. Genes Immun 2007;8(2):115–23.

6. Robinson WP, van der Linden SM, Khan MA, et al. HLA-Bw60 increases susceptibility to ankylosing spondylitis in HLA-B27+ patients. Arthritis Rheum 1989; 32(9):1135–41.

7. Brown MA, Pile KD, Kennedy LG, et al. HLA class I associations of ankylosing spondylitis in the white population in the United Kingdom. Ann Rheum Dis 1996;55(4):268–70.

8. Cortes A, Pulit SL, Leo PJ, et al. Major histocompatibility complex associations of ankylosing spondylitis are complex and involve further epistasis with ERAP1. Nat Commun 2015;6:7146.

9. Kim K, Bang SY, Lee S, et al. An HLA-C amino-acid variant in addition to HLA-B*27 confers risk for ankylosing spondylitis in the Korean population. Arthritis Res Ther 2015;17:342.

10. Taurog JD, Maika SD, Satumtira N, et al. Inflammatory disease in HLA-B27 transgenic rats. Immunol Rev 1999;169:209–23.

11. Raychaudhuri S, Sandor C, Stahl EA, et al. Five amino acids in three HLA proteins explain most of the association between MHC and seropositive rheumatoid arthritis. Nat Genet 2012;44(3):291–6.

12. Wellcome Trust Case Control Consortium, Australo-Anglo-American Spondylitis Consortium, Burton PR, Clayton DG, Cardon LR, et al. Association scan of 14,500 nonsynonymous SNPs in four diseases identifies autoimmunity variants. Nat Genet 2007;39(11):1329–37.

13. International Genetics of Ankylosing Spondylitis Consortium, Cortes A, Hadler J, Pointon JP, et al. Identification of multiple risk variants for ankylosing spondylitis through high-density genotyping of immune-related loci. Nat Genet 2013;45(7): 730–8.

14. Strange A, Capon F, Spencer CC, et al. A genome-wide association study identifies new psoriasis susceptibility loci and an interaction between HLA-C and ERAP1. Nat Genet 2010;42(11):985–90.

15. Kirino Y, Bertsias G, Ishigatsubo Y, et al. Genome-wide association analysis identifies new susceptibility loci for Behcet's disease and epistasis between HLA-B*51 and ERAP1. Nat Genet 2013;45(2):202–7.

16. Kuiper JJ, Van Setten J, Ripke S, et al. A genome-wide association study identifies a functional ERAP2 haplotype associated with birdshot chorioretinopathy. Hum Mol Genet 2014;23(22):6081–7.

17. Robinson PC, Costello ME, Leo P, et al. ERAP2 is associated with ankylosing spondylitis in HLA-B27-positive and HLA-B27-negative patients. Ann Rheum Dis 2015;74:1627–9.

18. Reeves E, Colebatch-Bourn A, Elliott T, et al. Functionally distinct ERAP1 allotype combinations distinguish individuals with Ankylosing Spondylitis. Proc Natl Acad Sci U S A 2014;111(49):17594–9.

19. Robinson PC, Brown MA. ERAP1 biology and assessment in Ankylosing Spondylitis. Proc Natl Acad Sci U S A 2015;112(15):E1816.

20. Tsui FW, Haroon N, Reveille JD, et al. Association of an ERAP1 ERAP2 haplotype with familial ankylosing spondylitis. Ann Rheum Dis 2010;69(4):733–6.

21. Davidson SI, Liu Y, Danoy PA, et al. Association of STAT3 and TNFRSF1A with ankylosing spondylitis in Han Chinese. Ann Rheum Dis 2011;70(2):289–92.

22. Pimentel-Santos FM, Ligeiro D, Matos M, et al. Association of IL23R and ERAP1 genes with ankylosing spondylitis in a Portuguese population. Clin Exp Rheumatol 2009;27(5):800–6.

23. Bang SY, Kim TH, Lee B, et al. Genetic Studies of ankylosing spondylitis in Koreans Confirm Associations with ERAP1 and 2p15 reported in white patients. J Rheumatol 2010;38(2):322–4.

24. Ellinghaus D, Jostins L, Spain SL, et al. Analysis of five chronic inflammatory diseases identifies 27 new associations and highlights disease-specific patterns at shared loci. Nat Genet 2016;48(5):510–8.

25. Chang SC, Momburg F, Bhutani N, et al. The ER aminopeptidase, ERAP1, trims precursors to lengths of MHC class I peptides by a "molecular ruler" mechanism. Proc Natl Acad Sci U S A 2005;102(47):17107–12.

26. Saveanu L, Carroll O, Lindo V, et al. Concerted peptide trimming by human ERAP1 and ERAP2 aminopeptidase complexes in the endoplasmic reticulum. Nat Immunol 2005;6(7):689–97.

27. Evnouchidou I, Weimershaus M, Saveanu L, et al. ERAP1-ERAP2 dimerization increases peptide-trimming efficiency. J Immunol 2014;193(2):901–8.

28. Sanz-Bravo A, Campos J, Mazariegos MS, et al. Dominant role of the ERAP1 polymorphism R528K in shaping the HLA-B27 Peptidome through differential processing determined by multiple peptide residues. Arthritis Rheumatol 2015; 67(3):692–701.

29. Benjamin R, Parham P. HLA-B27 and disease: a consequence of inadvertent antigen presentation? Rheum Dis Clin North Am 1992;18(1):11–21.

30. Kenna TJ, Brown MA. Immunopathogenesis of ankylosing spondylitis. Int J Clin Rheumatol 2013;8(2):265–74.

31. Chen L, Ridley A, Hammitzsch A, et al. Silencing or inhibition of endoplasmic reticulum aminopeptidase 1 (ERAP1) suppresses free heavy chain expression and Th17 responses in ankylosing spondylitis. Ann Rheum Dis 2016;75(5):916–23.

32. Kenna TJ, Lau MC, Keith P, et al. Disease-associated polymorphisms in ERAP1 do not alter endoplasmic reticulum stress in patients with ankylosing spondylitis. Genes Immun 2015;16(1):35–42.

33. Tran TM, Hong S, Edwan JH, et al. ERAP1 reduces accumulation of aberrant and disulfide-linked forms of HLA-B27 on the cell surface. Mol Immunol 2016;74:10–7.

34. Evnouchidou I, Kamal RP, Seregin SS, et al. Cutting edge: coding single nucleotide polymorphisms of endoplasmic reticulum aminopeptidase 1 can affect antigenic peptide generation in vitro by influencing basic enzymatic properties of the enzyme. J Immunol 2011;186(4):1909–13.

35. Kochan G, Krojer T, Harvey D, et al. Crystal structures of the endoplasmic reticulum aminopeptidase-1 (ERAP1) reveal the molecular basis for N-terminal peptide trimming. Proc Natl Acad Sci U S A 2011;108(19):7745–50.

36. Evans DM, Spencer CC, Pointon JJ, et al. Interaction between ERAP1 and HLA-B27 in ankylosing spondylitis implicates peptide handling in the mechanism for HLA-B27 in disease susceptibility. Nat Genet 2011;43(8):761–7.

37. Zervoudi E, Saridakis E, Birtley JR, et al. Rationally designed inhibitor targeting antigen-trimming aminopeptidases enhances antigen presentation and cytotoxic T-cell responses. Proc Natl Acad Sci U S A 2013;110(49):19890–5.

38. May E, Dulphy N, Frauendorf E, et al. Conserved TCR beta chain usage in reactive arthritis; evidence for selection by a putative HLA-B27-associated autoantigen. Tissue Antigens 2002;60(4):299–308.

39. de Paula Alves Sousa A, Johnson KR, Nicholas R, et al. Intrathecal T-cell clonal expansions in patients with multiple sclerosis. Ann Clin Transl Neurol 2016;3(6): 422–33.

40. Mamedov IZ, Britanova OV, Chkalina AV, et al. Individual characterization of stably expanded T cell clones in ankylosing spondylitis patients. Autoimmunity 2009; 42(6):525–36.

41. Dulphy N, Peyrat M-A, Tieng V, et al. Common Intra-Articular T Cell expansions in patients with reactive arthritis- identical b-chain junctional sequences and cytotoxicity toward HLA-B27. J Immunol 1998;162:3830–9.

42. DerSimonian H, Sugita M, Glass DN, et al. Clonal Vctl2.1 + T cell expansions in the peripheral blood of rheumatoid arthritis patients. J Exp Med 1993;177: 1623–31.

43. Duchmann R, Lambert C, May E, et al. CD4+ and CD8+ clonal T cell expansions indicate a role of antigens in ankylosing spondylitis; a study in HLA-B27+ monozygotic twins. Clin Exp Immunol 2001;123(2):315–22.

44. Frauendorf E, von Goessel H, May E, et al. HLA-B27-restricted T cells from patients with ankylosing spondylitis recognize peptides from B*2705 that are similar to bacteria-derived peptides. Clin Exp Immunol 2003;134(2):351–9.

45. Hohler T, Hug R, Schneider PM, et al. Ankylosing spondylitis in monozygotic twins: studies on immunological parameters. Ann Rheum Dis 1999;58(7):435–40.

46. Brown MA, Rudwaleit M, Pile KD, et al. The role of germline polymorphisms in the T-cell receptor in susceptibility to ankylosing spondylitis. Br J Rheumatol 1998; 37(4):454–8.

47. Henderson LA, Volpi S, Frugoni F, et al. Next generation sequencing reveals restriction and clonotypic expansion of regulatory T cells in juvenile idiopathic arthritis. Arthritis Rheumatol 2016;68(7):1758–68.

48. Cortes A, Brown MA. Promise and pitfalls of the immunochip. Arthritis Res Ther 2011;13(1):101.

49. Vecellio M, Roberts AR, Cohen CJ, et al. The genetic association of RUNX3 with ankylosing spondylitis can be explained by allele-specific effects on IRF4 recruitment that alter gene expression. Ann Rheum Dis 2015;75:1534–40.

50. Apel M, Uebe S, Bowes J, et al. Variants in RUNX3 contribute to susceptibility to psoriatic arthritis, exhibiting further common ground with ankylosing spondylitis. Arthritis Rheum 2013;65(5):1224–31.

51. Costello ME, Ciccia F, Willner D, et al. Intestinal dysbiosis in ankylosing spondylitis. Arthritis Rheumatol 2014;28:687–702.

52. van der Heijde D, Deodhar A, Wei J, et al. Tofacitinib in patients with ankylosing spondylitis: a phase 2, 16-week, randomized, placebo-controlled, dose-ranging study. Arthritis Rheumatol 2015;67(Suppl 10):5L.

53. Rajalingam R. Human diversity of killer cell immunoglobulin-like receptors and disease. Korean J Hematol 2011;46(4):216–28.

54. Kollnberger S, Bird L, Sun MY, et al. Cell-surface expression and immune receptor recognition of HLA-B27 homodimers. Arthritis Rheum 2002;46(11):2972–82.

55. Chan AT, Kollnberger SD, Wedderburn LR, et al. Expansion and enhanced survival of natural killer cells expressing the killer immunoglobulin-like receptor KIR3DL2 in spondylarthritis. Arthritis Rheum 2005;52(11):3586–95.

56. Rysnik O, McHugh K, van Duivenvoorde L, et al. Non-conventional forms of HLA-B27 are expressed in spondyloarthritis joints and gut tissue. J Autoimmun 2016;70:12–21.

57. Jansen DT, Hameetman M, van Bergen J, et al. IL-17-producing CD4+ T cells are increased in early, active axial spondyloarthritis including patients without imaging abnormalities. Rheumatology (Oxford) 2015;54(4):728–35.

58. Harvey D, Pointon JJ, Sleator C, et al. Analysis of killer immunoglobulin-like receptor genes in ankylosing spondylitis. Ann Rheum Dis 2009;68(4):595–8.

59. Diaz-Pena R, Blanco-Gelaz MA, Suarez-Alvarez B, et al. Activating KIR genes are associated with ankylosing spondylitis in Asian populations. Hum Immunol 2008; 69(7):437–42.
60. Lopez-Larrea C, Blanco-Gelaz MA, Torre-Alonso JC, et al. Contribution of KIR3DL1/3DS1 to ankylosing spondylitis in human leukocyte antigen-B27 Caucasian populations. Arthritis Res Ther 2006;8(4):R101.
61. Zvyagin IV, Mamedov IZ, Britanova OV, et al. Contribution of functional KIR3DL1 to ankylosing spondylitis. Cell Mol Immunol 2010;7(6):471–6.
62. Martin MP, Gao X, Lee JH, et al. Epistatic interaction between KIR3DS1 and HLA-B delays the progression to AIDS. Nat Genet 2002;31(4):429–34.
63. Jiao YL, Ma CY, Wang LC, et al. Polymorphisms of KIRs gene and HLA-C alleles in patients with ankylosing spondylitis: possible association with susceptibility to the disease. J Clin Immunol 2008;28(4):343–9.
64. Jiao YL, Zhang BC, You L, et al. Polymorphisms of KIR gene and HLA-C alleles: possible association with susceptibility to HLA-B27-positive patients with ankylosing spondylitis. J Clin Immunol 2010;30(6):840–4.
65. Mahmoudi M, Jamshidi AR, Karami J, et al. Analysis of Killer Cell Immunoglobulin-like Receptor Genes and Their HLA Ligands in Iranian Patients with Ankylosing Spondylitis. Iran J Allergy Asthma Immunol 2016;15(1):27–38.

Genomics of Systemic Lupus Erythematosus

Insights Gained by Studying Monogenic Young-Onset Systemic Lupus Erythematosus

Linda T. Hiraki, MD, FRCPC, ScD[a,b,c], Earl D. Silverman, MD, FRCPC[a,b,d],*

KEYWORDS

- Genetics • Systemic lupus erythematosus • Monogenic diseases
- Interferonopathies • DNA sensing • RNA sensing • Complement deficiency

KEY POINTS

- Monogenic systemic lupus erythematosus (SLE) should be considered in patients with very young onset SLE (<5 years of age), children of consanguineous parents' marriages, and in patients with severe or resistant skin disease.
- Genetic defects of the complement system are the main cause of monogenic SLE and are frequently associated with an increased risk of infection.
- Genetic defects in RNA and DNA sensing molecules, and RNases and DNases can lead to the production of autoantibodies and autoimmunity via the abnormal production of type 1 interferons.
- Mutations in DNA endonucleases can lead to a failure to clear self-DNA, resulting in a breaking of tolerance with the production of autoantibodies and autoimmunity, including SLE.

Genetics play an important role in systemic lupus erythematosus (SLE) susceptibility. There is a 10-fold increased concordance for SLE in monozygotic compared with dizygotic twins as well as familial aggregation of SLE, with heritability estimates up to 66%.[1–3] Genome-wide association studies (GWASs) have identified more than 50 SLE-associated risk loci, suggesting that SLE is a complex phenotype.[4,5] However, aside from genetic variants in the human leukocyte antigen (HLA) region, the SLE risk attributed to an individual single nucleotide polymorphism (SNP) is often less than 2-fold. These GWAS-significant loci, collectively, explain less than 30% of the heritability of SLE.[5]

Disclosure Statement: The authors have nothing to disclose.
^a Division of Rheumatology, SickKids Hospital, SickKids Research Institute, 555 University Avenue, Toronto, Ontario M5G 1X8, Canada; ^b Department of Paediatrics, University of Toronto, 555 University Avenue, Toronto, Ontario M5G 1X8, Canada; ^c Epidemiology, Dalla Lana School of Public Health, 155 College Street, Toronto, Ontario M5T 3M7, Canada; ^d Department of Medicine, University of Toronto, Toronto, Ontario, Canada
* Corresponding author. 555 University Avenue, Toronto, Ontario M5G 1X8, Canada.
E-mail address: Earl.silverman@sickkids.ca

Rheum Dis Clin N Am 43 (2017) 415–434
http://dx.doi.org/10.1016/j.rdc.2017.04.005
0889-857X/17/© 2017 Elsevier Inc. All rights reserved.

rheumatic.theclinics.com

It has been suggested that, because of the earlier onset of SLE in childhood-onset SLE (cSLE) with a generally more severe disease phenotype, it is likely that there is a higher genetic contribution to its development compared with adult-onset SLE (aSLE). Targeted SNP studies have not identified any unique genes associated with cSLE, although it has been shown that a higher genetic load was associated with young age of onset and cSLE (Dominez, unpublished data, 2017 and Ref.[6]) Few studies have estimated heritability or the proportion of variance explained in susceptibility to cSLE. A study of 252 cSLE subjects had a heritability estimate of 21% from autosomal SNPs.[7] This is much lower than the anticipated heritability estimate derived from epidemiologic studies. This small fraction of explained heritability may be because SLE is not a single, complex disease but a heterogeneous phenotype comprised of genetically distinct, monogenic diseases with overlapping clinical features, autoantibodies, and shared inflammatory pathways. It is increasingly recognized that these monogenic forms of SLE are generally enriched in the pediatric population due to young onset, and in families with multiple affected members (multiplex families).[8] This article focuses on the monogenic forms of SLE and their insights into the pathogenesis of SLE (**Table 1**).

COMPLEMENT DEFICIENCIES

The complement system comprises more than 30 proteins and is an important component of the innate and adaptive immune systems' defense against foreign pathogens. Genetic defects in the complement system can lead to increased susceptibility to infection, autoimmunity, and SLE. Genetic defects in the complement system are the most common cause of monogenic SLE. Complement is important in host defense and maintaining tolerance (see later discussion).

Removal of Apoptotic Cells and Immune Complexes

Complement components, in particular C1q, C4b, and C3b, are important in opsonization of apoptotic cells. Therefore, any defect in these complement components might prevent or hinder the removal or clearance of apoptotic cells or immune complexes, thus allowing these potential autoantigens to activate the immune system and lead to a loss of tolerance and SLE.

Complement Receptors are Important in Immune Tolerance

The interaction of the innate and adaptive immune systems is important to maintain self-tolerance. Complement receptors 1 (CR1/CD35) and 2 (CR2/CD21) on follicular dendritic cells are important in presenting complement-coated self-antigens to maintain autoreactive B cells in a state of anergy. Experimental evidence for this theory includes the demonstration that mice deficient in CD21/CD35 or C4 exhibit lupus-like disease.[9]

Control of Dendritic Cell Cytokine Production

C1q is important in toll-like receptor–induced cytokine production and immune complex–induced IFN-1 production by dendritic cells.[10] Therefore, abnormalities of C1q can lead to abnormal cytokine production, including type 1 interferon (IFN-1) and production of autoantibodies.

Monogenic defects in the complement activation proteins C1q, C1s, C1r, C2, and C4 have been described in patients with SLE and this is the focus instead of complement receptors.

Table 1
Reviewed proteins and genes associated with monogenic forms of systemic lupus erythematosus

Protein	Gene	Inheritance	Mechanism	Female to Male Patient Ratio	Associated Symptoms
C1q	C1QA, C1QB, C1QC	Autosomal recessive	Complement deficiency	1:1	SLE (cutaneous, renal, CNS, arthritis, ANA), young age onset, recurrent bacterial infections
C1r/s	C1R, C1S	Autosomal recessive	Complement deficiency	1:1	SLE (fever, cutaneous, arthritis, renal, ANA, ENA), recurrent infections - encapsulated bacteria
C2	C2	Autosomal recessive	Complement deficiency	7:1	SLE (cutaneous, arthritis), young age onset
C4	C4A, C4B	Autosomal recessive	Complement deficiency	1:1	SLE (severe photosensitive rash, renal, ANA, Ro), young age onset
TREX1	TREX1	Autosomal Dominant (FCL), Autosomal recessive and dominant (AGS)	Abnormal DNA clearance leading to IFN activation	Likely 1:1	FCL, AGS, SLE
MDA5	IFIH1	Autosomal Dominant	Activation IFN production	Likely 1:1	AGS, SLE, FCL
SAMHD1	SAMHD1	Autosomal recessive and dominant	Abnormal DNA or RNA clearance leading to IFN production	Likely 1:1	AGS, SLE, FCL
RNaseH2	RNASH2	Autosomal dominant and recessive	Abnormal RNA clearance leading to IFN production	Likely 1:1	AGS, SLE
ADAR1	ADAR1	Mainly autosomal dominant	Abnormal RNA clearance leading to IFN production	Likely 1:1	AGS, SLE
STING	TMEM173	Autosomal Dominant	Activation IFN production	1:1	SAVI, FCL, SLE
DNase I	DNASE1	Autosomal Dominant	Abnormal DNA clearance-break intolerance	Female	SLE (dsDNA), adolescent onset
Dnase1-like-3	DNASE1L3	Autosomal recessive	Abnormal DNA clearance-break intolerance	1:2	SLE (hypocomplementemia, dsDNA, cANCA, renal)

Abbreviations: AGS, Aicardi-Goutières syndrome; FCL, familial chilblain lupus; SAVI, STING-associated vasculopathy with onset in infancy.

C1q

C1q is encoded by 3 genes (C1QA, C1QB, and C1QC), which are present on chromosome 1p36. C1q is important in phagocytosis via opsonization of apoptotic cells. Therefore, variants in C1q genes can lead to C1q deficiency or loss of function that then allow autoantigen presentation with subsequent loss of tolerance. This is best demonstrated in the C1QA knockout $^{(-/-)}$ mouse. This mouse develops high titer autoantibodies and an immune complex glomerulonephritis that is associated with the presence of apoptotic bodies.[11] These results suggest that C1q is required to clear apoptotic cells and that this failure leads to autoimmunity.

In 1979, the first patient with C1q deficiency and an SLE-like syndrome was described.[12] It is now apparent that almost 90% of people with C1q deficiency, as a result of the complete absence of C1q or as a result of defective protein production, develop SLE.[13,14] Recent reviews of SLE in C1q deficiency have reported that clinical characteristics include photosensitive skin rash, nephritis, oral ulceration, and arthritis. Most of the patients had young-onset SLE (median age 6 years) with an equal frequency of male and female patients.[15] Recurrent bacterial infections were seen in 41%, and 17% died of sepsis. Patients with C1q deficiency–associated SLE generally had normal complement C3 and C4 levels with low total hemolytic complement levels, which is an important clue to the diagnosis. Anti-Ro antibodies were more commonly detected than anti-DNA antibodies. Evidence that C1q deficiency leads to SLE in these patients included (1) the demonstration that C1q infusions lead to resolution of symptoms and (2) amelioration of SLE symptoms and restoration of normal C1q activity by bone marrow transplantation.[16,17]

Most cases of C1q deficiency are in the offspring of consanguineous parents and are associated with homozygous variants.[14] However, multiple isolated cases of C1q deficiency leading to young-onset SLE have been described in offspring of non-consanguineous parents.[18–20] Genetic defects have been found in C1QA, C1QB, and C1QC genes. These genetic sequence variants usually result in a stop codon, leading to an absence of the protein, although cases of dysfunctional C1q have been reported secondary to a homozygous change in C1QC.[14,21] Multiple studies have examined the association of SNPs in C1q genes and SLE susceptibility with varying results depending on the ethnicity of the population.[22] The most consistent finding is the association of rs172378 SNP with disease susceptibility and, possibly, lupus nephritis among Europeans.[22]

C1s/C1r

C1s and C1r exist as a heterotetramer and along with C1q form the C1 complex. C1r is activated by C1q following the activation of C1q by immune complexes in the presence of calcium. Activated C1r then acts as a protease to cleave and activate C1s, which, as part of the C1 protease complex, activates C2 and C4 that, in turn, form the C3 convertase C4b2a.

Complete C1s deficiency and partial C1r deficiency are commonly inherited together. Both C1R and C1S genes consist of 12 exons located on chromosome 12p13. Genetic defects in both C1R and C1S genes are generally the result of sequence variants that lead to a premature stop codon and, less commonly, a missense changes. These variants either lead to a truncated protein or an abnormal protein without protease activity. C1R and C1S variants have been described in approximately 20 patients.[14]

Almost all patients have severe skin disease and glomerulonephritis is present in approximately 50% of cases. Similar to patients with C1q variants, most patients have very young-onset disease with recurrent bacterial infections. Patients with

C1s/C1r deficiency frequently have anti-Ro antibodies or other anti-extractable nuclear antigen (ENA) antibodies and, less frequently, anti-DNA antibodies. Antinuclear antibodies (ANAs) may be absent or only low titer. They usually have increased, not decreased, C3 and C4 levels and normal C1q levels. Only 13 cases of C1s/C1r deficiency have been reported, but most (approximately two-thirds) developed SLE.[23] Because C1s or C1r deficiency does not allow the formation of the C1 complex, the immunologic consequences are similar to those seen in C1q deficiency.

C4

One of the earliest associations of complement abnormalities and SLE was low C4 secondary to a genetic deficiency in C4 production. The C4 gene locus is located in chromosome 6p21.3 in the major histocompatibility complex (MHC) class III cluster and encodes 2 different C4 proteins (C4A and C4B). To further increase the complexity of C4 proteins, the genes can encode for either a long or a short protein due to copy number variation of C4 genes. Gene copy number (GCN) varies from 2 to 8 copies with most healthy individuals having 2 copies of each of C4A and C4B, resulting in a GCN of 4.

Homozygous deficiency of both C4A and C4B proteins is rare with less than 30 cases reported in the literature but is strongly associated with SLE.[14] Similar to genetic deficiencies of the early complement components, most patients have young age of onset, a male to female patient ratio of approximately 1, severe skin disease, glomerulonephritis, and the presence of anti-Ro antibodies. C4 knockout mice ($C4^{-/-}$) develop autoimmunity across multiple genetic backgrounds, whereas heterozygous mice ($C4^{+/-}$) develop autoreactivity but to a lesser degree.[24] These studies confirm a role for C4 gene dose in the development of autoimmunity.

More common than complete C4 deficiency is the association of SLE with low GCN.[25] Cohort studies of European populations showed that median GCNs were lower in SLE subjects than controls and this was usually the result of lower numbers of C4A rather than C4B genes. C4A gene deficiency, in combination with a C4B-short gene, was significantly associated with the risk of SLE. Although only 1% of East Asians with SLE had C4A deficiency, the odds ratio for disease susceptibility was 12.4 (95% CI 1.57–97.9).[26] Conversely, higher GCN was protective of SLE in both Europeans and Asian populations.[25,26] One study in cSLE suggested that the association of low GCN is found more frequently in cSLE than in aSLE.[27] It had been suggested that the association between lower number of C4 genes (single C4B-short gene) and C4A deficiency was the result of linkage disequilibrium to HLA A*01, B*08, and DRB1*0301 in Europeans. However, in East Asians the association of lower number of C4 genes and C4A deficiency was linked to HLA-DRB1*1501 and not the white haplotype (which is very rare in the Asian population). These results strongly suggest that low GCN in C4 with C4A deficiency is the true mechanism by which there is an increased SLE susceptibility and not the extended HLA A*01, B*08, and DRB1*0301 haplotypes. No specific clinical or laboratory features of SLE have been associated with low C4 GCN.

C2

It has been estimated that the prevalence of homozygous C2 deficiency in a European population is 1:10,000 to 20,000. However, most (>60%) of these individuals are asymptomatic with only 10% to 30% developing SLE. Individuals with C2 deficiency are at a lower risk for recurrent infections than people with C1q or C4 deficiencies.[28] It has been suggested that in C2-deficient individuals, a higher concentration of antibody than is usually required to activate the classic complement pathway allows activated C1 complex to activate C4 to C4b and interact with the alternative pathway to then cleave C3 to form C3 convertase without requiring C2.[28] Most cases of C2 deficiency are the result of a 28-bp deletion in exon 6, which is associated with HLA-B*18, S042, DRB1*15 haplotype (type I).[29] This variant prevents the translation of the C2 protein. In a minority of cases (approximately 10%), C2 deficiency is caused by a missense variant that results in a failure to secrete the protein (type II).[30]

Most commonly, SLE patients with C2 deficiency present during adulthood, although C2 deficiency has been reported in cSLE. C2-deficient SLE patients commonly have severe skin disease with cutaneous vasculitis, malar rash, discoid rash, and arthritis, as well as, less frequently, major organ involvement. Similar to patients with C1q deficiencies, anti-Ro antibodies are more frequently seen than anti-DNA antibodies but these patients also tend to have anticardiolipin antibodies.[31] In aSLE with C2 deficiency there is a slight increase in male patients (7:1) compared with aSLE without C2 deficiency (9:1).[32]

ABNORMAL TYPE 1 INTERFERON PRODUCTION (INTERFERONOPATHIES)
Type 1 Interferons

IFN-1 plays an important role in immunity by detecting viral nucleic acids and restricting viral replication. Type-1 IFNs can directly restrict viral replication, activate other cells, and expand lymphocytes to target viruses. Increased IFN-1 levels are observed in SLE patients across multiple ethnic backgrounds and seem to be more common in cSLE than in aSLE. Further evidence for the importance of IFN-1 in SLE is the observation that patients treated with recombinant IFN may rarely develop drug-induced SLE.

Before examining specific monogenetic defects, it is important to review the DNA- and RNA-sensing pathways.

DNA Sensing

The presence of DNA in the cytoplasm is an important danger signal that triggers host immune responses. DNA in the plasma, isolated or attached to microparticles (blebs), interacts with a cytosolic DNA sensor, GMP-AMP synthase (cGAS), which then sets in motion a signaling pathway leading to the production of IFN-1, proinflammatory cytokines, and then interferon-stimulated genes (ISGs) (**Fig. 1**). Specifically, the DNA-cGAS interaction induces the production of cyclic GMP-AMP (cGAMP). This then binds to and activates the adaptor protein receptor protein stimulator of interferon genes (STING), which then translocates to the endoplasmic reticulum (ER), leading to an interaction with TANK-binding kinase 1 (TBK1) and the subsequent phosphorylation of interferon-regulating factor-3 (IRF3). Phosphorylated IRF3 can then translocate to the nucleus and activate the production of IFN-1 and proinflammatory cytokines. This can then lead to the production of ISGs (interferon signature) (see **Fig. 1**). Importantly, although cGAS has a broad specificity for double-stranded DNA (dsDNA) so that it can recognize multiple pathogens (viruses, bacteria, and intracellular pathogens), it also can recognize self-dsDNA. Therefore, any defects in the structure or function of enzymes that degrade DNA (DNases) could lead to the accumulation of self-dsDNA, whether it is generated by apoptosis, necrosis, or NETosis (form of cell death, characterized by release of decondensed chromatin and granular contents to the extracellular space), then leading to a loss of self-tolerance.

RNA Sensing

Intracellular sensing of viral nucleic acids is important in detecting and eliminating viral infections. In addition, to maintain homeostasis, the cell must be able to differentiate self-RNA from nonself-RNA and DNA. Viral RNA is detected by members of retinoic acid inducible gene (RIG)-like receptors (RLRs) family: RIG-1, melanoma differentiation-associated gene 5 (MDA5), and Laboratory of Genetics and Physiology

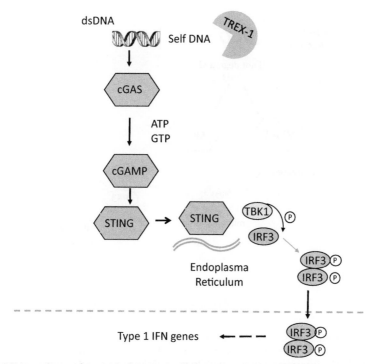

Fig. 1. DNA sensing pathway. Viral-DNA or self-dsDNA is a danger signal for the cell. Important to this process is cytosolic DNA sensor, cGAS. Specifically, the DNA-cGAS interaction induces the production of (cyclic GMP-AMP [cGAMP]). This then binds to and activates the adaptor protein stimulator of interferon genes (STING), which then translocates to the endoplasma reticulum (ER). Activated STING can interact with TBK1, resulting in the phosphorylation of IRF3 with subsequent nuclear translocation and production of IFN-1 and proinflammatory cytokines, and then interferon-regulated genes. cGAS is a very important DNA sensor and, as such, must recognize a very large number of different DNAs from multiple pathogens (viruses, bacteria, and intracellular pathogens). However, and important to autoimmunity, cGAS also can recognize self-dsDNA. In the case of self-dsDNA, the TREX-1 endonuclease leads to the degradation of self-DNA and thereby not allowing it to activate the IRF-3 signaling pathway resulting IFN-1 production. However, when TREX-1 is mutated and unable to function properly, it cannot degrade self-DNA, which leads to activation of the IRF-3 signaling pathway with abnormal IFN-1 production as seen in Aicardi-Goutières syndrome and familial chilblains lupus.

2 (LGP2) that are present in the cytosol (**Fig. 2**). Activated RIG-1 or MDA5 then translocates to the mitochondria to activate mitochondrial antiviral signaling (MAVS) protein, which is bound to the external mitochondrial membrane. Activated MAVS interacts with TBK1 to activate IRF3. IRF3 then activates NFκB, IRF3/7, and AP1, leading to transcription of IFN-1 and proinflammatory cytokine genes. IFN-1 then leads to ISG production (see **Fig. 2**). Therefore, it is not surprising that defects in RNases or gain of function variants in RLRs may lead to high levels of IFN-1 and autoimmunity.

Aicardi-Goutières Syndrome

Aicardi-Goutières syndrome (AGS), a genetic syndrome resembling congenital viral infection, is associated with high levels of IFN-1 in which many patients have evidence of autoimmunity.[33] AGS is characterized by early-onset encephalopathy that is usually associated with calcification of the basal ganglia and white matter changes on brain

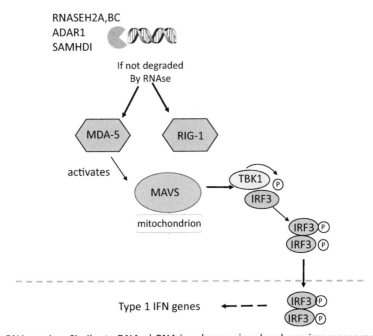

Fig. 2. RNA sensing. Similar to DNA, dsRNA is a danger signal and requires sensor molecules. Viral RNA sensors are collectively referred to as RIG-like receptors (RLRs). The RLRs are: RIG-1, MDA5 encoded by interferon induced with helicase C domain 1(IFIH1), and LGP2. However, how LGP2 signals is not well-known. The detection and interaction of RIG-1 or MDA5 with viral RNA leads to their translocation to the outside of the mitochondria, which allows them to activate membrane-bound MAVS protein. MAVS can now activate the kinases, TBK1 and IKK. Then TNK1 can phosphorylate IRF3, which now can translocate to the nucleus and produce IFN-1, leading to ISGs. MAVS activation also leads to the activation of NF-κB with the subsequent production of other proinflammatory cytokines. Failure to degrade viral-DNA or the abnormal detection of self-RNA would lead to abnormal MDA-5 activation and subsequent ISG production. Similarly, an activating mutation of MDA-5 will lead to ISG production.

imaging (the same changes seen in congenital viral infections). AGS patients almost universally have elevated IFN-1 levels in both serum and cerebral spinal fluid, and increased expression of ISGs in the peripheral blood. Frequently, there is cutaneous disease and, in particular, chilblains. To date, in order of descending frequency, the variants in the following genes have been found in patients with AGS: ribonuclease H2 subunit B (RNASEH2B), 3'repair exonuclease 1 (TREX1), ribonuclease H2 subunit C (RNASEH2C), SAM domain and HD domain-containing 1 (SAMHD1), RNA-specific adenosine deaminase (ADAR), ribonuclease H2 subunit A (RNASEH2A), and interferon-induced with helicase C domain 1 (IFIH1).[34] There is an almost 100% correlation of high IFN-1 production and the presence of the disease-causing variants in all AGS genes except for RNASEH2B in which only approximately two-thirds of patients have high IFN-1 production.[35] Patients with AGS have been shown to have multiple IgG autoantibodies particularly directed against nuclear antigens, basement membrane components, gliadin, and brain endothelial cells and astrocytes.[36] These observations suggest that genetic defects in RNA or DNA clearance result in increased

IFN-1 and ISGs, and then lead to autoimmunity. Each of these genes and their associated phenotypes are specifically reviewed.

TREX1

TREX1 is important in the immune response to single-stranded (ss)-DNA and dsDNA, including viral dsDNA. TREX1 is a major intracellular DNase that exists as a dimer and is capable of interacting and binding to the 3'end of DNA. It is a 314 amino acid protein that is encoded by 1 exon on 3p21.31. TREX1 knockout mice (Trex1 $^{-/-}$) die of autoimmunity via activation of the cytoplasmic DNA sensor cGAS leading to IFN-1 production via the IRF-3 pathway (see **Fig. 1**). Autoimmunity in these mice is IFN-1–dependent because TREX1/IFN receptor double knockout mice do not develop autoimmunity. Lymphocytes, with the production of autoantibodies, macrophages, as a result of increased tumor necrosis factor (TNF)-α and IFN-1 production, increased antigen presentation to CD4+ T cells, impaired clearance of apoptotic T cells, and dendritic cells are important in the development of autoimmunity in Trex1 $^{-/-}$ mice. B cells, cardiomyocytes, neurons, and astrocytes did not show increased IFN-1 production as a result of the inactivation of Trex1. Thus, individual cell types differentially responded to the loss of Trex1. Dendritic cells were shown to be essential in preventing the breakdown of self-tolerance by endogenous dsDNA.[37–39]

Approximately 25% of AGS patients have a disease-causing TREX1 variant that diminishes the nuclease activity of the enzyme.[34] A review of autoimmune features in AGS patients showed that approximately 60% of patients with a TREX1 variant had at least 1 autoimmune feature: thrombocytopenia, leukopenia, ANA, skin lesions, oral ulceration, arthritis, anti-dsDNA antibodies, or anti-ENA antibodies.[33] The largest study of AGS found that hypothyroidism, chilblains, SLE or antiphospholipid syndrome, familial chilblains lupus (FCL), inflammatory gastrointestinal disease (Crohn's disease, atrophic gastritis, celiac disease, autoimmune hepatitis, nonspecific colitis), cardiomyopathy, cerebrovascular disease, and demyelinating peripheral neuropathy were all present at much higher than expected rates.[40] Most patients with AGS have homozygous TREX1 variants, but some are heterozygous, which tends to be associated with early-onset chilblain lupus, a cold-induced severe discoloration of hands, feet, and ears, where the lesions frequently ulcerate.[33,41,42]

TREX1 and systemic lupus erythematosus Frameshift changes in the c-terminus coding region of TREX1 gene may interfere with exonuclease activity, subcellular localization, or interaction of TREX1 with other proteins.[43] A subject with SLE and central nervous system (CNS) disease with features of severe Raynaud phenomenon was shown to have a novel heterozygous variant (p.Arg128His) in the TREX1 gene.[44] This variant was not seen in more than 1700 healthy controls. Another study, of a cSLE subject with disease onset at age 4 years and CNS involvement, demonstrated a different TREX1 coding variant, p.Arg97His that was associated with a 20-fold reduction in enzyme activity and elevated ISGs.[45] A very large multiethnic study of SLE subjects showed that nonsynonymous TREX1 variants were present in approximately 0.5% of subjects across all ethnicities, although the specific sequence variants differed across ethnicities. One Asian subject with a young age of onset SLE had a homozygous (p.Arg114His) variant. This variant is the most common TREX1 variant associated with AGS. This subject did not have an AGS phenotype.[46] Therefore, it seems that TREX1 variants are implicated in the pathogenesis of SLE in a small number of patients both with and without neurologic involvement.

IFIH1 and MDA5

The human IFIH1 gene consists of 16 exons and is localized on chromosome 2q24. It encodes the 1025 amino acid MDA5 protein.[47] Disease-causing sequence variants in IFIH1 are seen in less than 5% of patients with AGS. Heterozygous variants in IFIH1 leading gain of function in MDA5 are seen in AGS and nonsyndromic spastic paraparesis.[48] Singleton-Merton syndrome, characterized by aortic calcification, delayed dentition with early loss of permanent teeth, osteopenia, acro-osteolysis, psoriasis, and glaucoma, is also due to variants in IFIH1 and elevated ISGs.

In mice, a gain of function mutation in MDA5 gene leads to a lupus-like syndrome with activated dendritic cells and macrophages. These cells produce IFN-1, which then leads to the activation T cells and plasma cells and the production of autoantibodies. These mice have glomerulonephritis with immune deposition and a skin rash.[49] The mutant protein lacks responsiveness to dsRNA but has constitutive activity.

It was initially shown that the IFIH1 rs1990760 coding change variant (p.Ala946Thr) was associated with an increased risk of SLE and these subjects had increased sensitivity to IFN signaling.[50] This led to more intensive investigation of this gene and it was shown that a sequence variant in the IFIH1 gene that resulted in a gain of function in MDA5 was associated with early-onset SLE. Serum IFN-1 levels were elevated and IFIHI gene expression in peripheral blood mononuclear cells (PBMCs) was markedly elevated. This variant is also seen in patients with AGS, suggesting that there may be modifying genes leading to different phenotypes.[51] Young-onset SLE with AGS-like disease was described in a 3-year-old with a heterozygous sequence variant (c1483G > A; p Gly495Arg) in IFIH1 who had been diagnosed with hereditary spastic paralysis (the patient's father had spastic paralysis and high ISGs) and then developed neuromyelitis optica with anti-aquaporin4 antibodies, positive ANA, and anti-dsDNA antibodies.[52] Two patients with heterozygous variants in IFIH and AGS, had immunologic abnormalities consist with SLE.[53] Examining a separate autoimmune disease, it is interesting that a subpopulation of patients with amyopathic dermatomyositis have anti-MDA5 antibodies.[54] However, the role these antibodies have in amyopathic dermatomyositis is not clear. A family has been described in which all 3 affected family members had severe, early-onset chilblains with associated elevated IFN-1 levels, and a c1465G > A; p.Ala489Thr sequence variant in the IFIH1 gene. Clinical features were (1) proband, malar rash and neurologically normal with a skin biopsy consistent with FCL or cutaneous lupus; (2) sibling, neurologic involvement, abnormal MRI, and glaucoma; and (3) father, photosensitivity and deforming.[48]

SAMHD1

SAMHD1 is a triphosphohydrolase that is important in cell-cycle progression and cell proliferation. It acts by controlling the intracellular level of deoxynucleoside triphosphates (dNTPs). It helps regulate retroviruses (thought to be important in controlling human immunodeficiency virus [HIV] infection) and DNA viruses requiring dNTPs. It is important in sensing of self-dsDNA but also binds to ssRNA and ssDNA.[55,56] SAMDH1-deficient mice have elevated ISGs but without evidence of autoimmune disease.[57] Truncating variants in SAMDH1 lead to its accumulation in the cytosol rather than in the nucleus where the unmutated protein resides.[58] SAMHD1 disease-causing variants are present in approximately 13% of AGS patients. One patient with a SAMHD1 variant met ACR classification criteria for SLE and 1 patient had FCL.[33,59]

RNaseH2

RNaseH2 is a ribonuclease complex expressed in all cells that function to degrade RNA:DNA hybrid complexes and is important in ribonucleotide excision repair.[60]

Each subunit is encoded by a RNASEH2 gene. Insights into the mechanism of mutant RNaseH2's signaling were hindered because RNASEH2 knockout ($^{-/-}$) mice have a lethal phenotype. However, with the development of an RnaseH2bA174T$^{(+/+)}$ knock-in mouse, it was shown that RNaseH2 works by RNA sensing and through cGAS/STING signaling with tissue-specific ISG upregulation.[60]

Approximately one-third of AGS patients with RNASEH2 variants had a positive ANA.[61] Sequencing of RNASEH2 (A, B, C) genes in 600 SLE subjects identified 18 rare variants in all 3 of the subunits (splice and nonsynonymous changes). The odds ratio for SLE was 2.0 and, clinically, these tended to have mild SLE without major organ involvement. Further examination of these RNASEH2 variants showed that 17 out of 18 resulted in impaired enzyme activity, altered stability of the complex, or altered subcellular localization. Subjects with RNASEH2 variants that severely altered RNaseH2 function had a 3.8-fold increased risk of SLE.[61] The sister of a child with AGS was noted to have severe chilblains of her fingers and toes beginning at age 2 years, arthralgias, and elevated anti-dsDNA antibodies but was neurologically normal with only mild MRI abnormalities and no calcifications. Both children had the same homozygous variant of the RNASEH2 gene. Both parents, heterozygous carriers, had weakly positive ANAs and anti-dsDNA antibodies but not chilblains. These cases demonstrate the variable phenotype associated with RNASEH variants ranging from typical AGS and no autoimmune features to chilblain lupus.[62]

ADAR1 (adenosine deaminase acting on RNA1)

As previously described, dsRNA in the cytoplasm can bind and activate the RNA sensor (RIG-I-like) proteins that can distinguish host from viral or pathogenic RNA.[63] ADAR1 enzyme is encoded by the ADAR1 gene on chromosome 1q21.1 and functions as an RNA-editing enzyme by deaminating dsRNA and altering its structure. It, therefore, can prevent dsRNA activation of the MDA5 pathway by acting as a negative regulator of MDA5 signaling and thereby can control IFN-1 and ISGs production (see **Fig. 2**).[64]

The ADAR1 knockout ($^{-/-}$) mouse has a lethal phenotype. The prevention of embryonic death in ADAR1 $^{-/-}$ mice by crossing with other mutant mouse strains demonstrated that ADAR1 defects result in impaired RNA editing, leading to production of ISGs.[63] These studies showed that ADAR1 works by degrading endogenous dsRNA and thereby prevents the activation of the MDA5 pathway and prevents autoimmunity.[65,66] ADAR1 is important for early fetal development and this may explain why documented ADAR1 sequence variants in humans are all heterozygous.[64] Nine different heterozygous variants in the ADAR1 gene have been described in AGS subjects.[67] A review of 28 subjects with ADAR1 variants and AGS found that 7/28 (25%) had features of an autoimmune disease: 2 met SLE criteria, 2 hypothyroidism, 1 isolated chilblains, 1 autoimmune gastritis, and 1 demyelinating peripheral neuropathy.[40]

Familial Chilblain Lupus (FCL)

Chilblain lesions are commonly seen in patients with AGS. FCL is an autosomal dominant form of SLE caused by variants in the TREX1 gene; c.52G > A of TREX1 leading to p.Asp18Asn is the most common missense variant, although other variants have been described.[68–70] The lesions usually start in early childhood and patients generally do not have an AGS phenotype. However, a family has been described in which the proband had severe chilblains and developmental delay with calcification of basal ganglia on CT scan, and 2 other family members with the same variant had chilblains only without neurologic or CT abnormalities.[70] Skin biopsies of patients with FCL are consistent with SLE, showing vacuolar degeneration of basal keratinocytes, a perivascular lymphocytic infiltrate with mucin deposition, and the deposition of complement and immunoglobulin in immunofluorescent studies.[71,72] IFN-1 is upregulated in FCL. FCL patients frequently have positive ANAs; arthritis; hematologic abnormalities; and, less commonly, specific autoantibodies. The direct effect of the p.Asp18Asn-TREX1 variant was tested in mice by replacing the wildtype TREX1 gene with TREX1 p.Asp18Asn allele. Homozygous TREX1 p.Asp18Asn had systemic inflammation, lymphadenopathy, vasculitis, and immune complex renal disease, as well as high titer anti-dsDNA antibodies.[69]

One family with FCL with early-onset chilblain lesions, photosensitivity, and skin biopsy consistent with SLE had a heterozygous at T > A transversion at c602 in the fifth exon of the SAMDH1 gene, resulting in a p.Arg201 Ile. A homozygous variant at this position in SAMDH1 gene is seen in some patients with AGS.[59] A RNASEH2 disease-causing variant has also been seen in FCL.[62]

Stimulator of Interferon Genes (STING) and Stimulator of Interferon Gene –Associated Vasculopathy with Onset in Infancy (SAVI)

The TMEM173 gene, chromosome 5q31.2, encodes STING (also called MITA, ERIS, MPYS), a 348 amino acid transmembrane protein that is present on the ER as a dimer. STING has an essential role as a sensor of cyclic dinucleotides (CDNs) and dsDNA in the cytosol leading to the production of IFN, and is present on multiple immune cells, including macrophages and dendritic cells (see **Fig. 1**).[73,74]

STING-associated vasculopathy with onset in infancy (SAVI) is an autoimmune or autoinflammatory disease caused by gain of function variants in the TMEM173, leading to constitutive activation of the STING-IFN-1 pathway.[75,76] STING normally resides in the cytosol and then, on activation, translocates to the Golgi and perinuclear punctate vesicles. However, a mutated STING protein, present in a subject with SAVI, was found to be localized mainly to the Golgi and in perinuclear punctiform vesicles, where it resided in an activated state leading to IFN-1 production.[76] This same variant and 2 different sequence changes nearby were reported in other subjects with SAVI, with all these subjects having elevated ISGs.[75]

The initial description of SAVI reported on 6 children (3 boys, 3 girls) who all developed symptoms between the age 2 to 6 weeks with rashes that progressed over time. All patients had a maculopapular, pustular, or blistering rash in the malar distribution associated with telangiectasia, as well as rashes on fingers, toes, and soles. Skin biopsy showed vasculitis limited to the capillaries characterized by a neutrophilic infiltrate and karyorrhexis with fibrin deposition. All subjects developed acral plaques and distal ulcers and lesions similar to chilblains as the lesions became worse in cold weather. Similar to subjects with AGS, lesions on the ears were also seen. All subjects developed paratracheal adenopathy and 5 had evidence of interstitial lung disease on CT scan. Two subjects developed an inflammatory myositis and 1 developed a rheumatoid factor (RF)-positive erosive arthritis. There was evidence of systemic inflammation with elevated acute phase reactants in all, and 5 had recurrent low-grade fever during flares. Low-titer ANAs were present in 50%, antiphospholipid antibodies in 5 out of 6, and c-ANCA in 1 subject.[75]

A second family with 4 members with SAVI was subsequently described. The proband presented at age 2 with fevers, malar rash, lung disease, failure to thrive, and elevated IFN-1 levels. Her father and uncle (monozygotic twins) had malar rash, alopecia, lung disease, polyarthritis, and recurrent fevers with onset as teenagers. They all had an elevated erythrocyte sedimentation rate (ESR) and C-reactive protein (CRP), higher titer ANAs, and RF, whereas the proband only had low titer anti-dsDNA antibodies (other autoantibodies not commented on). All 3 had a gain of STING function variant in TMEM173.[76] The founder variant was in the grandfather who had an elevated ESR and CRP with a positive RF but no other autoantibodies, and only arthralgia with chronically low weight. This same variant was seen in 1 of the subjects in the initial report.[75] The most recent report of SAVI described 5 family members over 4 generations who developed chilblain lesions on fingers, toes, nose, and ears between 2 months and 12 years of age. There was no internal organ involvement or evidence of systemic inflammation. ANA was positive in 4 out of 5, 1 had anti-C1q antibodies, and all had elevated ISGs. TMEM173 gene sequencing showed a heterozygous variant in the dimerization domain of STING, leading to gain of function.[77] This is the same domain but at a different location where disease-causing variants in SAVI subjects were described.[75,76] The results of these studies show significant autoimmunity in patients with SAVI.

In a murine model of SLE, abnormal STING signaling in dendritic cells can alter CD4+ follicular T-cell development, activate B-cells and plasma cells, and lead to anti-dsDNA antibody production, showing how STING signaling leads to autoimmunity.[78] cGAS gene expression was elevated in PBMCs of approximately 50% of SLE subjects, as was the product of its enzymatic activity, cGAMP, although in a lower proportion of subjects, demonstrating that this pathway is abnormally activated in some SLE patients.[79]

BREAKING TOLERANCE: DISEASE-CAUSING VARIANTS IN DNA ENDONUCLEASES
DNases

Serum endonucleases play an important function for maintenance of tolerance by recognizing and degrading DNA and chromatin produced by dead cells undergoing apoptosis, NETosis, or necrosis. A second function is the recognition and clearance of DNA from foreign pathogens. DNase1, encoded by the DNASE1 gene, is the major endonuclease, present in serum and urine, capable of cleaving both ssDNA and dsDNA. Both serum and urine DNase1 activity are lower in NZB/NZWF1 than in control mice and low DNase1 activity has been shown to be present in the serum of SLE subjects. This suggests that low DNase1 activity may be important in SLE by failing to degrade self-dsDNA, allowing it to stimulate dsDNA-specific B cells.[80,81] The protective effect of DNase1 is best demonstrated in the DNase1 knockout ($^{-/-}$) mice, which produced ANAs, anti-ssDNA antibodies, and anti-nucleosome antibodies. These mice developed an immune complex glomerulonephritis. Of note, female mice more commonly had autoantibodies and developed a glomerulonephritis than male mice, recapitulating human disease.[81]

DNASE1

In humans, to date, only 2 siblings with onset of SLE at ages 13 and 17 years were identified with variants in the DNASE1 gene. They both had heterozygous c.A > G172 transversion in exon 2 of DNASE1 gene that resulted in a truncated 5 amino acid rather than 282 amino acid protein with poor DNase1 function. They had significantly higher antinucleosome antibodies than other SLE patients, suggesting that the production of antinucleosome antibodies was driven by the poor clearance of self-dsDNA.[82]

DNases 1L3

DNase1L3 functions as an endonuclease capable of cleaving both ssDNA and dsDNA. DNases1L3 is generally present in the cytoplasm but can translocate to the nucleus to cleave DNA during apoptosis or necrosis. Important to autoimmunity, it is secreted by macrophages and dendritic cells and is present in liver cells.[83–85] Both MLR/lpr and NZB/W mice have a c438 C > T (p. Thr89Ile) mutation in DNASE1L3 gene that is presumed to alter the ability of these mice to detect and degrade apoptotic bodies.[86] A recently developed DNase1L3 knockout ($^{-/-}$) mouse rapidly developed anti-dsDNA and anti-chromatin antibodies. However, the onset of an SLE-like disease was delayed.[83] These studies suggested that the major function of DNase1L3 was to degrade DNA, generated by apoptosis, necrosis, or NETosis, from contacting potentially autoreactive DNA-specific B cells. Therefore, alterations of DNase1L3 structure or function can lead to autoimmunity (**Fig. 3**).

Defective DNase1L3 function has been shown to be present in 2 groups of subjects with autoimmunity: (1) hypocomplementemic urticarial vasculitis (HUVS) and (2) young-onset SLE.

Hypocomplementemic urticarial vasculitis

HUVS is a clinical syndrome characterized by recurrent or persistent urticarial with evidence of serum hypocomplementemia. Lesional biopsies show evidence of leukocytoclastic vasculitis. Many of these patients have other clinical features of SLE, including malar rash, photosensitivity, glomerulonephritis as seen in SLE, Raynaud phenomenon, arthritis, and multiple autoantibodies.[87] Angioedema and episcleritis or conjunctivitis, features not commonly seen in patients with SLE, are commonly seen in HUVS patients.[88] Of particular interest is that many of the patients with HUVS and SLE had young-onset SLE and multiplex families with HUVS and SLE features have been described.[89] This raised the possibility that at least some cases of HUVS with SLE

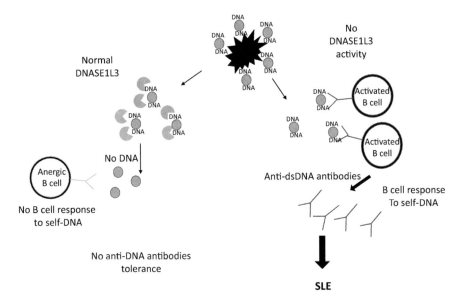

Fig. 3. How abnormal DNase1L3 activity leads to autoimmunity. During cell death, nuclear dsDNA will attach to microparticles and then be released into the surrounding area. The left side of the figure demonstrates normal tolerance. In the presence of normal DNas1L3, the endonucleases will digest DNA from the microparticle and, therefore, potentially self-reactive B-cells remain in anergic state and do not produce anti-dsDNA antibodies. The right side of the figure shows how SLE can develop when DNase1L3 is abnormal. Now circulating B-cells can contact dsDNA on microparticles and normal tolerance is broken with the production of anti-dsDNA antibodies and SLE.

may be a monogenic disease. However, it was not until 2013 that disease-causing variants in DNase1L3 gene were detected in 2 separate multiplex families. One family with 3 affected children had a frameshift variant, c.289_290delAC (p.Thr97 Ilefs*2), leading to a truncated protein. In the other family, there were 2 affected members who had a homozygous DNase1L3 4 base-pair deletion (c.320+4delAGTA), leading to exon skipping. Both deletion variants were associated with loss of DNase1L3 function.[90] In 2016, a third multiplex family with varying phenotype was described with the same DNase1L3 c.289_290delAC (p.Thr97 Ilefs*2).[90] The proband had SLE with HUVS, his mother (homozygous for the deletion) had renal failure with hypocomplementemia, a deceased (unrelated causes) sibling had juvenile idiopathic arthritis, and another homozygous sibling had rheumatoid arthritis with a malar rash. The parents were consanguineous and the well father was a heterozygous carrier.[91]

Before the demonstration that young-onset HUVS with SLE can be the result of variants in the DNase1L3 gene, 7 different multiplex consanguineous families with young-onset SLE were shown to have the same deletion in the DNase1L3 gene (c.643delT; p.Trp215GlyfsX2). Clinically, the subjects had nephritis with hypocomplementemia and the presence of ANAs and anti-DNA antibodies. Unusual features in the cohort were the male predominance (11 out of 18 patients) and the young-onset of symptoms (all <12 years of age, with onset in most <5 years of age).[92]

SUMMARY

The study of monogenic forms of SLE provides insights into the mechanisms leading to autoimmunity and SLE. Different single-gene defects can lead to common inflammatory pathways, resulting in autoimmunity and SLE. The main pathways in which these genes are involved are reviewed (see **Table 1**) and some of the key, distinguishing, associated clinical and laboratory features identified.

Abnormalities of the early complement components (C1q complex, C2 and C4) lead to the development of autoimmunity with or without an associated immune deficiency. These patients tend to have severe skin disease, young onset (except for C2 deficiency), and anti-Ro antibodies with equal male to female ratio. Deficiencies of each of the C1q complex proteins (C1q, C1r, and C1s) have the common features of severe early-onset, skin disease with photosensitivity that is difficult to treat, and the production of multiple autoantibodies, in particular anti-Ro antibodies. The most common deficiency is C1q.

To date, several single gene variants resulting in abnormal regulation and activation of sensing pathways of dsDNA or dsRNA within the cytosol can lead to abnormal IFN-1 production with subsequent autoimmunity and the production of autoantibodies. The implicated genes encode proteins involved in DNA or RNA sensing, endonuclease, and exonuclease activity. Despite the common end result of abnormal IFN-1 and ISGs production, the clinical phenotype differ between and within the same pathways. The studies of DNASE1L3 variants demonstrate that tolerance to self-DNA can be broken by a single gene variant in enzymes that fail to clear extracellular DNA produced by apoptosis, necrosis, or NETosis. Much work still needs to be done to discover defects in new pathways and genes that lead to autoimmunity and SLE.

REFERENCES

1. Alarcon-Segovia D, Alarcon-Riquelme ME, Cardiel MH, et al. Familial aggregation of systemic lupus erythematosus, rheumatoid arthritis, and other autoimmune diseases in 1,177 lupus patients from the GLADEL cohort. Arthritis Rheum 2005; 52(4):1138–47.

2. Deapen D, Escalante A, Weinrib L, et al. A revised estimate of twin concordance in systemic lupus erythematosus. Arthritis Rheum 1992;35(3):311–8.

3. Block SR, Winfield JB, Lockshin MD, et al. Studies of twins with systemic lupus erythematosus. A review of the literature and presentation of 12 additional sets. Am J Med 1975;59(4):533–52.

4. Bentham J, Morris DL, Cunninghame Graham DS, et al. Genetic association analyses implicate aberrant regulation of innate and adaptive immunity genes in the pathogenesis of systemic lupus erythematosus. Nat Genet 2015;47(12):1457–64.

5. Morris DL, Sheng Y, Zhang Y, et al. Genome-wide association meta-analysis in Chinese and European individuals identifies ten new loci associated with systemic lupus erythematosus. Nat Genet 2016;48(8):940–6.

6. Webb R, Kelly JA, Somers EC, et al. Early disease onset is predicted by a higher genetic risk for lupus and is associated with a more severe phenotype in lupus patients. Ann Rheum Dis 2011;70(1):151–6.

7. Li YR, Zhao SD, Li J, et al. Genetic sharing and heritability of paediatric age of onset autoimmune diseases. Nat Commun 2015;6:8442.

8. Ghodke-Puranik Y, Niewold TB. Immunogenetics of systemic lupus erythematosus: a comprehensive review. J Autoimmun 2015;64:125–36.

9. Prodeus AP, Goerg S, Shen LM, et al. A critical role for complement in maintenance of self-tolerance. Immunity 1998;9(5):721–31.

10. Lood C, Gullstrand B, Truedsson L, et al. C1q inhibits immune complex-induced interferon-alpha production in plasmacytoid dendritic cells: a novel link between C1q deficiency and systemic lupus erythematosus pathogenesis. Arthritis Rheum 2009;60(10):3081–90.

11. Botto M, Dell'Agnola C, Bygrave AE, et al. Homozygous C1q deficiency causes glomerulonephritis associated with multiple apoptotic bodies. Nat Genet 1998; 19(1):56–9.

12. Berkel AI, Loos M, Sanal O, et al. Clinical and immunological studies in a case of selective complete C1q deficiency. Clin Exp Immunol 1979;38(1):52–63.

13. Hannema AJ, Kluin-Nelemans JC, Hack CE, et al. SLE like syndrome and functional deficiency of C1q in members of a large family. Clin Exp Immunol 1984; 55(1):106–14.

14. Lintner KE, Wu YL, Yang Y, et al. Early components of the complement classical activation pathway in human systemic autoimmune diseases. Front Immunol 2016;7:36.

15. Leffler J, Bengtsson AA, Blom AM. The complement system in systemic lupus erythematosus: an update. Ann Rheum Dis 2014;73(9):1601–6.

16. Mehta P, Norsworthy PJ, Hall AE, et al. SLE with C1q deficiency treated with fresh frozen plasma: a 10-year experience. Rheumatology (Oxford) 2010;49(4):823–4.

17. Arkwright PD, Riley P, Hughes SM, et al. Successful cure of C1q deficiency in human subjects treated with hematopoietic stem cell transplantation. J Allergy Clin Immunol 2014;133(1):265–7.

18. Higuchi Y, Shimizu J, Hatanaka M, et al. The identification of a novel splicing mutation in C1qB in a Japanese family with C1q deficiency: a case report. Pediatr Rheumatol Online J 2013;11(1):41.

19. Stone NM, Williams A, Wilkinson JD, et al. Systemic lupus erythematosus with C1q deficiency. Br J Dermatol 2000;142(3):521–4.

20. Bowness P, Davies KA, Norsworthy PJ, et al. Hereditary C1q deficiency and systemic lupus erythematosus. QJM 1994;87(8):455–64.

21. Topaloglu R, Bakkaloglu A, Slingsby JH, et al. Molecular basis of hereditary C1q deficiency associated with SLE and IgA nephropathy in a Turkish family. Kidney Int 1996;50(2):635–42.

22. Radanova M, Vasilev V, Dimitrov T, et al. Association of rs172378 C1q gene cluster polymorphism with lupus nephritis in Bulgarian patients. Lupus 2015;24(3): 280–9.

23. Wu YL, Brookshire BP, Verani RR, et al. Clinical presentations and molecular basis of complement C1r deficiency in a male African-American patient with systemic lupus erythematosus. Lupus 2011;20(11):1126–34.

24. Paul E, Pozdnyakova OO, Mitchell E, et al. Anti-DNA autoreactivity in C4-deficient mice. Eur J Immunol 2002;32(9):2672–9.

25. Yang Y, Chung EK, Wu YL, et al. Gene copy-number variation and associated polymorphisms of complement component C4 in human systemic lupus erythematosus (SLE): low copy number is a risk factor for and high copy number is a protective factor against SLE susceptibility in European Americans. Am J Hum Genet 2007;80(6):1037–54.

26. Yih Chen J, Ling Wu Y, Yin Mok M, et al. Effects of complement C4 gene copy number variations, size dichotomy, and C4A deficiency on genetic risk and clinical presentation of systemic lupus erythematosus in East Asian populations. Arthritis Rheumatol 2016;68(6):1442–53.

27. Pereira KM, Faria AG, Liphaus BL, et al. Low C4, C4A and C4B gene copy numbers are stronger risk factors for juvenile-onset than for adult-onset systemic lupus erythematosus. Rheumatology (Oxford) 2016;55(5):869–73.

28. Miller EC, Atkinson JP. Overcoming C2 deficiency. Clin Immunol 2012;144(3): 269–71.

29. Jonsson G, Sjoholm AG, Truedsson L, et al. Rheumatological manifestations, organ damage and autoimmunity in hereditary C2 deficiency. Rheumatology (Oxford) 2007;46(7):1133–9.

30. Zhu ZB, Atkinson TP, Volanakis JE. A novel type II complement C2 deficiency allele in an African-American family. J Immunol 1998;161(2):578–84.

31. Hauck F, Lee-kirsch MA, Aust D, et al. Complement C2 deficiency disarranging innate and adaptive humoral immune responses in a pediatric patient: treatment with rituximab. Arthritis Care Res (Hoboken) 2011;63(3):454–9.

32. Macedo AC, Isaac L. Systemic lupus erythematosus and deficiencies of early components of the complement classical pathway. Front Immunol 2016;7:55.

33. Ramantani G, Kohlhase J, Hertzberg C, et al. Expanding the phenotypic spectrum of lupus erythematosus in Aicardi-Goutières syndrome. Arthritis Rheum 2010;62(5):1469–77.

34. Rice GI, Rodero MP, Crow YJ. Human disease phenotypes associated with mutations in TREX1. J Clin Immunol 2015;35(3):235–43.

35. Rice GI, Forte GM, Szynkiewicz M, et al. Assessment of interferon-related biomarkers in Aicardi-Goutières syndrome associated with mutations in TREX1, RNASEH2A, RNASEH2B, RNASEH2C, SAMHD1, and ADAR: a case-control study. Lancet Neurol 2013;12(12):1159–69.

36. Cuadrado E, Vanderver A, Brown KJ, et al. Aicardi-Goutières syndrome harbours abundant systemic and brain-reactive autoantibodies. Ann Rheum Dis 2015; 74(10):1931–9.

37. Stetson DB, Ko JS, Heidmann T, et al. Trex1 prevents cell-intrinsic initiation of autoimmunity. Cell 2008;134(4):587–98.

38. Pereira-Lopes S, Celhar T, Sans-Fons G, et al. The exonuclease Trex1 restrains macrophage proinflammatory activation. J Immunol 2013;191(12):6128–35.

39. Peschke K, Achleitner M, Frenzel K, et al. Loss of Trex1 in dendritic cells is sufficient to trigger systemic autoimmunity. J Immunol 2016;197(6):2157–66.

40. Crow YJ, Chase DS, Lowenstein Schmidt J, et al. Characterization of human disease phenotypes associated with mutations in TREX1, RNASEH2A, RNASEH2B, RNASEH2C, SAMHD1, ADAR, and IFIH1. Am J Med Genet A 2015;167A(2): 296–312.

41. Haaxma CA, Crow YJ, van Steensel MA, et al. A de novo p.Asp18Asn mutation in TREX1 in a patient with Aicardi-Goutieres syndrome. Am J Med Genet A 2010; 152a(10):2612–7.

42. Rice G, Patrick T, Parmar R, et al. Clinical and molecular phenotype of Aicardi-Goutieres syndrome. Am J Hum Genet 2007;81(4):713–25.

43. Lee-Kirsch MA, Gong M, Chowdhury D, et al. Mutations in the gene encoding the 3′-5′ DNA exonuclease TREX1 are associated with systemic lupus erythematosus. Nat Genet 2007;39(9):1065–7.

44. de Vries B, Steup-Beekman GM, Haan J, et al. TREX1 gene variant in neuropsychiatric systemic lupus erythematosus. Ann Rheum Dis 2010;69(10):1886–7.

45. Ellyard JI, Jerjen R, Martin JL, et al. Identification of a pathogenic variant in TREX1 in early-onset cerebral systemic lupus erythematosus by Whole-exome sequencing. Arthritis Rheumatol 2014;66(12):3382–6.

46. Namjou B, Kothari PH, Kelly JA, et al. Evaluation of the TREX1 gene in a large multi-ancestral lupus cohort. Genes Immun 2011;12(4):270–9.

47. Buers I, Nitschke Y, Rutsch F. Novel interferonopathies associated with mutations in RIG-I like receptors. Cytokine Growth Factor Rev 2016;29:101–7.

48. Bursztejn AC, Briggs TA, del Toro Duany Y, et al. Unusual cutaneous features associated with a heterozygous gain-of-function mutation in IFIH1: overlap between Aicardi-Goutières and Singleton-Merten syndromes. Br J Dermatol 2015; 173(6):1505–13.

49. Funabiki M, Kato H, Miyachi Y, et al. Autoimmune disorders associated with gain of function of the intracellular sensor MDA5. Immunity 2014;40(2):199–212.

50. Robinson T, Kariuki SN, Franek BS, et al. Autoimmune disease risk variant of IFIH1 is associated with increased sensitivity to IFN-{alpha} and serologic autoimmunity in lupus patients. J Immunol 2011;187(3):1298–303.

51. Van Eyck L, De Somer L, Pombal D, et al. Brief report: IFIH1 mutation causes systemic lupus erythematosus with selective IgA deficiency. Arthritis Rheumatol 2015;67(6):1592–7.

52. Hacohen Y, Zuberi S, Vincent A, et al. Neuromyelitis optica in a child with Aicardi-Goutières syndrome. Neurology 2015;85(4):381–3.

53. Rice GI, del Toro Duany Y, Jenkinson EM, et al. Gain-of-function mutations in IFIH1 cause a spectrum of human disease phenotypes associated with upregulated type I interferon signaling. Nat Genet 2014;46(5):503–9.

54. Sato S, Hoshino K, Satoh T, et al. RNA helicase encoded by melanoma differentiation-associated gene 5 is a major autoantigen in patients with clinically amyopathic dermatomyositis: association with rapidly progressive interstitial lung disease. Arthritis Rheum 2009;60(7):2193–200.

55. Tungler V, Staroske W, Kind B, et al. Single-stranded nucleic acids promote SAMHD1 complex formation. J Mol Med (Berl) 2013;91(6):759–70.

56. Ballana E, Este JA. SAMHD1: at the crossroads of cell proliferation, immune responses, and virus restriction. Trends Microbiol 2015;23(11):680–92.

57. Rehwinkel J, Maelfait J, Bridgeman A, et al. SAMHD1-dependent retroviral control and escape in mice. EMBO J 2013;32(18):2454–62.

58. Goncalves A, Karayel E, Rice GI, et al. SAMHD1 is a nucleic-acid binding protein that is mislocalized due to Aicardi-Goutières syndrome-associated mutations. Hum Mutat 2012;33(7):1116–22.

59. Ravenscroft JC, Suri M, Rice GI, et al. Autosomal dominant inheritance of a heterozygous mutation in SAMHD1 causing familial chilblain lupus. Am J Med Genet A 2011;155A(1):235–7.

60. Mackenzie KJ, Carroll P, Lettice L, et al. Ribonuclease H2 mutations induce a cGAS/STING-dependent innate immune response. EMBO J 2016;35(8):831–44.

61. Gunther C, Kind B, Reijns MA, et al. Defective removal of ribonucleotides from DNA promotes systemic autoimmunity. J Clin Invest 2015;125(1):413–24.

62. Vogt J, Agrawal S, Ibrahim Z, et al. Striking intrafamilial phenotypic variability in Aicardi-Goutières syndrome associated with the recurrent Asian founder mutation in RNASEH2C. Am J Med Genet A 2013;161a(2):338–42.

63. Mannion NM, Greenwood SM, Young R, et al. The RNA-editing enzyme ADAR1 controls innate immune responses to RNA. Cell Rep 2014;9(4):1482–94.

64. Pestal K, Funk CC, Snyder JM, et al. Isoforms of RNA-editing enzyme ADAR1 independently control nucleic acid sensor MDA5-driven autoimmunity and multi-organ development. Immunity 2015;43(5):933–44.

65. Liddicoat BJ, Piskol R, Chalk AM, et al. RNA editing by ADAR1 prevents MDA5 sensing of endogenous dsRNA as nonself. Science 2015;349(6252):1115–20.

66. Heraud-Farlow JE, Walkley CR. The role of RNA editing by ADAR1 in prevention of innate immune sensing of self-RNA. J Mol Med (Berl) 2016;94(10):1095–102.

67. Rice GI, Kasher PR, Forte GM, et al. Mutations in ADAR1 cause Aicardi-Goutières syndrome associated with a type I interferon signature. Nat Genet 2012;44(11):1243–8.

68. Gunther C, Berndt N, Wolf C, et al. Familial chilblain lupus due to a novel mutation in the exonuclease III domain of 3' repair exonuclease 1 (TREX1). JAMA Dermatol 2015;151(4):426–31.

69. Grieves JL, Fye JM, Harvey S, et al. Exonuclease TREX1 degrades double-stranded DNA to prevent spontaneous lupus-like inflammatory disease. Proc Natl Acad Sci U S A 2015;112(16):5117–22.

70. Abe J, Izawa K, Nishikomori R, et al. Heterozygous TREX1 p.Asp18Asn mutation can cause variable neurological symptoms in a family with Aicardi-Goutieres syndrome/familial chilblain lupus. Rheumatology (Oxford) 2013;52(2):406–8.

71. Sugiura K, Takeichi T, Kono M, et al. Severe chilblain lupus is associated with heterozygous missense mutations of catalytic amino acids or their adjacent mutations in the exonuclease domains of 3'-repair exonuclease 1. J Invest Dermatol 2012;132(12):2855–7.

72. Gunther C, Meurer M, Stein A, et al. Familial chilblain lupus–a monogenic form of cutaneous lupus erythematosus due to a heterozygous mutation in TREX1. Dermatology 2009;219(2):162–6.

73. Ahn J, Barber GN. Self-DNA, STING-dependent signaling and the origins of auto-inflammatory disease. Curr Opin Immunol 2014;31:121–6.

74. Burdette DL, Monroe KM, Sotelo-Troha K, et al. STING is a direct innate immune sensor of cyclic di-GMP. Nature 2011;478(7370):515–8.

75. Liu Y, Jesus AA, Marrero B, et al. Activated STING in a vascular and pulmonary syndrome. N Engl J Med 2014;371(6):507–18.

76. Jeremiah N, Neven B, Gentili M, et al. Inherited STING-activating mutation underlies a familial inflammatory syndrome with lupus-like manifestations. J Clin Invest 2014;124(12):5516–20.

77. Konig N, Fiehn C, Wolf C, et al. Familial chilblain lupus due to a gain-of-function mutation in STING. Ann Rheum Dis 2017;76(2):468–72.
78. Klarquist J, Hennies CM, Lehn MA, et al. STING-mediated DNA sensing promotes antitumor and autoimmune responses to dying cells. J Immunol 2014; 193(12):6124–34.
79. An J, Durcan L, Karr RM, et al. Expression of cyclic GMP-AMP synthase in patients with systemic lupus erythematosus. Arthritis Rheumatol 2017;69(4):800–7.
80. Macanovic M, Lachmann PJ. Measurement of deoxyribonuclease I (DNase) in the serum and urine of systemic lupus erythematosus (SLE)-prone NZB/NZW mice by a new radial enzyme diffusion assay. Clin Exp Immunol 1997;108(2): 220–6.
81. Napirei M, Karsunky H, Zevnik B, et al. Features of systemic lupus erythematosus in Dnase1-deficient mice. Nat Genet 2000;25(2):177–81.
82. Yasutomo K, Horiuchi T, Kagami S, et al. Mutation of DNASE1 in people with systemic lupus erythematosus. Nat Genet 2001;28(4):313–4.
83. Sisirak V, Sally B, D'Agati V, et al. Digestion of chromatin in apoptotic cell microparticles prevents autoimmunity. Cell 2016;166(1):88–101.
84. Koyama R, Arai T, Kijima M, et al. DNase gamma, DNase I and caspase-activated DNase cooperate to degrade dead cells. Genes Cells 2016;21(11):1150–63.
85. Shiokawa D, Tanuma S. Characterization of human DNase I family endonucleases and activation of DNase gamma during apoptosis. Biochemistry 2001;40(1): 143–52.
86. Wilber A, O'Connor TP, Lu ML, et al. Dnase1l3 deficiency in lupus-prone MRL and NZB/W F1 mice. Clin Exp Immunol 2003;134(1):46–52.
87. Yamazaki-Nakashimada MA, Duran-McKinster C, Ramirez-Vargas N, et al. Intravenous immunoglobulin therapy for hypocomplementemic urticarial vasculitis associated with systemic lupus erythematosus in a child. Pediatr Dermatol 2009;26(4):445–7.
88. Her MY, Song JY, Kim DY. Hypocomplementemic urticarial vasculitis in systemic lupus erythematosus. J Korean Med Sci 2009;24(1):184–6.
89. Ozcakar ZB, Yalcinkaya F, Altugan FS, et al. Hypocomplementemic urticarial vasculitis syndrome in three siblings. Rheumatol Int 2013;33(3):763–6.
90. Ozcakar ZB, Foster J 2nd, Diaz-Horta O, et al. DNASE1L3 mutations in hypocomplementemic urticarial vasculitis syndrome. Arthritis Rheum 2013;65(8):2183–9.
91. Carbonella A, Mancano G, Gremese E, et al. An autosomal recessive DNASE1L3-related autoimmune disease with unusual clinical presentation mimicking systemic lupus erythematosus. Lupus 2017;26(7):768–72.
92. Al-Mayouf SM, Sunker A, Abdwani R, et al. Loss-of-function variant in DNASE1L3 causes a familial form of systemic lupus erythematosus. Nat Genet 2011;43(12): 1186–8.

Genetics of Juvenile Idiopathic Arthritis

 CrossMark

Aimee O. Hersh, MD[a], Sampath Prahalad, MD, MS[b,c,*]

KEYWORDS

- Juvenile idiopathic arthritis • Genetics • Association • Genomewide

KEY POINTS

- Juvenile idiopathic arthritis (JIA) is a complex heterogeneous phenotype with different clinical features, and genetic associations.
- Several variants underlying susceptibility to oligoarticular and rheumatoid factor (RF)-negative polyarticular JIA have been identified through genomewide association studies, including HLA, PTPN22, and STAT4 loci.
- Genomewide association studies of systemic onset JIA have identified that HLA DRB1:11 is strongly associated with it.

INTRODUCTION

Juvenile idiopathic arthritis (JIA) is among most common autoimmune or inflammatory conditions of childhood, affecting approximately 1 in 1000 children in the United States. The cause of JIA remains unknown but, as with most autoimmune conditions, it is thought to be multifactorial with a strong interplay between genetic susceptibility and environmental factors.

Over the last 2 decades, knowledge regarding the genetic basis of JIA has grown exponentially, highlighted by the publication of a genomewide association study (GWAS) in 2012 and an Immunochip study in 2013 that identified several new susceptibility loci for JIA.[1–4] This article summarizes results from the recent GWAS, which

Disclosure Statement: The authors have nothing to disclose.
Dr S. Prahalad is supported by The Marcus Foundation Inc. Dr A.O. Hersh is supported by a grant from the National Institutes of Arthritis and Musculoskeletal and Skin Diseases (NIAMS: K23-AR066064). The content is solely the responsibility of the authors and does not necessarily represent the official views of the NIAMS or the National Institutes of Health.
^a Pediatric Rheumatology, University of Utah School of Medicine, 81 Mario Capecchi Drive, 4th Floor, Salt Lake City, UT 84113, USA; ^b Department of Pediatrics, Children's Healthcare of Atlanta, Emory University School of Medicine, 1760 Haygood Drive Northeast, Atlanta, GA 30322, USA; ^c Department of Human Genetics, Children's Healthcare of Atlanta, Emory University School of Medicine, 1760 Haygood Drive Northeast, Atlanta, GA 30322, USA
* Corresponding author. Emory University School of Medicine, 1760 Haygood Drive Northeast, Atlanta, GA 30322.
E-mail address: sprahal@emory.edu

provide evidence for the genetic contribution to JIA, highlight several genetic loci that have been implicated in its pathogenesis, and summarize the literature regarding JIA pharmacogenomics.

GENETICS OF JUVENILE IDIOPATHIC ARTHRITIS

JIA has several categories, including oligoarticular (persistent or extended oligoarticular subcategories), rheumatoid factor (RF)-positive polyarthritis, RF-negative polyarthritis, enthesitis-related arthritis (ERA; usually associated with HLAB27 positivity), systemic onset, psoriatic, and undifferentiated JIA.[5] Extending from the clinical diversity, there also seem to be differences in genetics among the categories of JIA. For example, there are distinct shared polymorphisms between patients with oligoarticular and polyarticular seronegative JIA versus patients with systemic onset JIA. The genetics of JIA is also complicated by genetic differences due to ethnicity and gender. The clinical diversity of JIA contributes to the challenges noted with identifying genetic risk factors for this group of related conditions.

FAMILIAL AGGREGATION OF JUVENILE IDIOPATHIC ARTHRITIS

Despite the heterogeneity of JIA, there is a growing body of evidence of a genetic contribution to JIA, particularly based on findings from twin and affected sibling pair studies. The concordance rates for JIA among monozygotic twins ranges from 25% to 40%.[6] In studies of both twin and sibling pairs with JIA, the disease phenotypes were strikingly similar for onset and disease course.[7,8]

Some of the strongest evidence to suggest a genetic predisposition to JIA comes from familial studies, including the use of population databases to identify extended multiplex pedigrees with multiple affected individuals.[9,10] A study using the Utah Population Database identified 22 founders who had a higher than expected number of descendants with JIA. Siblings of probands with JIA had an 11.6-fold increase in the risk of JIA compared with the general population, whereas first cousins had a 5.6-fold risk. In a recent study using nationwide registries in Sweden, Frisell and colleagues[11] performed a case-control study designed to estimate the risk of arthritis among first-degree relatives of probands with seropositive or seronegative rheumatoid arthritis (RA). There was an almost 4-fold higher risk of developing JIA if the proband had seropositive RA (odds ratio [OR] 3.98 [3.01–5.26]). If they had seronegative RA, the OR was 5.70 (3.47–9.36). Taken together these studies suggest a familial link between RA and JIA.

There seems to be an increased prevalence of familial autoimmunity, such as autoimmune thyroid disease, among probands of patients with JIA.[12] Similarly, a recent study using the Childhood Arthritis and Rheumatology Research Alliance (CARRA) registry found that subjects with JIA and systemic lupus erythematosus (SLE) had a higher proportion of first-degree relatives with an autoimmune disease compared with subjects with juvenile dermatomyositis.[13]

GENOMEWIDE STUDIES OF JUVENILE IDIOPATHIC ARTHRITIS

For some complex traits, traditional linkage studies have been helpful in the identification of causative variants. However, to be successful, linkage studies require ascertainment of many families with multiple affected individuals. This has been a limitation for JIA in which multiply affected families are rarely described. Affected sibling pairs can be used for nonparametric linkage studies when large collections of multiplex families are unavailable for traditional genomewide linkage studies. The availability of a modest number of JIA-affected sibling pairs has led to nonparametric linkage studies. A genomewide linkage study involving 121 JIA-affected sibpair families suggested that genes in the HLA and other regions influence risk of JIA.[14] However, most results were not statistically significant, suggesting lack of statistical power to identify most of the causal variants despite using the largest collection of sibpairs at the time.

GWAS have resulted in the successful identification of genetic variants predisposing to susceptibility of several autoimmune diseases. The first GWAS in JIA was reported by Hinks and colleagues,[15] in 2009. The investigators performed a GWAS using a microarray with 100,000 single nucleotide polymorphism (SNP) markers. Not surprisingly, the strongest signal of association was in the HLA region. The next strongest signal or association was seen with an SNP in the VTCN1 gene. VTCN1 encodes the costimulatory molecule B7-H4. A US based genetic association study using 809 cases and 531 controls did not replicate the association between JIA and VTCN1 variants.[16] In a subsequent study of 272 Dutch subjects with persistent oligoarthritis, extended oligoarthritis, and RF-negative polyarticular JIA, Albers and colleagues[17] found that VTCN1 rs10923223 and JIA subtype were the strongest independent factors for disease course. This suggests that VTCN1 variants might influence the course of disease (remitting, unremitting, or intermediate) in JIA. Further supporting an important role for this gene in inflammatory arthritis, variants in VTCN1 were found to be associated with RA in a Dutch cohort.[18] Of particular interest was that VTCN1 rs4376721 was associated with anticitrullinated peptide antigen (ACPA)-negative subset of RA, whereas another variant (rs10923217) was associated with both ACPA-positive and ACPA-negative subsets of RA.

Another GWAS of 814 children with oligoarticular and RF-negative polyarticular JIA, 658 local controls, and 2400 out-of-study controls followed by meta-analysis using 5 independent cohorts has been reported by Thompson and colleagues.[4] This study confirmed the HLA association at genomewide level of significance, and provided evidence of association at 3q13 within C3orf1 and near several genes, including CD80. This association was verified in a replication cohort as well as in the meta-analysis of the discovery and replication cohorts. Variants in a second novel non-HLA region were found to be associated with JIA at 10q21 near JMJD1C. Replication supported association of only 1 of 5 SNPS in this region. A third region of interest was the 4q31 region, which included the gene-encoding interleukin 15 (IL-15). However, although the initial association was not replicated, a nearby SNP in linkage disequilibrium showed modest association in the discovery and replication cohorts. To identify the putative causative variants, gene expression quantitative trait locus (eQTL) analysis was performed by the investigators using 68 JIA cases and 23 controls. eQTL data showed cis-associations for SNPs from the 3q31 and 10q21 loci. (See Vincent A. Laufer and colleagues' article, "Integrative Approaches to Understanding the Pathogenic Role of Genetic Variation in Rheumatic Diseases," in this issue.) Thus, this study suggested a role for novel candidate genes in disease pathogenesis.

The Immunochip Consortium was established with a goal to investigate shared loci identified in GWAS across multiple autoimmune disorders.[19] The Immunochip genotyping array contains about 200,000 SNPs, including dense coverage of the major histocompatibility complex (MHC) region, and approximately 180 loci that have shown genomewide evidence of association with 1 or more of 12 autoimmune diseases.[19] The Immunochip consortium has been successful at identifying loci associated with many autoimmune disorders including, celiac disease,[20] inflammatory bowel disease,[21] RA,[22] and ankylosing spondylitis.[23]

The International JIA Immunochip consortium published the results of the analysis in 2816 cases with oligoarticular and RF-negative polyarticular JIA and 13,056 controls.

In addition to confirming the 3 loci that have previously been associated at genome-wide level of significance, 14 new loci were discovered (**Table 1**). In addition, 11 loci were found at suggestive levels of significance. Many of the loci were shared with RA, type 1 diabetes (T1D), and celiac disease. This study also highlighted crucial pathways, including IL-2 pathway in JIA pathogenesis.

A third GWAS of JIA was published recently by Finkel and colleagues.[24] The initial GWAS was done using 388 children with JIA and 2500 controls. Three additional cohorts were used for replication, with the discovery and replication cohort totaling 1166 JIA cases and 9500 unrelated controls. It should be noted that this study

Table 1
Regions showing genomewide or suggestive association with oligoarticular and rheumatoid factor–negative polyarticular juvenile idiopathic arthritis

Gene Region	Chr	Most Significant SNP	Best P Value	OR	SNP Position
PTPN22[a]	1	rs6679677	3.2×10^{-25}	1.59	Intergenic
ATP8B2-IL6R	1	rs11265608	2.8×10^{-8}	1.33	Intergenic
RUNX3	1	rs464881	4.66×10^{-7}	1.16	Intergenic
STAT4	2	rs10174238	1.3×10^{-13}	1.29	Intron
AFF3-LONRF2	2	rs6740838	8.83×10^{-7}	1.25	Intergenic
CCR1-CCR3	3	rs79893749	1.88×10^{-7}	0.78	Intergenic
TIMMDC1-CD80	3	rs4688013	6.30×10^{-7}	1.20	Intron
IL2-IL21	4	rs1479924	6.2×10^{-11}	0.79	Intergenic
ANKRD55	5	rs71624119	4.4×10^{-11}	0.78	Intron
ERAP2-LNPEP	5	rs27290	7.5×10^{-9}	1.32	Intron
C5orf56-IRF1	5	rs4705862	1.0×10^{-8}	0.84	Intergenic
HLA DQB1-DQA2[a]	6	rs7775055	3.1×10^{-174}	6.01	Intergenic
IL6	7	rs7808122	5.8×10^{-8}	1.19	intergenic
JAZF1	7	rs10280937	6.60×10^{-7}	1.25	intron
IL2RA	10	rs7909519	8.0×10^{-10}	0.72	Intron
FAS	10	rs7069750	2.9×10^{-8}	1.18	Intron
PRR5L	11	rs4755450	3.35×10^{-7}	0.80	Intergenic
SH2B3-ATXN2	12	rs3184504	2.6×10^{-9}	1.20	Coding
LTBR	12	rs2364480	5.1×10^{-8}	1.20	Coding NS
COG6	13	rs7993214	1.6×10^{-7}	0.84	Intergenic
13q14	13	rs34132030	1.77×10^{-7}	1.18	Intergenic
ZFP36L1	14	rs12434551	1.6×10^{-8}	0.77	Intergenic
PRM1-RM12	16	rs66718203	4.46×10^{-7}	0.81	Intergenic
PTPN2[a]	18	rs2847293	1.4×10^{-12}	1.31	Intergenic
TYK2	19	rs34536443	1.0×10^{-10}	0.56	Coding
RUNX1	21	rs9979383	1.1×10^{-8}	0.78	Intergenic
UBE2L3	22	rs2266959	6.2×10^{-9}	1.24	Intron
Il2RB	22	rs2284033	1.6×10^{-8}	0.84	Intron

Bold indicates genomewide significance.

Abbreviations: Chr, chromosome; NS, nonsynonymous.

[a] Genetic associations previously shown to be genomewide significant before JIA Immunochip consortium study.

included all JIA categories, and of the 1166 JIA cases in the final analysis, 399 (34%) were in the systemic, psoriatic, ERA, or undifferentiated JIA categories. A strong association at the *HLA* locus on 6p21 was observed. Three other loci were found to be nominally significant: *PTPN22* ($P<1.77^{-05}$), *IL2RA* ($P<.022$), and *ANTXR2* ($P<.004$). The novel association discovered in this study was in the region 2q221.1, implicating the *CXCR4* gene. However, because this is known to be near the lactase gene, which is well known for being affected by population stratification, the original results were inflated due to subpopulation stratification. After adjusting for principal components, the association remained nominally significant ($P<10^{-4}$). Gene expression studies showed that expression of CXCR4 was correlated with *CXCR4* rs953387 genotypes in lymphoblastoid cell lines and T cells. The study team also sequenced this gene in a subset of 480 cases and controls and found significant enrichment for rare putatively damaging variants. Due to the concern for population stratification, additional replication of this locus in independent cohorts is needed.

Of the 3 GWAS studies described above, 2 used subjects with all JIA categories.[15,24] Due to the heterogeneity in the disease phenotype, as well as known HLA associations and family history of associated disorders, analyses of these phenotypes in aggregate is challenging. In contrast, Ombrello and colleagues[25] performed a multinational GWAS focusing on only 1 homogeneous JIA category, systemic onset JIA. A total of 770 cases of systemic JIA and 6947 controls from 9 countries were analyzed following imputation of more than 5.6 million SNPs. The strongest systemic JIA risk locus identified in this study was in the MHC locus. A previous report by the same consortium in 2015 focused on only the MHC region from the multinational cohort.[26] That study showed that *HLA DRB1*11* and its defining amino acid (glutamate 58) were strongly associated with systemic JIA. Association testing conditioned for the *HLA DRB1*11* effect showed no residual HLA associations. These observations support a relationship between systemic JIA and the class II HLA region, suggesting the involvement of adaptive immune system in the pathogenesis of systemic JIA. In the study by Ombrello and colleagues,[25] a non-MHC locus on 1p36.32 also demonstrated an association above the genomewide threshold of significance, with rs72632736 showing the peak association ($P<2.9 \times 10^{-9}$). The association peak is located upstream of a long intergenic noncoding RNA and 260 kb upstream of the nearest protein coding gene, *AJAP1*. In addition, 23 other SNPs showed at least suggestive evidence of association with JIA. Genetic and statistical approaches found no evidence of shared genetic architecture between systemic JIA and other JIA categories.

The cumulative data from genetic studies of rheumatic disease show that very strong genetic associations are rare (eg, HLA variants provide ~13% of genetic risk in RA compared with ~4% of the validated alleles outside the MHC).[27] Most risk alleles identified in GWAS are common in the general population, have only a modest effect on risk, and explain only a small part of the variance in disease risk. (See Vincent A. Laufer and colleagues' article, "Integrative Approaches to Understanding the Pathogenic Role of Genetic Variation in Rheumatic Diseases," in this issue.) Whereas the actual causal variants for many of the risk loci identified to date have not been discovered, several themes can be inferred: most variants are located in intronic or intergenic regions, many risk loci and variants are associated with more than 1 autoimmune disease, and many genes are associated with discrete biological pathways.[28] Finally, it is clear that identifying the numerous risk factors for rheumatic diseases in general, and pediatric rheumatic diseases in particular requires multinational collaborations to be successful.

REPLICATED GENETIC ASSOCIATIONS WITH JUVENILE IDIOPATHIC ARTHRITIS
Genes Associated with Multiple Autoimmune Conditions, Including Juvenile Idiopathic Arthritis

The familial clustering of autoimmune conditions may be due to genetic variants that predispose to multiple autoimmune disorders. One of the best characterized multiple autoimmunity genes is protein tyrosine phosphatase nonreceptor 22 (PTPN22). PTPN22 is located on chromosome 1p13.3 to 13.1 and encodes lymphoid protein tyrosine kinase, an enzyme that negatively regulates T cells. Mutations in PTPN22 may lead to T-cell activation and the subsequent development of autoimmune disease. The association between PTPN22 polymorphisms, specifically rs2476601 and rs6679677, and JIA was identified by a candidate gene case control study.[29] These findings were replicated in the subsequent JIA GWAS and Immunochip Consortium studies and in numerous other studies of specific ethnic populations.[30–36] In some groups, however, there was no link found between PTPN22 polymorphisms and JIA risk.[37,38] PTPN22 polymorphisms have also been associated with RA, Crohn disease (CD) and T1D, although it should be noted that the direction of association is opposite in CD compared with the other diseases.

Several other genes have been associated multiple autoimmune conditions. Early GWAS studies also noted an association between PTPN2 and JIA. PTPN2 encodes a protein tyrosine phosphatase involved in T-cell regulation.[16] PTPN2 is also associated with TID and ulcerative colitis (UC). Variants in the gene encoding signal transducer and activator of transcription factor 4 (STAT 4), particularly variant rs7574865, is associated with JIA, as well as other autoimmune conditions, including RA, SLE, Sjögren syndrome, and systemic sclerosis.[16,33,39–41] Ankyrin Repeat Domain 55 (ANKRD55) is a protein coding gene that may play a role in messenger RNA transcription in CD4+ T cells, and has been associated with JIA, RA, CD, and multiple sclerosis.[42–45] Ubiquitin conjugating enzyme E2L3 (UBE2L3) plays a functional role in the degradation of short-lived and abnormal proteins. Polymorphisms in the UBE2L3 gene have been associated with JIA, CD, and UC.[31] IL-2 promotes inflammation in autoimmune disease via binding to the IL-2 receptor. SNP rs2104286 in the interleukin receptor alpha (IL2RA) gene is associated with JIA, RA, and other autoimmune conditions.[46]

Genes Primarily Associated with Juvenile Idiopathic Arthritis Categories

When describing the gene polymorphisms associated specifically with juvenile arthritis, it is helpful to consider the individual category of JIA because each category has a distinct clinical presentation and specific genetic associations. Given the genetic overlap between RF-positive polyarticular JIA and adult RA, the genetics of RF-positive polyarticular JIA are not specifically discussed in this article.

Oligoarticular juvenile idiopathic arthritis or polyarticular rheumatoid factor–negative juvenile idiopathic arthritis

Together, oligoarticular JIA and polyarticular RF-negative JIA are the most common JIA subtypes, affecting up to 70% of JIA patients. Patients with oligoarticular JIA have 4 or fewer joints affected during the first 6 months of the disease. If they continue to have fewer than 4 joints involved, they are considered persistent. If they develop involvement of more than 4 joints, they are referred to as extended oligoarticular JIA. Extended oligoarticular JIA has a similar disease course and treatment response as RF-negative polyarticular JIA. Among primary distinctions is that patients with polyarticular JIA present with 5 or more joints involved. Both oligoarticular JIA and polyarticular JIA typically start in early childhood and have a female predominance. These patients are also uniquely at risk for developing anterior uveitis, particularly if they are antinuclear antibody positive.

Several HLA alleles have been associated with oligoarticular and polyarticular RF-negative JIA. Susceptibility to oligoarticular JIA is associated with HLA DRB1:01, DRB1:08, DRB1:11, DRB1:13, DPB1:02, and DQB1:04.[47] HLA DRB1:04 and DRB1:07 are less frequent in children with oligoarticular JIA than controls, suggesting a protective effect.[48] Polyarticular RF-negative JIA is associated with DRB1:08 and DPB1:03.[49] A 2010 study by Hollenbach and colleagues,[50] which included 820 children with JIA and 273 healthy controls, used high-resolution HLA typing for class I and class II loci. This study demonstrated age-specific effects of disease susceptibility based on HLA alleles. HLA DRB1:11:03/11:04 was associated with increased risk of JIA in both oligoarticular and younger polyarticular subjects, but not with older subjects with polyarticular disease. HLA DRB1:08:01 conferred an increased risk of JIA in younger and older subjects with both oligoarticular and polyarticular RF-negative JIA. HLA DRB1:15:01 was associated with a very strong protective effect for both oligoarticular and polyarticular RF-negative JIA subjects. HLA variants also demonstrated the strongest association in the JIA GWAS studies and the more recent Immunochip study in which the SNP rs7775055 located in the HLA-DQ region was associated with oligoarticular or polyarticular RF-negative JIA (OR 6.01, 95% CI 5.30–6.81, $P<3.1 \times 10^{-174}$).[3,16,40]

Several non-HLA alleles have been associated with oligoarticular or polyarticular RF-negative JIA, including several loci that were identified from the Immunochip Consortium study in which 14 loci reached genomewide level of significance for the first time and an additional 11 loci reached suggestive level of significance.[3] Six of these novel loci, C5orf56-IRF1 (rs4705862), ERAP2-LNPEP (rs27290), PRR5L (rs4755450), RUNX1 (rs9979383), RUNX3 (rs4648881), and UBE2L3 (rs2266959) were independently replicated in a genotyping study using the Australian Childhood Arthritis Risk Factor Identification Study (CLARITY) JIA case-control sample, which included 404 JIA cases and 676 healthy child controls.[51]

Genetic polymorphisms that may have a more direct link to disease pathogenesis include mutations in the TNFA and TRAF1 genes. TNFA encodes the proinflammatory cytokine tumor necrosis factor (TNF), among primary proinflammatory cytokines involved in the pathogenesis of JIA and among primary targets of therapy for JIA and other forms of inflammatory arthritis. The TNFA G-308a allele (rs1800629) is significantly associated with JIA.[52] A polymorphism in the IL2RA/CD25 gene (rs2104286), which encodes the alpha chain of the Interleukin 2 receptor was demonstrated to be a risk factor for JIA.[46] The TRAF-1 gene encodes TNF receptor-associated factor 1, a regulator in the TNF pathway. The TRAF1-C5 locus on chromosome 9 has been associated with JIA, as well as RA.[53]

Macrophage migration inhibitory factor (MIF) is a protein cofactor in T-cell activation that plays a role in the secretion of proinflammatory cytokines, leading to increased inflammatory activity. Several polymorphisms in the MIF gene, including the MIF -173*C allele, have been associated with JIA.[35,54,55]

Systemic-onset juvenile idiopathic arthritis
Systemic-onset JIA accounts for approximately 10% of all JIA cases in North America and Europe. In addition to arthritis, systemic JIA is characterized by the presence of systemic symptoms, including high spiking fevers, a characteristic rash, hepatosplenomegaly, lymphadenopathy, and serositis. In addition, patients with systemic JIA have significantly elevated inflammatory markers. These unique features have led some investigators to consider systemic JIA an autoinflammatory, versus an

autoimmune, condition. Not surprisingly then, genes associated with autoinflamma-tory conditions, including SNPs in the IL-1 ligand cluster, *TNFRSF1A*, *MVK*, and *MEFV* genes have been associated with systemic JIA.[56,57]

Several other genetic polymorphisms have been identified related to pathways implicated in systemic JIA pathogenesis. Polymorphisms in the *TNFA* gene have been identified in Japanese and Spanish cohorts of JIA subjects.[58,59] The *MIF-173*C* allele has been identified at a higher frequency in systemic JIA subjects versus controls and has been associated with worse outcome.[60,61]

Enthesitis-related arthritis

The association between *HLAB27* and ERA is well characterized. Depending on the population studies, up to 90% of patients with ERA are HLAB27 positive. ERA patients who are HLAB27 positive tend to have axial disease and a more persistent disease course, in contrast ERA to patients who are HLAB27 negative.[62] There have also been associations identified between ERA and class II HLA alleles.[63,64] In a cohort of 34 pediatric subjects, ERA was associated with HLA *DRB1*:01 (OR 3.6), *DQA1*:01:01 (OR 2.8), and *DQB1*:05 (OR 3.5), and a haplotype carrying these alleles (OR 4.9, 95% CI 2–12.1).[64] *DRB1*:07 (OR 0.3) and *DPB1*:02:01 (OR 0.1) was protective against ERA;[64] the protective association of *DPB1*:02 was also reported by Flato and colleagues.[63]

Susceptibility loci in the endoplasmic reticulum aminopeptidase 1 (*ERAP 1*) gene have been associated with ERA. A 2011 study by Hinks and colleagues,[65] which included 74 ERA cases, identified an association between the *ERAP1* SNP rs30187, which is associated with ankylosing spondylitis in adults, and ERA (p trend = 0.005). The same investigators identified a polymorphism in the *IL12A* gene (rs17810546) that was uniquely associated with ERA (p trend = 0.005, OR 1.88).[66] A higher frequency of mutations in the *MEFV* gene have also been found with ERA, although the clinical sig-nificance of this remains unknown.[67,68]

Psoriatic arthritis

Similar to ERA, the strongest HLA association with psoriatic arthritis is the *HLAB27* allele. Initial studies suggested an increased frequency of HLA A2 in psoriatic JIA pa-tients, but this association was not proven in subsequent studies.[69,70] Several HLA class II alleles have been associated with psoriatic JIA (*DRB1*:01 (OR 2.7), *DQA1*:01:01 (OR 4.2), and *DQB1*:05 (OR 4.4); and at least 3 HLA variants protective against psoriatic JIA (*DRB1*:01 (OR 0.3), *DQA1*:03 (OR 0.3), and *DQB1*:03 (OR 0.5).[64]

Polymorphisms in the *IL23R* gene have been associated with both adult psoriatic arthritis and psoriatic JIA. In a study including 93 subjects with psoriatic JIA, there was an association between the *IL23R* SNP rs11209026 and psoriatic JIA (OR 0.4 95%, CI 0.16–0.98, *P* = .04).[65] Similar to ERA, mutations in genes more commonly associated with autoinflammatory syndromes, such as *MEFV* and *NLRP3*, have been associated with psoriatic JIA.[71]

PHARMACOGENOMICS

With the discovery of candidate genes suggesting increased susceptibility to JIA, there has been an interest in understanding if these genetic differences could explain the variation in response to treatment and outcomes, and potentially predict treatment response.

Several studies have examined genetic polymorphisms and the response to treatment with methotrexate (MTX).[72] Approximately 30% of JIA patients fail to respond to MTX but it is difficult to determine who will and who will not respond a priori. In addition, the mechanism of action of MTX is not fully understood. Some of the initial work in this area focused on polymorphisms in the methylenetetrahy-drofolate reductase (*MTHFR*) gene and correlation with response to therapy. In a 2005 study of 85 subjects with JIA there was an association identified between the 1298 A/A *MTHFR* SNP and lower efficacy of MTX.[73] This finding was also noted in a study examining multiple clinical and genetic factors contributing to MTX response. JIA subjects with 2 copies of the *MTHFR* 1298A-677 C SNP were more likely to response to MTX than subjects with 0 or 1 copies of the haplotype (*P* = .039).

As a part of the Childhood Arthritis Response to Medication Study (CHARMS), Hinks and colleagues[74] performed SNP genotyping for 13 genes in the MTX pathway on 197 children with all JIA subtypes. Their findings were replicated in a cohort of 210 US children. They found 1 SNP within the inosine triphosphate pyro-phosphatase gene (*ITPA*) and 2 SNPs within the 5-aminoimidazole-4-carboxamide ribonucleotide transformylase gene (*ATIC*) that were associated with a poor response to MTX, as well as 1 *ATIC* SNP that showed a trend toward association with MTX response. The *ATIC* gene encodes the ATIC enzyme, which is inhibited by MTX polyglutamates and leads to an accumulation of adenosine, which is thought to be a potent anti-inflammatory mediator. A study using an Italian cohort of 69 subjects also found that the *ITPA* rs1127354 variant was associated with poor response, whereas the *ATIC* rs2372536 SNP was associated with achievement of remission.[75]

In a longitudinal cohort study of 287 JIA subjects treated with MTX, SNPs in the adenosine triphosphate-binding cassette transporter B1 (*ABCB1*) gene rs1045642 and the *ABCC3* gene polymorphism rs4793665 were associated with higher response to MTX, whereas the presence of the solute carrier 19A1 (*SLC19A1*) gene polymor-phism rs1051266 was associated with a lower likelihood of response to MTX.[76]

In a 2014 study, Cobb and colleagues[77] use a genomewide approach to identify novel genes for MTX response in a large cohort of 759 subjects with JIA from the United Kingdom, Netherlands, and Czech Republic, also a part the CHARMS con-sortium. After quality control, 694 JIA cases were genotyped and through a 2-phase analysis process the investigators identified 14 regions and 3 genes of biologic interest (*ZMIZ1*, *TGIF1*, and *CFTR*), which may represent novel potential pathways for MTX response.

Several studies have examined the association between JIA-associated TNF-α gene polymorphisms and response to treatment with TNF inhibitors. Using a cohort of 107 subjects with JIA, Cimaz and colleagues[78] compared genetic polymorphisms for *IL1B*+3954, *IL1RA* +2018, *TNF-α* −238, and *TNF-α* −308 and found no associa-tion between the frequency of the genetic polymorphisms and response to anti-TNF therapy. In a study of 74 white JIA subjects, those carrying the *TNF-α* −308 GA/AA and −238 GA genotypes had higher disease activity and a decreased response to anti-TNF treatment.[79]

Recent advances in molecular genetics, analytical approaches, and international consortia have resulted in significant improvements in the understanding of the ge-netic underpinnings of JIA and its categories. Although variants in the HLA region confer a significant risk of JIA, several non-HLA loci also show convincing evidence of association with JIA categories. Many of these loci are shared with other autoim-mune phenotypes. Identified variants still do not explain the genetic risk of JIA, sug-gesting other variants exist. Investigations of well-phenotyped cases, using whole exome and whole genome sequencing, will likely help fill the gaps in missing heritability.

REFERENCES

1. Mellins ED, Macaubas C, Grom AA. Pathogenesis of systemic juvenile idiopathic arthritis: some answers, more questions. Nat Rev Rheumatol 2011;7(7):416–26.
2. Hersh AO, Prahalad S. Immunogenetics of juvenile idiopathic arthritis: a comprehensive review. J Autoimmun 2015;64:113–24.
3. Hinks A, Cobb J, Marion MC, et al. Dense genotyping of immune-related disease regions identifies 14 new susceptibility loci for juvenile idiopathic arthritis. Nat Genet 2013;45(6):664–9.
4. Thompson SD, Marion MC, Sudman M, et al. Genome-wide association analysis of juvenile idiopathic arthritis identifies a new susceptibility locus at chromosomal region 3q13. Arthritis Rheum 2012;64(8):2781–91.
5. Petty RE, Southwood TR, Manners P, et al. International League of Associations for Rheumatology classification of juvenile idiopathic arthritis: second revision, Edmonton, 2001. J Rheumatol 2004;31(2):390–2.
6. Prahalad S, Ryan MH, Shear ES, et al. Twins concordant for juvenile rheumatoid arthritis. Arthritis Rheum 2000;43(11):2611–2.
7. Moroldo MB, Chaudhari M, Shear E, et al. Juvenile rheumatoid arthritis affected sibpairs: extent of clinical phenotype concordance. Arthritis Rheum 2004;50(6): 1928–34.
8. Moroldo MB, Tague BL, Shear ES, et al. Juvenile rheumatoid arthritis in affected sibpairs. Arthritis Rheum 1997;40(11):1962–6.
9. Prahalad S, O'Brien E, Fraser AM, et al. Familial aggregation of juvenile idiopathic arthritis. Arthritis Rheum 2004;50(12):4022–7.
10. Prahalad S, Zeft AS, Pimentel R, et al. Quantification of the familial contribution to juvenile idiopathic arthritis. Arthritis Rheum 2010;62(8):2525–9.
11. Frisell T, Hellgren K, Alfredsson L, et al. Familial aggregation of arthritis-related diseases in seropositive and seronegative rheumatoid arthritis: a register-based case-control study in Sweden. Ann Rheum Dis 2016;75(1):183–9.
12. Prahalad S, Shear ES, Thompson SD, et al. Increased prevalence of familial autoimmunity in simplex and multiplex families with juvenile rheumatoid arthritis. Arthritis Rheum 2002;46(7):1851–6.
13. Prahalad S, McCracken CE, Ponder LA, et al. Familial autoimmunity in the Childhood Arthritis and Rheumatology Research Alliance registry. Pediatr Rheumatol Online J 2016;14(1):14.
14. Thompson SD, Moroldo MB, Guyer L, et al. A genome-wide scan for juvenile rheumatoid arthritis in affected sibpair families provides evidence of linkage. Arthritis Rheum 2004;50(9):2920–30.
15. Hinks A, Barton A, Shephard N, et al. Identification of a novel susceptibility locus for juvenile idiopathic arthritis by genome-wide association analysis. Arthritis Rheum 2009;60(1):258–63.
16. Thompson SD, Sudman M, Ramos PS, et al. The susceptibility loci juvenile idiopathic arthritis shares with other autoimmune diseases extend to PTPN2, COG6, and ANGPT1. Arthritis Rheum 2010;62(11):3265–76.
17. Albers HM, Reinards TH, Brinkman DM, et al. Genetic variation in VTCN1 (B7-H4) is associated with course of disease in juvenile idiopathic arthritis. Ann Rheum Dis 2014;73(6):1198–201.
18. Daha NA, Lie BA, Trouw LA, et al. Novel genetic association of the VTCN1 region with rheumatoid arthritis. Ann Rheum Dis 2012;71(4):567–71.
19. Cortes A, Brown MA. Promise and pitfalls of the Immunochip. Arthritis Res Ther 2011;13(1):101.

20. Trynka G, Hunt KA, Bockett NA, et al. Dense genotyping identifies and localizes multiple common and rare variant association signals in celiac disease. Nat Genet 2011;43(12):1193–201.
21. Jostins L, Ripke S, Weersma RK, et al. Host-microbe interactions have shaped the genetic architecture of inflammatory bowel disease. Nature 2012; 491(7422):119–24.
22. Eyre S, Bowes J, Diogo D, et al. High-density genetic mapping identifies new susceptibility loci for rheumatoid arthritis. Nat Genet 2012;44(12):1336–40.
23. International Genetics of Ankylosing Spondylitis Consortium (IGAS), Cortes A, Hadler J, Pointon JP, et al. Identification of multiple risk variants for ankylosing spondylitis through high-density genotyping of immune-related loci. Nat Genet 2013;45(7):730–8.
24. Finkel TH, Li J, Wei Z, et al. Variants in CXCR4 associate with juvenile idiopathic arthritis susceptibility. BMC Med Genet 2016;17:24.
25. Ombrello MJ, Arthur VL, Remmers EF, et al. Genetic architecture distinguishes systemic juvenile idiopathic arthritis from other forms of juvenile idiopathic arthritis: clinical and therapeutic implications. Ann Rheum Dis 2016;76:906–13.
26. Ombrello MJ, Remmers EF, Tachmazidou I, et al. HLA-DRB1*11 and variants of the MHC class II locus are strong risk factors for systemic juvenile idiopathic arthritis. Proc Natl Acad Sci U S A 2015;112(52):15970–5.
27. Raychaudhuri S, Sandor C, Stahl EA, et al. Five amino acids in three HLA proteins explain most of the association between MHC and seropositive rheumatoid arthritis. Nat Genet 2012;44(3):291–6.
28. Gregersen PK. Closing the gap between genotype and phenotype. Nat Genet 2009;41(9):958–9.
29. Hinks A, Barton A, John S, et al. Association between the PTPN22 gene and rheumatoid arthritis and juvenile idiopathic arthritis in a UK population: further support that PTPN22 is an autoimmunity gene. Arthritis Rheum 2005;52(6):1694–9.
30. Bahrami T, Soltani S, Moazzami K, et al. Association of PTPN22 gene polymorphisms with susceptibility to juvenile idiopathic arthritis in Iranian population. Fetal Pediatr Pathol 2017;36(1):42–8.
31. Chiaroni-Clarke RC, Li YR, Munro JE, et al. The association of PTPN22 rs2476601 with juvenile idiopathic arthritis is specific to females. Genes Immun 2015;16(7): 495–8.
32. Di Y, Zhong S, Wu L, et al. The association between PTPN22 Genetic Polymorphism and Juvenile Idiopathic Arthritis (JIA) susceptibility: an updated meta-analysis. Iran J Public Health 2015;44(9):1169–75.
33. Fan ZD, Wang FF, Huang H, et al. STAT4 rs7574865 G/T and PTPN22 rs2488457 G/C polymorphisms influence the risk of developing juvenile idiopathic arthritis in Han Chinese patients. PLoS One 2015;10(3):e0117389.
34. Goulielmos GN, Chiaroni-Clarke RC, Dimopoulou DG, et al. Association of juvenile idiopathic arthritis with PTPN22 rs2476601 is specific to females in a Greek population. Pediatr Rheumatol Online J 2016;14(1):25.
35. Lee YH, Bae SC, Song GG. The association between the functional PTPN22 1858 C/T and MIF -173 C/G polymorphisms and juvenile idiopathic arthritis: a meta-analysis. Inflamm Res 2012;61(5):411–5.
36. Pazar B, Gergely P Jr, Nagy ZB, et al. Role of HLA-DRB1 and PTPN22 genes in susceptibility to juvenile idiopathic arthritis in Hungarian patients. Clin Exp Rheumatol 2008;26(6):1146–52.
37. Cinek O, Hradsky O, Ahmedov G, et al. No independent role of the -1123 G>C and+2740 A>G variants in the association of PTPN22 with type 1 diabetes and

juvenile idiopathic arthritis in two Caucasian populations. Diabetes Res Clin Pract 2007;76(2):297–303.

38. Seldin MF, Shigeta R, Laiho K, et al. Finnish case-control and family studies support PTPN22 R620W polymorphism as a risk factor in rheumatoid arthritis, but suggest only minimal or no effect in juvenile idiopathic arthritis. Genes Immun 2005;6(8):720–2.

39. Prahalad S, Hansen S, Whiting A, et al. Variants in TNFAIP3, STAT4, and C12orf30 loci associated with multiple autoimmune diseases are also associated with juvenile idiopathic arthritis. Arthritis Rheum 2009;60(7):2124–30.

40. Hinks A, Eyre S, Ke X, et al. Overlap of disease susceptibility loci for rheumatoid arthritis and juvenile idiopathic arthritis. Ann Rheum Dis 2010;69(6):1049–53.

41. Liang YL, Wu H, Shen X, et al. Association of STAT4 rs7574865 polymorphism with autoimmune diseases: a meta-analysis. Mol Biol Rep 2012;39(9):8873–82.

42. Burr ML, Naseem H, Hinks A, et al. PADI4 genotype is not associated with rheumatoid arthritis in a large UK Caucasian population. Ann Rheum Dis 2010;69(4): 666–70.

43. Lopez de Lapuente A, Feliu A, Ugidos N, et al. Novel insights into the multiple sclerosis risk gene ANKRD55. J Immunol 2016;196(11):4553–65.

44. Reinards TH, Albers HM, Brinkman DM, et al. CD226 (DNAM-1) is associated with susceptibility to juvenile idiopathic arthritis. Ann Rheum Dis 2015;74(12): 2193–8.

45. Viatte S, Massey J, Bowes J, et al. Replication of associations of genetic loci outside the HLA region with susceptibility to anti-cyclic citrullinated peptide-negative rheumatoid arthritis. Arthritis Rheumatol 2016;68(7):1603–13.

46. Hinks A, Ke X, Barton A, et al. Association of the IL2RA/CD25 gene with juvenile idiopathic arthritis. Arthritis Rheum 2009;60(1):251–7.

47. Vicario JL, Martinez-Laso J, Gomez-Reino JJ, et al. Both HLA class II and class III DNA polymorphisms are linked to juvenile rheumatoid arthritis susceptibility. Clin Immunol Immunopathol 1990;56(1):22–8.

48. Paul C, Schoenwald U, Truckenbrodt H, et al. HLA-DP/DR interaction in early onset pauciarticular juvenile chronic arthritis. Immunogenetics 1993;37(6):442–8.

49. Arnaiz-Villena A, Gomez-Reino JJ, Gamir ML, et al. DR, C4, and Bf allotypes in juvenile rheumatoid arthritis. Arthritis Rheum 1984;27(11):1281–5.

50. Hollenbach JA, Thompson SD, Bugawan TL, et al. Juvenile idiopathic arthritis and HLA class I and class II interactions and age-at-onset effects. Arthritis Rheum 2010;62(6):1781–91.

51. Chiaroni-Clarke RC, Munro JE, Chavez RA, et al. Independent confirmation of juvenile idiopathic arthritis genetic risk loci previously identified by immunochip array analysis. Pediatr Rheumatol Online J 2014;12:53.

52. Kaalla MJ, Broadaway KA, Rohani-Pichavant M, et al. Meta-analysis confirms association between TNFA-G238A variant and JIA, and between PTPN22-C1858T variant and oligoarticular, RF-polyarticular and RF-positive polyarticular JIA. Pediatr Rheumatol Online J 2013;11(1):40.

53. Albers HM, Kurreeman FA, Houwing-Duistermaat JJ, et al. The TRAF1/C5 region is a risk factor for polyarthritis in juvenile idiopathic arthritis. Ann Rheum Dis 2008; 67(11):1578–80.

54. Donn R, Alourfi Z, Zeggini E, et al. A functional promoter haplotype of macrophage migration inhibitory factor is linked and associated with juvenile idiopathic arthritis. Arthritis Rheum 2004;50(5):1604–10.

55. Berdeli A, Ozyurek AR, Ulger Z, et al. Association of macrophage migration inhibitory factor gene -173 G/C polymorphism with prognosis in Turkish children with juvenile rheumatoid arthritis. Rheumatol Int 2006;26(8):726–31.

56. Hinks A, Martin P, Thompson SD, et al. Autoinflammatory gene polymorphisms and susceptibility to UK juvenile idiopathic arthritis. Pediatr Rheumatol Online J 2013;11(1):14.

57. Lotfy HM, Kandil ME, Issac MS, et al. MEFV mutations in Egyptian children with systemic-onset juvenile idiopathic arthritis. Mol Diagn Ther 2014;18(5):549–57.

58. Modesto C, Patino-Garcia A, Sotillo-Pineiro E, et al. TNF-alpha promoter gene polymorphisms in Spanish children with persistent oligoarticular and systemic-onset juvenile idiopathic arthritis. Scand J Rheumatol 2005;34(6):451–4.

59. Date Y, Seki N, Kamizono S, et al. Identification of a genetic risk factor for systemic juvenile rheumatoid arthritis in the 5'-flanking region of the TNFalpha gene and HLA genes. Arthritis Rheum 1999;42(12):2577–82.

60. De Benedetti F, Meazza C, Vivarelli M, et al. Functional and prognostic relevance of the -173 polymorphism of the macrophage migration inhibitory factor gene in systemic-onset juvenile idiopathic arthritis. Arthritis Rheum 2003;48(5):1398–407.

61. Donn RP, Shelley E, Ollier WE, et al, British Paediatric Rheumatology Study Group. A novel 5'-flanking region polymorphism of macrophage migration inhibitory factor is associated with systemic-onset juvenile idiopathic arthritis. Arthritis Rheum 2001;44(8):1782–5.

62. Colbert RA. Classification of juvenile spondyloarthritis: enthesitis-related arthritis and beyond. Nat Rev Rheumatol 2010;6(8):477–85.

63. Flato B, Hoffmann-Vold AM, Reiff A, et al. Long-term outcome and prognostic factors in enthesitis-related arthritis: a case-control study. Arthritis Rheum 2006; 54(11):3573–82.

64. Thomson W, Barrett JH, Donn R, et al. Juvenile idiopathic arthritis classified by the ILAR criteria: HLA associations in UK patients. Rheumatology (Oxford) 2002;41(10):1183–9.

65. Hinks A, Martin P, Flynn E, et al, Childhood Arthritis Prospective Study CAPS. Subtype specific genetic associations for juvenile idiopathic arthritis: ERAP1 with the enthesitis related arthritis subtype and IL23R with juvenile psoriatic arthritis. Arthritis Res Ther 2011;13(1):R12.

66. Hinks A, Martin P, Flynn E, et al. Investigation of type 1 diabetes and coeliac disease susceptibility loci for association with juvenile idiopathic arthritis. Ann Rheum Dis 2010;69(12):2169–72.

67. Comak E, Dogan CS, Akman S, et al. MEFV gene mutations in Turkish children with juvenile idiopathic arthritis. Eur J Pediatr 2013;172(8):1061–7.

68. Gulhan B, Akkus A, Ozcakar L, et al. Are MEFV mutations susceptibility factors in enthesitis-related arthritis patients in the eastern Mediterranean? Clin Exp Rheumatol 2014;32(4 Suppl 84):S160–4.

69. Hamilton ML, Gladman DD, Shore A, et al. Juvenile psoriatic arthritis and HLA antigens. Ann Rheum Dis 1990;49(9):694–7.

70. Ansell B, Beeson M, Hall P, et al. HLA and juvenile psoriatic arthritis. Br J Rheumatol 1993;32(9):836–7.

71. Day TG, Ramanan AV, Hinks A, et al. Autoinflammatory genes and susceptibility to psoriatic juvenile idiopathic arthritis. Arthritis Rheum 2008;58(7):2142–6.

72. Pastore S, Stocco G, Favretto D, et al. Genetic determinants for methotrexate response in juvenile idiopathic arthritis. Front Pharmacol 2015;6:52.

73. Schmeling H, Biber D, Heins S, et al. Influence of methylenetetrahydrofolate reductase polymorphisms on efficacy and toxicity of methotrexate in patients with juvenile idiopathic arthritis. J Rheumatol 2005;32(9):1832–6.

74. Hinks A, Moncrieffe H, Martin P, et al. Association of the 5-aminoimidazole-4-carboxamide ribonucleotide transformylase gene with response to methotrexate in juvenile idiopathic arthritis. Ann Rheum Dis 2011;70(8):1395–400.

75. Pastore S, Stocco G, Moressa V, et al. 5-Aminoimidazole-4-carboxamide ribonucleotide-transformylase and inosine-triphosphate-pyrophosphatase genes variants predict remission rate during methotrexate therapy in patients with juvenile idiopathic arthritis. Rheumatol Int 2015;35(4):619–27.

76. de Rotte MC, Bulatovic M, Heijstek MW, et al. ABCB1 and ABCC3 gene polymorphisms are associated with first-year response to methotrexate in juvenile idiopathic arthritis. J Rheumatol 2012;39(10):2032–40.

77. Cobb J, Cule E, Moncrieffe H, et al. Genome-wide data reveal novel genes for methotrexate response in a large cohort of juvenile idiopathic arthritis cases. Pharmacogenomics J 2014;14(4):356–64.

78. Cimaz R, Cazalis MA, Reynaud C, et al. IL1 and TNF gene polymorphisms in patients with juvenile idiopathic arthritis treated with TNF inhibitors. Ann Rheum Dis 2007;66(7):900–4.

79. Scardapane A, Ferrante R, Nozzi M, et al. TNF-alpha gene polymorphisms and juvenile idiopathic arthritis: Influence on disease outcome and therapeutic response. Semin Arthritis Rheum 2015;45(1):35–41.

Integrative Approaches to Understanding the Pathogenic Role of Genetic Variation in Rheumatic Diseases

Vincent A. Laufer, BA[a], Jake Y. Chen, PhD[b],
Carl D. Langefeld, PhD[c,d], S. Louis Bridges, Jr., MD, PhD[e,*]

KEYWORDS

- Rheumatic disease • Integrative genomics • Systems biology • Precision medicine
- Genetics • GWAS

KEY POINTS

- Large genetic studies of rheumatic diseases have implicated many risk loci.
- Within risk loci, the identity and function of the pathogenic variants that underlie rheumatic diseases remain largely unknown, but methods in development will address these gaps in knowledge.
- Integrative analysis of omics datasets will yield new insights into the molecules, cells, tissues, and pathways that initiate and perpetuate rheumatic diseases.
- Functional characterization of prioritized genetic variants will pave the way for better diagnosis, treatment, and prevention of rheumatic diseases.

Disclosure Statement: J.Y. Chen discloses that he is also the founder of MedeoLinx, LLC, an Indianapolis startup biotech company providing novel drug discovery products and services based on translational systems biology. Other authors have nothing to disclose.
[a] Division of Clinical Immunology and Rheumatology, School of Medicine, University of Alabama at Birmingham, 1720 2nd Avenue South, SHEL 236, Birmingham, AL 35294-2182, USA; [b] The Informatics Institute, School of Medicine, University of Alabama at Birmingham, 1720 2nd Avenue South, THT 137, Birmingham, AL 35294-0006, USA; [c] Department of Biostatistical Sciences, Wake Forest University School of Medicine, Winston-Salem, NC 27101, USA; [d] Public Health Genomics, Division of Public Health Sciences, Department of Biostatistical Sciences, Wake Forest School of Medicine, Medical Center Boulevard, Winston-Salem, NC 27157, USA; [e] Division of Clinical Immunology and Rheumatology, School of Medicine, University of Alabama at Birmingham, 1720 2nd Avenue South, SHEL 178, Birmingham, AL 35294-2182, USA
* Corresponding author.
E-mail address: lbridges@uab.edu

INTRODUCTION

The study of rheumatic diseases draws on many genome-scale technologies. **Box 1** defines relevant terms that will be used in this discussion. Genome-wide association studies (GWAS) and other genetic studies have identified and replicated numerous loci associated with rheumatic diseases. Although these findings have led to increased awareness of particular pathogenetic pathways, there are multiple impediments to the translation of these results to the clinic. First, and as expected, the variants identified thus far do not account for the entirety of the heritable basis of any given rheumatic disease. Second, genetic variants in close physical proximity tend to be inherited together (linkage disequilibrium, or LD, see **Box 1**). As a result, a rheumatic disease risk locus usually contains multiple associated variants, from which the actual pathogenic variants are difficult to separate. This is most pronounced in the major histocompatibility complex region, where there are hundreds of associated variants, many of which are in strong LD. However, new techniques that leverage transethnic and annotation data will help narrow the search for single-nucleotide polymorphisms (SNPs) that are directly pathogenic. Finally, determining the mechanisms of action of pathogenic variants is challenging, due to interaction effects, cell type–specific gene expression, the local tissue milieu, the temporal course of gene expression, and complicating environmental factors.

There is hope, however. Although rheumatic diseases are complex and have considerable differences in etiology, clinical presentation, and treatment, there is overlap in the pathogenic mechanisms involved. For example, pathobiology involving the adaptive immune system (eg, autoantibodies) is similar among rheumatoid arthritis (RA), systemic lupus erythematosus (SLE), inflammatory myositis, and Sjögren syndrome. In these conditions, failure of adaptive immune cells (B and T lymphocytes) to maintain self-tolerance opens the way to several aspects of autoimmune pathogenesis, such as autoantibody production. These commonalities stem in part from genetic variants that affect multiple rheumatic diseases and similar conditions; for instance, dysregulation of autoantibody production characterizes patients with a risk variant in *PTPN22*, and this variant is associated with many rheumatic conditions, including RA, SLE, type 1 diabetes, and others.[1] Identifying such shared risk factors may provide insights into causes of rheumatic diseases. Furthermore, ongoing technological and bioinformatic advancements have enabled increasingly accurate and sensitive characterization of cells, tissues, organisms, and diseases through analyses of the genome, transcriptome, epigenome, proteome, and metabolome (see **Box 1** for definitions). This review discusses how integration of data can help characterize and prioritize genetic variants for laboratory-based studies of their functional and biological consequences that will lead to better understanding of the mechanisms of human rheumatic diseases.

HERITABILITY OF RHEUMATIC DISEASES

Historical evidence for the heritability of rheumatic diseases comes from studies of familial clustering, sibling recurrence risk ratios, twin studies, and parent-child trio studies.[2] More recently, a large number of advanced methodologies based on genome-wide assays for estimating heritability have been devised.[3–5] Heritability estimates for rheumatic diseases are often approximately 0.5,[2] but this is highly variable. GWAS (see **Box 1**) conducted to date have identified hundreds of risk loci for autoimmune diseases and thousands of associations with disease and traits.[1,2]

Although in aggregate these studies explain a meaningful proportion of disease risk, much of the heritable basis of rheumatic disease remains unexplained. There are

Box 1
A glossary of relevant terms

- 5' untranslated region (5'-UTR): The region directly upstream of the initiation codon and translation start site. In mRNA, the sequence of this region strongly influences translation, and likewise the corresponding regions of template DNA contain many elements that can produce a marked effect on transcription.

- ATAC-Seq (Assay for Transposase-Accessible Chromatin with high-throughput sequencing): This technique is used to study chromatin accessibility (accessible or protected), which is related to transcription factor binding and gene expression.

- Copy number variation (CNV): A form of genetic variation resulting in a change in the number of copies of a gene or genomic element. Deletion and insertion of DNA by a variety of mechanisms can produce genetic variants affecting as little as a few kilobases (kb) or as much as an entire chromosome. CNVs have been difficult to assay using common technologies, affect a substantial portion of the genome, and influence a variety of diseases, including rheumatic diseases.

- CpG site: A DNA sequence consisting of a 5' guanine nucleotide joined to a cytosine residue by a phosphate group. Cytosines in CpG sites can be methylated to form 5-methylcytosine, which can change its expression.

- DNA methylation: Modification of DNA by attachment of a methyl group to DNA nucleotides. One common site of methylation is CpG sites (see previous definition).

- Epigenetics: The study of genetic effects produced by mechanisms that do not alter the primary sequence of DNA. For instance, methylation of DNA (see previous definition) or of histones producing differences in gene regulation are examples of epigenetic effects. Epigenetic modifications may result in changes to gene expression and regulation.

- Extrinsic filtering: Data filtering based on information outside of the dataset, such as the inclusion of genomic annotations from the National Institutes of Health Roadmap Epigenomics Mapping Consortium (ROADMAP) or the Encyclopedia of DNA elements (ENCODE).

- Genome-wide association study (GWAS): Examination of a genome-wide set of genetic variants (typically single-nucleotide polymorphisms [SNPs]) to uncover associations between genotypic variation and a phenotype or trait. Similarly, epigenetic variation such as DNA methylation can be investigated in epigenome-wide association studies.

- Haplotype: A set of SNPs on the same DNA strand that are inherited together due to linkage to one another (see definition later in this glossary).

- Heritability: The proportion of phenotypic variation that can be accounted for based on genotypic variation.

- Imputation: Statistical inference of unobserved data, such as predicting the most likely allele of a particular SNP due to known linkage disequilibrium (LD)/haplotype structure. Imputation methods are most well established for genotyping data.

- Intrinsic filtering: Filtering of data based on information calculated from the dataset itself, such as filtering genetic variants based on linkage to another variant strongly associated in that dataset.

- Linkage disequilibrium (LD): The nonrandom association of 2 or more genetic variants. Genetic recombination during meiosis allows for independent assortment of alleles and genetic variants. Genomic proximity, as well as forces like selection, population structure, and genetic drift, can maintain the association of 2 variants over a considerable period.

- Long noncoding RNAs (lncRNA): lncRNAs are molecules of RNA greater than 200 nucleotides in length that do not code for protein products. These RNAs interact with several levels of gene-specific transcription, splicing, translation, posttranslational modification, and gene regulation. RNA-Seq studies have mostly targeted a genomic locus and having high depth can identify associated these lncRNAs for further analysis.

- Mendelian randomization: An epidemiologic method in which genetic variation in genes of known function is used to examine whether a modifiable exposure has a causal effect relationship to disease in nonexperimental studies. This method can be used to test for causal effects among 2 phenotypes (often an intermediate phenotype and a disease outcome) without conducting a randomized controlled trial.

- Metaorganism: A community of organisms including the host and others that is indicated by the metagenome. The metagenome comprises all the genetic material associated with a human being, including, for example, host DNA, microbial DNA, and the virome.

- Multiple enhancer variant hypothesis: The hypothesis based on the observation that multiple variants in linkage may act cooperatively to regulate the expression of a target gene, and in diseases such as RA, SLE, and multiple sclerosis.

- Nonadditive genetic effects: Effects for which the contribution of alleles influencing a trait are not independent of one another, or not independent of the environment.

- Metabolomics: The study of metabolites (small molecules left behind as part of specific cellular processes) within cells, fluids, or tissues or organisms. Collectively, these small molecules are referred to as the metabolome.

- Pathogenic variant: A variant that contributes to the pathogenesis of a specified disease state. Such variants also may contribute to or protect against other phenotypes. Pathogenic variants need be neither necessary nor sufficient to produce a disease state due to incomplete penetrance.

- Phased haplotype: With short read sequencing, it is uncertain whether variants are inherited from the maternal or paternal copy of a given chromosome. Algorithms have been devised to deduce phased haplotypes, or the most likely assignment of variants in a region to one or the other parental copy of a chromosome, enabling inference of haplotypes.

- Phenome: The phenome refers to the set of all phenotypic states for a given biological unit of interest, such as an organism or population.

- Polygenic traits: Traits influenced by genetic variation in several or many genes or genetic loci. Recent studies of rheumatic diseases suggest that thousands of genetic variants of small effect may modify disease risk.

- Proteomics: Analysis of the full complement of proteins produced by a given biological entity of interest, such as a cell, tissue, or organism, including those modified through splicing or posttranslational modification.

- Quantitative trait locus: A genetic variant that is associated with a quantitative difference in the measurement of a phenotype or trait. For instance, an expression quantitative trait locus is a genetic variant correlated with expression level of either local genes (<5 Mb; a cis-eQTL) or faraway genes (>5 Mb; a trans-eQTL). The presence of an SNP that correlates with the methylation state of 1 or more genomic elements, such as nearby CpG sites, is referred to as a methylQTL or meQTL.

- RNA-Seq: A next-generation sequencing technology that allows quantitative profiling of the transcriptome (eg, identifying the presence and amount of messenger RNA in a sample of cells, tissues).

- Single-nucleotide polymorphism (SNP): A DNA sequence variation affecting only 1 nucleotide, typically present in at least 1% of a given population. For instance, in the hypothetical sequence AGT(C)TA, the substitution of cytosine by thymine resulting in a sequence of AGT(T)TA would define an SNP.

- Structural variation (SV): Large-scale DNA sequence variants. Copy number variants (see previous definition) producing deletion or duplication of a genomic segment are structural variants, as are genomic rearrangements not resulting in a gain or loss of genetic material, such as an inversion or translocation.

- Transcriptomics: Study of the set of all RNA transcripts produced by the genome, usually studied in particular tissues or organs (eg, blood) or cell types (eg, CD4+ T lymphocytes).

many possible explanations for this problem, which is referred to as "missing herita-bility"[6] (**Box 2**). In some cases, it is possible that the estimate of heritability is inflated. Recent studies of the heritability of RA reported only 12% of phenotypic variance in the susceptibility to RA due to additive genetic effects,[7] whereas typical estimates from previous studies ranged between 50% and 60%.[8] This study instead found a 50% contribution from shared environmental effects and 38% from nonshared envi-ronmental effects.[7]

Alternatively, methodological factors may be implicated. For example, a recent GWAS of RA identified thousands of variants, which individually do not meet the threshold of association, but collectively constitute a substantial fraction (~20%) of disease risk.[9] Cohort design, study design, and disease definition also may contribute to this problem. For instance, transethnic meta-analyses of a disease performed by many groups in collaboration often include different disease subtypes or include patients using different diagnostic criteria, leading to failure to capture available heri-tability through inclusion of heterogeneous subtypes of patients.

Box 2
Possible reasons for missing heritability in large-scale genomic studies

- Polygenicity and nonadditive genetic effects: Nonadditive genetic effects (see **Box 1** for definition) are not well measured by traditional methods of estimating heritability, and therefore might represent sources of missing heritability. For instance, haplotypes of common SNPs could explain a fraction of the missing heritability, which could be related to epistasis (the interaction of genes, which changes their effect) or better tagging of pathogenetic variants. Recent studies of complex diseases suggest that thousands of variants may each contribute a small fraction of disease risk. However, the contributions of marginally associated variants are often not included in the heritability accounted for in a given study. Thus, estimates of heritability based only on highly significant SNPs would not include such effects, resulting in inability to account for disease heritability. This appears to be a major source of missing heritability.

- Rare variants and structural variants: Many kinds of genetic variants (eg, short insertions and deletions), structural variants (eg, copy number variants), and rare variants are not well assayed by current genotyping arrays. There are several reports of structural variant association with rheumatic diseases, but these associations have generally been difficult to reproduce. Current NGS technology can capture information on these variants, but with much lower accuracy than on common variants, making their contribution difficult to assess. Despite this limited accuracy, several large sequencing studies have been performed with the goal of identifying rare variants implicated in autoimmune disease, and often conclude they do not account for a substantial fraction of missing heritability. It will be necessary to obtain very large studies of long-read sequencing data to accurately assess the contribution of rare and structural variants.

- Inflated heritability estimates: If heritability is overestimated, then the amount of missing heritability also will be high. It is possible that many estimates in the literature misattribute environmental effects on disease risk as genetic liability. Although debate continues, many experts do not expect inflated heritability estimates to be a major contributor to the problem of missing heritability.

- Epigenetic effects: Because some forms of epigenetic variation are inherited, phenotypic variance incorrectly attributed to genetic rather than epigenetic mechanisms could produce artificially high heritability estimates. Such effects may account for a moderate or large portion of missing heritability.

- Biotechnology effects: The use of different platforms and technologies, superimposed on other effects, may lead to errors in heritability estimates. With sound analytical practices, such effects on estimation of missing heritability should be minor.

Other studies indicate that some missing heritability may reside in genetic variants not readily identifiable with current technologies. For instance, the genetic association of *FCGR3B* with SLE may be caused by structural variation (SV) (see **Box 1**),[10] although to our knowledge there are no conclusive data that a pathogenic SV produces a specific rheumatic disease association indexed in the National Human Genome Research Institute GWAS Catalog.[1] Advances in technology, such as the ability to infer "phased haplotypes" (see **Box 1**) from genomic DNA using long-read next-generation sequencing (NGS)[11,12] technology platforms, could enable better identification of contributions of SVs and haplotypes to missing heritability than current NGS platforms.

Many recent functional studies have shown that rare variants (genetic variants having an allele frequency of <5%) contribute to a spectrum of phenotypes, including rheumatic diseases.[13,14] Several studies have sought to quantify the contribution of rare variants to missing heritability of complex diseases. For instance, 1 large exome-sequencing study examined risk loci from 6 autoimmune diseases and found that rare variants contributed less than 3% of the heritability explained by common variants at known risk loci.[15] However, more recent studies have found that most autoimmune risk variants lie in noncoding elements ($\sim$90%), greatly limiting the value of an exome-based approach for autoimmune applications. Indeed, until very large, high-depth, whole-genome sequencing studies are widely available, quantifying the contribution of rare variants in rheumatic disease will remain problematic. Further description of likely sources of missing heritability is provided in **Box 2**.

HIGH-THROUGHPUT OMICS APPROACHES THAT CAN BE INTEGRATED WITH GENETIC DATA TO UNDERSTAND RHEUMATIC DISEASES
Gene Expression

RNA-seq
Advances in biotechnology have led to high-throughput studies of gene expression (the transcriptome) that can lend insight into the pathogenesis of rheumatic diseases. RNA-Seq (see **Box 1**) is a method of interrogating the transcriptome that uses NGS to identify and quantify RNA transcripts, and offers several advantages over array-based technologies.[16] Notably, this includes the ability to identify allelic imbalance, to quantify gene expression in a transcript-specific manner, and to capture unexpected alternative splicing, truncation, and post-transcriptional modification events.[17] RNA-Seq has been used to perform biomarker discovery in peripheral blood monocytes in RA, and to study differential expression in synovial fibroblasts[18] in RA and monocytes in SLE.[19] Focused analyses of a single locus using RNA-Seq can provide a detailed picture of mRNA and noncoding RNA.[20] A recent study of the *TRAF1-C5* locus revealed a long noncoding RNA (lncRNA) (see **Box 1**) that influences C5 levels in RA.[21] In SLE, single-gene profiling of *IRF5* was performed to assess the well-known population-specific diversity and genetic associations in the locus. Notably, this study identified 14 new differentially spliced *IRF5* transcript variants and found that one of the risk haplotypes for SLE is among the most abundant transcripts produced in the disease.[22] RNA-Seq has also been used to study microRNA in the salivary glands of patients with SS[23] and to investigate gene regulation in RA as a part of an integrative bioinformatics approach.[24]

Typically, RNA-Seq measures a bulk sample of cells of a given type. However, individual cells isolated from samples of whole blood are frequently in different states producing different amounts of transcript.[25] Single-cell RNA-Seq may detect differences in transcript splicing or transcript isoform expression between cells that are lost on aggregation even among seemingly phenotypically similar cells isolated from the same tissue.[25,26] This rapidly maturing technology has been used to analyze expanded CD4+ T cells in the peripheral blood and synovium of patients with RA.[27] This study revealed that skewing of phenotypes of expanded CD4+ T-cell clones is likely due to nonspecific expansion of naïve and memory T-cell subsets. RNA-Seq is also well-suited to studying regulatory variants found in rheumatic diseases.[28]

Expression quantitative trait loci

Integration of genetic/genomic data with expression data has provided important insights. SNPs (see **Box 1**) that influence gene expression are called expression quantitative trait loci (eQTL); these may affect the expression of nearby genes (*cis*-eQTLs) or distant genes (*trans*-eQTLs) (see QTL in **Box 1**). eQTLs are enriched among suspected pathogenic variants in autoimmune risk loci. A recent study used eQTLs to quantify the contribution of gene expression to heritability and found that, on average, 21% of disease heritability was attributable to the cis-genetic component of gene expression levels for many complex phenotypes, including rheumatic diseases.[29] In general, *cis*-eQTLs are more commonly associated with complex disease and tend to have a greater impact on gene expression compared with *trans*-eQTLs.[30]

Although there is much evidence that eQTLs are important in rheumatic diseases, relatively few variants have well-characterized pathogenic effects. rs140490, a cis-eQTL associated with SLE, is one such example.[2,31] rs140490 is just upstream of the 5' untranslated region (see **Box 1**) of *UBE2L3*, and is associated with increased expression and translation of *UBE2L3*, probably through diminished degradation of the nuclear factor (NF)-κB inhibitor-α (IκBα).[32] The resulting activation of NF-κB leads to increased B-cell survival in both healthy controls and patients with SLE. Patients with SLE with the risk genotype have elevated *UBE2L3* within proliferating and activated B cells, as well as increased counts of antibody-producing plasmablasts. This example demonstrates the complexity of characterizing pathogenic variants in SLE: the variant is located in a regulatory region affecting only some disease-relevant cell types (B cells and monocytes) and functions in a temporally variable and an activation-state–dependent manner.

Recent studies have integrated genetic and eQTL data on a massive scale. An approach called summary data–based Mendelian randomization (see **Box 1**) used genome-wide genetic data from more than 338,000 people and eQTL data from more than 5000 people to link genes in 126 risk loci to 5 different phenotypes, including RA.[33] This finding highlights the ability of this technique to identify novel disease associations. Methods of imputation (see **Box 1**) of gene expression based on reference panels are being devised. Such advancement will allow identification of expression-trait associations of small effect[34] while avoiding the high cost of obtaining eQTL data.

Epigenetics/Epigenomics

Several major classes of epigenetic regulation are relevant to human disease,[35] and are assayed using a growing number of technologies.[36] Analogous to eQTLs,[37] methylQTLs (meQTLs; see Quantitative trait locus in **Box 1**) are CpG sites the methylation state of which correlates with a genetic variant. Such methylated DNA impedes transcriptional proteins and increases affinity for proteins that alter DNA accessibility. Thus, cellular outcomes, such as transcription and cell fate, are altered in ways that can impact rheumatic disease. For example, in a study of SLE among twins, DNA methylation differences are associated with twin discordance,[38] and a study of 24 patients with SLE and controls showed evidence of differential DNA methylation in CD4+

T cells.[39] Many meQTLs are found in tight LD with risk variants for rheumatic diseases,[40] although the possibility that both independently affect transcription cannot be excluded. Other epigenetic assays, such as ATAC-Seq (see **Box 1**), have been used to investigate the correlation of nucleosome modifications with functional elements genome-wide, for instance in naïve B cells in SLE,[41] whereas DNAse-seq pairs DNAse hypersensitivity methodology with deep sequencing to identify portions of the genome accessible to transcriptional machinery and transcription factors. One methodology integrating epigenomic and other assays, RASQUAL (Robust Allele Specific QUAntification and quality controL), has been applied to autoimmune risk loci and is described in further detail later in this article.

Epigenetic factors likely contribute to the heritability of rheumatic diseases,[42] and may alter heritability estimates derived from genetic data. Because epigenetic modifications can be inherited across generations, but are not assayed by genotyping chips or by whole genome sequencing,[43] it is difficult to exclude the possibility that epigenetic alterations could account for a proportion of disease risk normally attributed to genetics. This assertion gains further support from studies suggesting that such alterations affect human disease phenotypes.[44] In SLE, there is an association between DNA methylation patterns and twin discordance.[38] Several mechanisms, including imprinting, incomplete erasure of DNA methylation, and persistence of histone markings,[42,43,45] could produce such an effect. Nevertheless, at this time, estimates of epigenetic missing heredity are not widespread for complex diseases.

Proteomics and Metabolomics

Proteomic studies typically profile a tissue or fluid important to the disease process, such as synovial fluid in RA, often with the goal of finding biomarkers to enable early diagnosis or identification of common pathways.[46] Other common applications in RA include monitoring disease activity, disease severity, and treatment efficacy.[47] Importantly, levels of a particular protein (for example in serum, plasma, or synovial fluid) cannot be inferred from gene expression data,[48] due in part to the presence of uncoupled posttranslational protein regulatory mechanisms,[49] and in part to the aggregation of proteins from various nearby tissues and bodily fluids. Advances in mass spectrometry[3] have enabled proteomic assays to evolve beyond simple catalogs of protein abundance by capturing the rates of protein synthesis, degradation, and turnover. Incorporation of subcellular localization and tissue abundance of the proteins being studied[3,4] adds a further dimensionality to these increasingly rich datasets. Therefore, proteomic technology is becoming more useful in determining biological effects (eg, increased protein levels) of upstream events (eg, gene expression levels influenced by genetic variants and epigenetic factors) in rheumatic diseases.

Informatics-based approaches to characterizing protein interaction networks have also been useful to understand rheumatic diseases. Current evidence suggests genetic risk variants for rheumatic diseases are organized in pathways, physically interact with one another,[50] and are enriched for protein-protein interaction network modules.[51] Recognition of this pattern in complex diseases has already led to identification of drug targets,[52] and has been used to prioritize gene relevancy within risk loci.[53,54] Such interaction network modeling techniques have been used to perform functional characterization of pathogenic variants among genomic, transcriptomic, and proteomic data.[55]

Techniques used in large-scale metabolomics studies include proton nuclear magnetic resonance and mass spectrometry. These have been used to profile small molecules in rheumatic diseases and have been reviewed in detail recently.[56] Integration of the metabolome with GWAS data has enabled detection of genetic variation that affects metabolite levels (referred to as metabolome QTLs) in several organisms,[57–60] but continued improvements to modeling and methodology are needed before application to human rheumatic diseases becomes widespread.

Cell-Specific and Tissue-Specific Gene Expression: Influence on Integrated Multi-Omic Analysis of Rheumatic Diseases

One crucial consideration in the interpretation of transcriptomic, epigenomic, and proteomic analyses is the cell-based or tissue-based specificity of expression of variants that may exert pathogenic effects. Consortia such as Encyclopedia of DNA elements (ENCODE) provide a catalog of functional elements across the human genome.[61] More recently, the National Institutes of Health Roadmap Epigenomics Mapping Consortium provided a publically available catalog of methylation, histone modification, chromatin accessibility, and other data.[62] Drawing heavily on such datasets, a recent study fine mapped pathogenic autoimmune disease variants. There was markedly different enrichment in acetylation of cis-regulatory elements of 33 different cell types across 39 autoimmune diseases and related traits.[30] The investigators of another variant prioritization methodology provide more than 8000 genome-wide annotations to aid investigators in study of risk loci.[63] Thus, although it can be daunting to isolate the effect of a genetic variant to the appropriate tissue, the increasingly comprehensive annotation of the human genome can aid investigators in selecting the appropriate tissues and focusing hypotheses.

One recent study combined an impressive array of publically available data and tools for analysis of microRNA, transcription factor binding sites, epigenetic data, data from ENCODE, and chromatin immunoprecipitation data. By analyzing these aggregated data, the investigators were able to frame and test the hypothesis that a variant in the autoimmune risk locus *ETS1* increases *pSTAT1* binding and decreases *ETS1* expression in Asian individuals, but not other populations, with SLE.[64] Thus, tissue-specific effects are often also subject to additional complicating factors, such as activation state dependency, transethnic differences, and temporal variability, necessitating careful design of follow-up functional studies. The emergence of large datasets to provide reference points that can be used to interpret data from cells and tissues from diseases will be critical to these future studies.

APPROACHES TO DATA INTEGRATION

Integration of high-throughput data for analysis of rheumatic diseases is a complicated topic reviewed in detail elsewhere.[65] We include a brief summary of 2 types of techniques (multistage analysis and metadimensional analysis) and 2 forms of data filtering (intrinsic and extrinsic) to provide helpful context. Intrinsic data filtering uses information from the dataset itself, such as filtering genetic variants based on linkage to other variants of interest in that dataset. Extrinsic data filtering is based on information outside of the dataset, such as the inclusion of genomic annotations from separate studies such as ENCODE. Currently, both intrinsic and extrinsic data filtering are essential for efficient characterization of complex disease genetics.

Multistage Analysis

Multistage analysis sequentially examines relationships between each dataset and the other datasets, and also between each dataset and the trait. For instance, the correlation of a genetic variant with gene expression level is performed in 1 analytical step, then correlation of such a variant or gene expression level with a disease state like RA is performed in a subsequent step. Such designs are common in rheumatic disease genetic research, such as the analysis of eQTLs, which includes analysis of genetic variants (eg, SNPs) and gene expression levels.

Multistage analyses have much greater power to detect the effect of a single SNP on gene expression than several weak independent effects that together lead to important changes in gene expression.[65–67] Although multistaged analyses are useful, they also have limitations. In rheumatic disease research, the combined effects of multiple variants on gene regulation may be critical (the multiple enhancer variant hypothesis), therefore making them difficult to discover in multistage analysis.[68]

Metadimensional Analysis

For complex multivariate data sets from different platforms, metadimensional analysis may perform well.[57] This technique takes advantage of simultaneous combination of multiple data types into a single search space to construct a final model. Metadimensional analysis can use 3 types of integration strategies; that is, to combine raw or processed data sets by directly "concatenation" of them before modeling and analysis, to perform data mapping or "transformation" first before modeling and analysis, and to model the data independently before merging all models toward the final analysis. Metadimensional analysis approaches can draw on a variety of techniques, such as regression trees,[69] Bayesian networks,[70] and evolutionary computation.[71] These algorithms may be tuned to search for known conventional relationships, or could be relaxed to search for new or unexpected complex relationships, but are often computationally intensive.

Selected Insights Gleaned from Integrative Analyses

In the following section, we describe several examples in which integrative analyses of large datasets have been used to provide novel insights into the pathogenesis of rheumatic diseases. For example, a recent study noted genetic and epigenetic interactions affect the expression of the gene *LBH* and potentially risk for diseases such as RA, SLE, and celiac disease.[72] Making use of intrinsic and extrinsic data filtering, this study integrated GWAS, gene expression, and DNA methylation data in RA with publically available data from the ENCODE project. Using reporter constructs methylated in vitro and transfected into synovial fibroblasts, the investigators showed that the RA-associated SNP in *LBH* decreased *LBH* transcription. This study illustrates how confluence of data from multiple genomic assays, specifically a GWAS risk variant for RA, a differentially methylated locus, and open DNA regulatory elements, can aid in characterization of RA pathobiology by showing how a functional SNP and a differentially methylated enhancer regulate aggressiveness of RA fibroblast-like synoviocyte(s).

Another recent study presented a method to integrate transcriptomic data and epigenetic data in a highly novel way. The RASQUAL method[73] was used to combine expression and chromatin conformation data (from ATAC-Seq) and led to significant findings within RA risk loci. Strikingly, an SNP identified by previous GWAS of RA, rs909685 in *SYNGR1*, may act to alter gene expression by altering chromatin structure and accessibility. The finding that a genetic variant affects the 3-dimensional conformation of DNA and histone folding illustrates the utility of integrative analysis by offering an example of how these methods naturally provide a springboard for future studies compared with association analysis alone.

Integrated proteomics approaches are becoming more common as well. The COMBINE (Controlling chronic inflammatory diseases with combined efforts) study integrated DNA, RNA, flow cytometry, and proteomic data to predict clinical response to tumor necrosis factor (TNF) inhibitors (TNFi) in RA.[74] Specifically, results from commercial protein biomarker panels, DNA microarrays, and RNA-Seq were filtered based on publically available datasets on TNFi responsiveness. Measurements of these biomarkers, genetic variants, and expression levels were then fit into a linear regression model with treatment response 3 months after initiation of TNFi as the primary outcome. This approach replicated 11 biomarkers for anti-TNF treatment in RA and successfully combined multiple levels of omics data into a predictive model with a sensitivity of 73% and a specificity of 78%. Studies such as these are early indicators of the potential of integrative approaches in precision medicine.

PRIORITIZATION OF GENOMIC VARIANTS/PATHWAYS FOR FUNCTIONAL ANALYSIS

One of the problems arising from the analyses of large numbers of patients with rheumatic diseases using high-throughput methodologies is the generation of a very large number of candidate risk loci to be examined. The expense and logistics of analyzing a large number of loci is daunting, and there is a need for systematic, rational, and biology-based approaches to identify variants with the highest likelihood of clinically relevant effects. Numerous methodologically distinct approaches to variant prioritization have been developed and several have been applied to rheumatic diseases. Prioritization approaches using intrinsic or extrinsic data filtering, or both (see **Box 1**) are routinely used, and leverage enrichment of variants bearing certain functional annotations,[63,75,76] transethnic differences in genetic variation,[63,77] and association strength of genetic variants.[30,63,76–78] Other tools, such as OMIM Explorer, integrate high-dimensional clinical phenotyping data with genotype information, and offer powerful frameworks for variant prioritization as well.[79] Due to the number, complexity, and size of the datasets used to filter variants, we anticipate these increasingly sophisticated methods will be critical to guiding optimal variant prioritization based on empirical classifiers. Here, we discuss a few variant prioritization tools that have been calibrated on, or applied to, rheumatic diseases. Many other variant prioritization tools are available and under development but are not discussed in this review.[75,79–81]

The Probabilistically Identified Causal Single-Nucleotide Polymorphism Algorithm

A study of dense genotyping of a large number of patients with different autoimmune diseases and controls was used to develop an algorithm called Probabilistically Identified Causal SNPs (PICS).[30] This algorithm estimates the likelihood that each variant is pathogenic, using the strength of association and LD values of variants in a locus. Application of this algorithm to genetic data from 21 autoimmune diseases, including Sjögren syndrome, RA, SLE, and seronegative spondyloarthritis (SNSA), resulted in identification of approximately 9000 candidate causal variants called PICS. Nearly 90% of these "autoimmune" PICS mapped outside of coding regions, and 60% to immune-cell enhancers. Strikingly, these PICS tended to be near to, but outside of, canonical binding sites of regulators of immune differentiation, in less well-characterized regions of the enhancer. Therefore, in addition to providing a prioritization tool, and identifying a large list of candidate SNPs, this study is significant for its suggestion that current gene regulatory models may be incomplete.

The Probabilistic Annotation INTegratOR Algorithm

The Probabilistic Annotation INTegratOR (PAINTOR) algorithm is an open-source fine-mapping program that integrates association summary statistics (Z-scores) from GWAS, LD scores, and functional annotation information. It was developed to model the likelihood of causality of 1 or more SNPs in a risk locus. One of the strengths of this algorithm is that it can leverage transethnic studies to better prioritize variants.

PAINTOR2 was recently used to perform a meta-analysis of a large genetic dataset from RA.[53] The algorithm assigned a very high posterior probability value of causality to rs2476601, a missense variant in *PTPN22*. Given that the effects of rs2476601 are relatively well studied and that it underlies risk of many autoimmune and rheumatic conditions, this finding might be regarded as a positive control. Intriguingly, it also assigned a very high posterior probability to variants in 4 other RA risk loci, *ANKRD55*, *TNFRSF14*, *UBASH3A*, and *TYK2*, the functional roles of which are not well established. Identification of variants such as these increases cost efficacy by reducing the number of likely candidates (the credible set), thereby increasing the likelihood of studying a pathogenic variant. PAINTOR 3.0, the most recently released version of the software, extends the PAINTOR framework to multiple traits across transethnic studies, and is capable of modeling 1 or more causal variants per locus (http://bogdan.bioinformatics.ucla.edu/2016/11/03/paintor-3-0/, accessed December 26, 2016). PAINTOR uses functional annotation as input to enable better prioritization of candidate variants, or output enrichment of candidate causal variants within functional classes.[63]

A distinct Bayesian approach to accomplish the latter goal was recently described.[82] It uses association statistics computed across the genome to identify classes of genomic elements that are enriched with (or depleted of) loci influencing a trait. Thus, this approach incorporates internal filtering to make inferences about the relative importance of annotation data. Reweighting each GWAS by using information from functional genomics increased the number of loci with high-confidence associations by approximately 5%.

The Molecular Interaction Network-Based Ranking Algorithm

There is a need for developing systems biology approaches to integrate comprehensive genetic information and provide new insight on complex disease biology. We took such an approach[54] to study type 2 diabetes (T2D); however, the method is readily applicable to the study of other rheumatic diseases, such as RA. The method works by bringing in protein-protein interaction data to construct a disease-specific molecular interaction network, which consists of disease-specific genetic risk genes and all their direct interacting gene partners. Then, network centrality measures using "network topological features," such as hubs and clustering coefficients are used to rank genes from the network or network modules. These genes can be further ranked based on additional GWAS association hazard ratio data and related pathway enrichment and gene set enrichments results. We found that *PI3KR1*, *ESR1*, and *ENPP1* were the interconnected T2D disease network "hub" genes most strongly associated to T2D genetic risks.[54] Contrary to expectations, the well-characterized gene *TCF7L2* was not among the highest-ranked genes in the T2D gene list. However, many highly relevant pathways were reaffirmed from the integrated data sets, including pathways involved in insulin signaling, T2D, mature-onset diabetes, adipocytokine signaling pathways, and cancer-related pathways. Similar pathway and network analysis approaches based on this framework[83] are critical for improving interpretations of genetic variations and genetic risk factors. These approaches may facilitate attribution of complex disease genetic risk to the summative genetic effects of many genes involved in a broad range of signaling pathways and functional networks.

METHODS FOR EXPLORATION OF RELATIONSHIPS BETWEEN CLINICAL PHENOTYPES

Given the overlap between autoimmune diseases, techniques that can be used to study relationships between phenotypes are of intense interest. The principles of Mendelian randomization (see **Box 1**) can be applied in a variety of ways to make inferences about environmental determinants of disease, among other applications.[84] An innovative algorithm was used to examine 43 GWAS on 42 human traits to identify pairs of traits sharing association of multiple (common; minor allele frequency >5%) genetic variants.[85] This analysis found that variants that increase risk of coronary artery disease (CAD) tend to decrease risk of RA, whereas variants affecting RA appear to have little effect on CAD risk. This can be interpreted as evidence of a causal link between CAD and RA, but this result could not be confirmed in a larger study despite other successes of the algorithm.[85] The results obtained in this detailed study generally agree with data from randomized controlled trials and Mendelian randomization studies.[85] Importantly, inferred causal relationships obtained from Mendelian randomization frameworks such as these may be used even if the studies paired share no common subjects. Therefore, given the paucity of high-quality comprehensive phenomic datasets,[85–87] these methodologies are exceedingly valuable because they can provide information that would otherwise be available only through costly trials. Equally important are the implications to the paradigm of personalized medicine: if pleiotropic effects are widespread in the phenome, then even a targeted intervention aimed at a single pathogenic variant is likely to affect other phenotypes. Alternatively, if legal and organizational obstacles can be overcome, high-dimensional phenomic data may ultimately become available through the electronic medical record, curated by clinical centers, enabling exploration of the extent of pleiotropy and genome-phenome interactions. Early steps toward this goal have been made in the form of phenome-wide association studies.[88]

FUNCTIONAL VALIDATION OF PATHOGENIC REGULATORY VARIATION IN COMPLEX DISEASE

We have argued that the integration of multiple omics technologies can be used to frame specific hypotheses and design experiments to test them. However, even when such analysis is done well, functional validation of findings from omic assays remains a crucial limiting step to advancement of our understanding. This may be particularly difficult if the distribution and concentration of multiple genetic variants in noncoding elements, such as enhancers, is critical to autoimmune disease risk, as is currently expected.[68] Nevertheless, there are several promising technologies that are currently used for functional validation of regulatory variants, and that are potentially scalable. The creation of multiple distinct Cas9 mutant enzymes facilitates different functions, such as gene silencing, gene activation, or site-specific DNA recognition and cleavage and enables study of complex disease variants.[89] Certain Cas9 mutants can introduce precise mutations or knock-ins such as those found in immune enhancer regions. A recent review covers developments in CRISPR/Cas9 relevant for rheumatologists.[90] Combining reporter assays with DNA synthesis,[91] DNAse-seq,[92] and barcoding[93] has substantially increased throughput of these assays, even allowing massively parallel interrogation of regulatory variants in human cells.[94,95] RNAi-based screens, which could recapitulate loss-of-function analyses produced by pathogenic risk variants in regulatory regions in vivo,[96] also could be used to study rheumatic diseases. Continued refinement of these technologies and others may eventually prove commensurate to the challenge presented by integrated omics data; namely, understanding the context and biologic roles of thousands of pathogenic risk variants acting in concert to produce rheumatic disease.

SUMMARY

In summary, we begin by providing an overview of heritability of rheumatic diseases and describing potential explanations for why much of genetic risk remains unknown.

We then highlight how the use of high-throughput omics approaches, such as RNA-Seq, expression (and other forms) of QTLs, epigenetics, and proteomics can help understand the genetic basis for the pathogenesis of rheumatic diseases. Having outlined several genomic technologies, we then describe approaches to integrating multiple forms of data, including multistage and metadimensional analytical designs (using extrinsic and intrinsic data filtering) and provide specific examples of novel insights into the mechanisms of rheumatic diseases that these analyses provide. We also describe statistical approaches to prioritizing genomic variants for functional analysis. We provide examples showing that these integrative analytical approaches are valuable because they are better at providing context necessary for researchers to frame targeted hypotheses. Overall, we believe coordinated study of human biology alongside programs to analyze large datasets in detail raise hope for better approaches to the diagnosis, treatment, and prevention of complex conditions such as the rheumatic diseases.

REFERENCES

1. Welter D, MacArthur J, Morales J, et al. The NHGRI GWAS catalog, a curated resource of SNP-trait associations. Nucleic Acids Res 2014;42:D1001-6.
2. Gutierrez-Arcelus M, Rich SS, Raychaudhuri S. Autoimmune diseases—connecting risk alleles with molecular traits of the immune system. Nat Rev Genet 2016; 17:160-74.
3. Visscher PM, Macgregor S, Benyamin B, et al. Genome partitioning of genetic variation for height from 11,214 sibling pairs. Am J Hum Genet 2007;81:1104-10.
4. Vinkhuyzen AA, Wray NR, Yang J, et al. Estimation and partition of heritability in human populations using whole-genome analysis methods. Ann Rev Genet 2013; 47:75-95.
5. Visscher PM, Goddard ME. A general unified framework to assess the sampling variance of heritability estimates using pedigree or marker-based relationships. Genetics 2015;199:223-32.
6. Manolio TA, Collins FS, Cox NJ, et al. Finding the missing heritability of complex diseases. Nature 2009;461:747-53.
7. Svendsen AJ, Kyvik KO, Houen G, et al. On the origin of rheumatoid arthritis: the impact of environment and genes–a population based twin study. PLoS One 2013;8(2):e57304.
8. Kurkó J, Besenyei T, Laki J, et al. Genetics of rheumatoid arthritis - a comprehensive review. Clin Rev Allergy Immunol 2013;45(2):170-9.
9. Stahl EA, Wegmann D, Trynka G, et al. Bayesian inference analyses of the polygenic architecture of rheumatoid arthritis. Nat Genet 2012;44:483-9.
10. Ptacek T, Li X, Kelley JM, et al. Copy number variants in genetic susceptibility and severity of systemic lupus erythematosus. Cytogenet Genome Res 2008;123: 142-7.
11. Chaisson MJ, Huddleston J, Dennis MY, et al. Resolving the complexity of the human genome using single-molecule sequencing. Nature 2015;517:608-11.
12. Zheng GX, Lau BT, Schnall-Levin M, et al. Haplotyping germline and cancer genomes with high-throughput linked-read sequencing. Nat Biotechnol 2016;34: 303-11.
13. Rieux-Laucat F, Casanova JL. Immunology. Autoimmunity by haploinsufficiency. Science 2014;345:1560-1.

14. Rice GI, del Toro Duany Y, Jenkinson EM, et al. Gain-of-function mutations in IFIH1 cause a spectrum of human disease phenotypes associated with upregulated type I interferon signaling. Nat Genet 2014;46:503–9.
15. Hunt KA, Mistry V, Bockett NA, et al. Negligible impact of rare autoimmune-locus coding-region variants on missing heritability. Nature 2013;498:232–5.
16. Giannopoulou EG, Elemento O, Ivashkiv LB. Use of RNA sequencing to evaluate rheumatic disease patients. Arthritis Res Ther 2015;17:167.
17. Maher CA, Kumar-Sinha C, Cao X, et al. Transcriptome sequencing to detect gene fusions in cancer. Nature 2009;458:97–101.
18. Heruth DP, Gibson M, Grigoryev DN, et al. RNA-seq analysis of synovial fibroblasts brings new insights into rheumatoid arthritis. Cell Biosci 2012;2:43.
19. Shi L, Zhang Z, Yu AM, et al. The SLE transcriptome exhibits evidence of chronic endotoxin exposure and has widespread dysregulation of non-coding and coding RNAs. PLoS One 2014;9:e93846.
20. Clark MB, Mercer TR, Bussotti G, et al. Quantitative gene profiling of long non-coding RNAs with targeted RNA sequencing. Nat Methods 2015;12:339–42.
21. Messemaker TC, Frank-Bertoncelj M, Marques RB, et al. A novel long non-coding RNA in the rheumatoid arthritis risk locus TRAF1-C5 influences C5 mRNA levels. Genes Immun 2016;17:85–92.
22. Stone RC, Du P, Feng D, et al. RNA-Seq for enrichment and analysis of IRF5 transcript expression in SLE. PLoS One 2013;8:e54487.
23. Tandon M, Gallo A, Jang SI, et al. Deep sequencing of short RNAs reveals novel microRNAs in minor salivary glands of patients with Sjogren's syndrome. Oral Dis 2012;18:127–31.
24. Song YJ, Li G, He JH, et al. Bioinformatics-based identification of microRNA-regulated and rheumatoid arthritis-associated genes. PloS One 2015;10:e0137551.
25. Vieira Braga FA, Teichmann SA, Chen X. Genetics and immunity in the era of single-cell genomics. Hum Mol Genet 2016;25(R2):R141–8.
26. Stubbington MJ, Lonnberg T, Proserpio V, et al. T cell fate and clonality inference from single-cell transcriptomes. Nat Methods 2016;13:329–32.
27. Ishigaki K, Shoda H, Kochi Y, et al. Quantitative and qualitative characterization of expanded CD4+ T cell clones in rheumatoid arthritis patients. Sci Rep 2015;5:12937.
28. Lappalainen T, Sammeth M, Friedlander MR, et al. Transcriptome and genome sequencing uncovers functional variation in humans. Nature 2013;501:506–11.
29. Luke J, O'Connor AG, Liu X, et al. Estimating the proportion of disease heritability mediated by gene expression levels. New York: Cold Spring Harbor Laboratory; 2017. p. 118018.
30. Farh KK, Marson A, Zhu J, et al. Genetic and epigenetic fine mapping of causal autoimmune disease variants. Nature 2015;518:337–43.
31. Harley JB, Alarcon-Riquelme ME, Criswell LA, et al. Genome-wide association scan in women with systemic lupus erythematosus identifies susceptibility variants in ITGAM, PXK, KIAA1542 and other loci. Nat Genet 2008;40:204–10.
32. Lewis MJ, Vyse S, Shields AM, et al. UBE2L3 polymorphism amplifies NF-kappaB activation and promotes plasma cell development, linking linear ubiquitination to multiple autoimmune diseases. Am J Hum Genet 2015;96:221–34.
33. Zhu Z, Zhang F, Hu H, et al. Integration of summary data from GWAS and eQTL studies predicts complex trait gene targets. Nat Genet 2016;48:481–7.
34. Gusev A, Ko A, Shi H, et al. Integrative approaches for large-scale transcriptome-wide association studies. Nat Genet 2016;48:245–52.

35. Brookes E, Shi Y. Diverse epigenetic mechanisms of human disease. Annu Rev Genet 2014;48:237–68.
36. Greenleaf WJ. Assaying the epigenome in limited numbers of cells. Methods 2015;72:51–6.
37. Gibbs JR, van der Brug MP, Hernandez DG, et al. Abundant quantitative trait loci exist for DNA methylation and gene expression in human brain. PLoS Genet 2010;6:e1000952.
38. Javierre BM, Fernandez AF, Richter J, et al. Changes in the pattern of DNA methylation associate with twin discordance in systemic lupus erythematosus. Genome Res 2010;20:170–9.
39. Jeffries MA, Dozmorov M, Tang Y, et al. Genome-wide DNA methylation patterns in CD4+ T cells from patients with systemic lupus erythematosus. Epigenetics 2011;6:593–601.
40. Lemire M, Zaidi SH, Ban M, et al. Long-range epigenetic regulation is conferred by genetic variation located at thousands of independent loci. Nat Commun 2015;6:6326.
41. Scharer CD, Blalock EL, Barwick BG, et al. ATAC-seq on biobanked specimens defines a unique chromatin accessibility structure in naive SLE B cells. Scientific Rep 2016;6:27030.
42. Zhou Y, Simpson S Jr, Holloway AF, et al. The potential role of epigenetic modifications in the heritability of multiple sclerosis. Mult Scler 2014;20:135–40.
43. Trerotola M, Relli V, Simeone P, et al. Epigenetic inheritance and the missing heritability. Hum genomics 2015;9:17.
44. Yehuda R, Daskalakis NP, Bierer LM, et al. Holocaust exposure induced intergenerational effects on FKBP5 methylation. Biol Psychiatry 2016;80:372–80.
45. Connolly S, Heron EA. Review of statistical methodologies for the detection of parent-of-origin effects in family trio genome-wide association data with binary disease traits. Brief Bioinformatics 2015;16:429–48.
46. Bhattacharjee M, Balakrishnan L, Renuse S, et al. Synovial fluid proteome in rheumatoid arthritis. Clin Proteomics 2016;13:12.
47. Park YJ, Chung MK, Hwang D, et al. Proteomics in rheumatoid arthritis research. Immune Netw 2015;15:177–85.
48. Hillenmeyer ME, Fung E, Wildenhain J, et al. The chemical genomic portrait of yeast: uncovering a phenotype for all genes. Science 2008;320:362–5.
49. Breker M, Schuldiner M. The emergence of proteome-wide technologies: systematic analysis of proteins comes of age. Nat Rev Mol Cel Biol 2014;15:453–64.
50. Rossin EJ, Lage K, Raychaudhuri S, et al. Proteins encoded in genomic regions associated with immune-mediated disease physically interact and suggest underlying biology. PLoS Genet 2011;7:e1001273.
51. Marson A, Housley WJ, Hafler DA. Genetic basis of autoimmunity. J Clin Invest 2015;125:2234–41.
52. Chen JY, Pinkerton SL, Shen C, et al. An integrated computational proteomics method to extract protein targets for Fanconi anemia studies. 21st annual ACM symposium on applied computing. Dijon, France, April 23–27, 2006. 173–9.
53. Okada Y, Wu D, Trynka G, et al. Genetics of rheumatoid arthritis contributes to biology and drug discovery. Nature 2014;506:376–81.
54. Hale PJ, Lopez-Yunez AM, Chen JY. Genome-wide meta-analysis of genetic susceptible genes for type 2 diabetes. BMC Syst Biol 2012;6(Suppl 3):S16.
55. Wu X, Chen JY. Molecular Interaction Networks: Topological and Functional Characterizations. In: Alterovitz G, Benson R, Ramoni M, editors. Automation in

Proteomics and Genomics: An Engineering Case-Based Approach. Chichester (UK): John Wiley & Sons Ltd.

56. Guma M, Tiziani S, Firestein GS. Metabolomics in rheumatic diseases: desperately seeking biomarkers. Nat Rev Rheumatol 2016;12:269–81.

57. Joseph B, Corwin JA, Li B, et al. Cytoplasmic genetic variation and extensive cytonuclear interactions influence natural variation in the metabolome. ELife 2013;2: e00776.

58. Reed LK, Lee K, Zhang Z, et al. Systems genomics of metabolic phenotypes in wild-type *Drosophila melanogaster*. Genetics 2014;197:781–93.

59. Nicholson G, Rantalainen M, Li JV, et al. A genome-wide metabolic QTL analysis in Europeans implicates two loci shaped by recent positive selection. PLoS Genet 2011;7:e1002270.

60. Shin SY, Fauman EB, Petersen AK, et al. An atlas of genetic influences on human blood metabolites. Nat Genet 2014;46:543–50.

61. An integrated encyclopedia of DNA elements in the human genome. Nature 2012;489:57–74.

62. Bernstein BE, Stamatoyannopoulos JA, Costello JF, et al. The NIH Roadmap Epigenomics Mapping Consortium. Nat Biotechnol 2010;28:1045–8.

63. Kichaev G, Pasaniuc B. Leveraging functional-annotation data in trans-ethnic fine-mapping studies. Am J Hum Genet 2015;97:260–71.

64. Lu X, Zoller EE, Weirauch MT, et al. Lupus risk variant increases pSTAT1 binding and decreases ETS1 expression. Am J Hum Genet 2015;96:731–9.

65. Holzinger ER, Ritchie MD. Integrating heterogeneous high-throughput data for meta-dimensional pharmacogenomics and disease-related studies. Pharmacogenomics 2012;13:213–22.

66. Culverhouse R, Suarez BK, Lin J, et al. A perspective on epistasis: limits of models displaying no main effect. Am J Hum Genet 2002;70:461–71.

67. Ritchie MD, Holzinger ER, Li R, et al. Methods of integrating data to uncover genotype-phenotype interactions. Nat Rev Genet 2015;16:85–97.

68. Corradin O, Saiakhova A, Akhtar-Zaidi B, et al. Combinatorial effects of multiple enhancer variants in linkage disequilibrium dictate levels of gene expression to confer susceptibility to common traits. Genome Res 2014;24:1–13.

69. Schwarz DF, Konig IR, Ziegler A. On safari to random jungle: a fast implementation of random forests for high-dimensional data. Bioinformatics 2010;26:1752–8.

70. Jiang X, Barmada MM, Visweswaran S. Identifying genetic interactions in genome-wide data using Bayesian networks. Genet Epidemiol 2010;34:575–81.

71. Turner SD, Dudek SM, Ritchie MD. ATHENA: a knowledge-based hybrid backpropagation-grammatical evolution neural network algorithm for discovering epistasis among quantitative trait loci. BioData Min 2010;3:5.

72. Hammaker D, Whitaker JW, Maeshima K, et al. LBH gene transcription regulation by the interplay of an enhancer risk allele and DNA methylation in rheumatoid arthritis. Arthritis Rheumatol 2016;68:2637–45.

73. Kumasaka N, Knights AJ, Gaffney DJ. Fine-mapping cellular QTLs with RASQUAL and ATAC-seq. Nat Genet 2016;48:206–13.

74. Folkersen L, Brynedal B, Diaz-Gallo LM, et al. Integration of known DNA, RNA and protein biomarkers provides prediction of anti-TNF response in rheumatoid arthritis: results from the COMBINE study. Mol Med 2016;22:322–8.

75. Hou L, Zhao H. A review of post-GWAS prioritization approaches. Front Genet 2013;4:280.

76. Kichaev G, Yang WY, Lindstrom S, et al. Integrating functional data to prioritize causal variants in statistical fine-mapping studies. PLoS Genet 2014;10:e1004722.

77. Zaitlen N, Pasaniuc B, Gur T, et al. Leveraging genetic variability across populations for the identification of causal variants. Am J Hum Genet 2010;86:23–33.

78. Chen W, Larrabee BR, Ovsyannikova IG, et al. Fine mapping causal variants with an approximate Bayesian method using marginal test statistics. Genetics 2015; 200:719–36.

79. James RA, Campbell IM, Chen ES, et al. A visual and curatorial approach to clinical variant prioritization and disease gene discovery in genome-wide diagnostics. Genome Med 2016;8:13.

80. Salatino S, Ramraj V. BrowseVCF: a web-based application and workflow to quickly prioritize disease-causative variants in VCF files. Brief Bioinformatics 2016. [Epub ahead of print].

81. Glanzmann B, Herbst H, Kinnear CJ, et al. A new tool for prioritization of sequence variants from whole exome sequencing data. Source code Biol Med 2016;11:10.

82. Pickrell JK. Joint analysis of functional genomic data and genome-wide association studies of 18 human traits. Am J Hum Genet 2014;94:559–73.

83. Wu X, Hasan MA, Chen JY. Pathway and network analysis in proteomics. J Theor Biol 2014;362:44–52.

84. Smith GD, Ebrahim S. Mendelian randomization: prospects, potentials, and limitations. Int J Epidemiol 2004;33:30–42.

85. Pickrell JK, Berisa T, Liu JZ, et al. Detection and interpretation of shared genetic influences on 42 human traits. Nat Genet 2016;48:709–17.

86. Gratten J, Visscher PM. Genetic pleiotropy in complex traits and diseases: implications for genomic medicine. Genome Med 2016;8:78.

87. Visscher PM, Yang J. A plethora of pleiotropy across complex traits. Nat Genet 2016;48:707–8.

88. Denny JC, Ritchie MD, Basford MA, et al. PheWAS: demonstrating the feasibility of a phenome-wide scan to discover gene-disease associations. Bioinformatics 2010;26:1205–10.

89. Hilton IB, D'Ippolito AM, Vockley CM, et al. Epigenome editing by a CRISPR-Cas9-based acetyltransferase activates genes from promoters and enhancers. Nat Biotechnol 2015;33:510–7.

90. Gibson GJ, Yang M. What rheumatologists need to know about CRISPR/Cas9. Nat Rev Rheumatol 2017;13(4):205–16.

91. Patwardhan RP, Hiatt JB, Witten DM, et al. Massively parallel functional dissection of mammalian enhancers in vivo. Nat Biotechnol 2012;30:265–70.

92. Murtha M, Tokcaer-Keskin Z, Tang Z, et al. FIREWACh: high-throughput functional detection of transcriptional regulatory modules in mammalian cells. Nat Methods 2014;11:559–65.

93. Arnold CD, Gerlach D, Spies D, et al. Quantitative genome-wide enhancer activity maps for five *Drosophila* species show functional enhancer conservation and turnover during cis-regulatory evolution. Nat Genet 2014;46:685–92.

94. Vockley CM, Guo C, Majoros WH, et al. Massively parallel quantification of the regulatory effects of noncoding genetic variation in a human cohort. Genome Res 2015;25:1206–14.

95. Vanhille L, Griffon A, Maqbool MA, et al. High-throughput and quantitative assessment of enhancer activity in mammals by CapStarr-seq. Nat Commun 2015;6:6905.

96. Crotty S, Pipkin ME. In vivo RNAi screens: concepts and applications. Trends Immunol 2015;36:315–22.

Drug Repositioning Strategies for the Identification of Novel Therapies for Rheumatic Autoimmune Inflammatory Diseases

Amrie C. Grammer, PhD*, Peter E. Lipsky, MD

KEYWORDS

- SLE • Lupus • Rheumatic autoimmune inflammatory disease (RAID)
- Drug repositioning • Drug repurposing • Bioinformatics

KEY POINTS

- RAID such as systemic sclerosis, myositis, Sjögren's syndrome and systemic lupus erythematosus (SLE) have had few new treatments developed over the past half century.
- Of the 82 drugs approved by the FDA from 2014 to mid-2016, only three had a RAID indication (http://www.centerwatch.com/drug-information/fda-approved-drugs/year/).
- There are four major approaches to drug repositioning: computational modeling, disease mechanism-of-action based approaches, genetic profiling and translational bioinformatics.
- Artificial intelligence cognitive computer systems (AICCS) or human bioinformaticians narrow down drug repositioning candidates using similar tools but the background and experience of human biologists inform the bioinformatic analysis in a way that a machine cannot replicate.

INTRODUCTION

There are many and varied approaches to drug repositioning that have been used in the search for effective treatments for patients with a variety of different diseases[1,2] (**Box 1**). Methodologies typically use information from one of the following: structural similarity, adverse events, literature mining, clinical trials, gene expression, genome-wide association studies (GWAS), pathways, and/or the interactome.[3,4] Drug

---

Declaration of Conflicting Interests: The authors declared no potential conflicts of interest with respect to the research, authorship, and/or publication of this article.
AMPEL BioSolutions and RILITE Research Institute, 250 West Main Street, Suite 300, Charlottesville, VA 22902, USA
* Corresponding author.
E-mail address: amriegrammer@comcast.net

Rheum Dis Clin N Am 43 (2017) 467–480
http://dx.doi.org/10.1016/j.rdc.2017.04.010
0889-857X/17/© 2017 Elsevier Inc. All rights reserved.

Box 1
Strategies to identify novel therapies for rheumatic autoimmune inflammatory diseases

Predicting drugs that bind protein products of genes abnormally expressed in disease
  Molecular docking
    PharmMAPPER   http://59.78.96.61/pharmmapper/help.php
  Computational modeling
    CANDO   http://ram.org/compbio/protinfo/cando/
    SDTNBI   http://lmmd.ecust.edu.cn/methods/bsdtnbi/
Using molecular activity similarity to predict drugs from differentially expressed gene profiles
  cMAP/LINCS   http://www.lincscloud.org/l1000/
  D-GEX   https://github.com/uci-cbcl/D-GEX
  Cogena   https://bioconductor.org/packages/release/bioc/html/cogena.html
  QUADrATiC   https://omictools.com/qub-accelerated-drug-and-transcriptomic-
                           connectivity-tool
  DTome   https://bioinfo.uth.edu/DTome/
Translational bioinformatics
  HumanDiseaseNetwork https://exploringdata.github.io/info/human-disease-network/
  eMERGE   https://emerge.mc.vanderbilt.edu/
  RE:fineDrugs   http://drug-repurposing.nationwidechildrens.org/search
Identifying disease-drug and gene-drug relationships
  Protein-protein interactions
    BioGRID   http://thebiogrid.org/
  Domain-domain interactions
    PFam   http://pfam.xfam.org/
  Integrates interaction networks
    Consensus DB   http://consensuspathdb.org/
  Machine learning drug prediction
    GOPredict   http://csblcanges.fimm.fi/GOPredict/

Abbreviations: cMAP, Connectivity Map; CANDO, computational analysis of novel drug opportunities; D-GEX, Deep machine learning-Gene EXpression; DTome, Drug-Target Interactome; LINCS, Library of Integrated Network-Based Cellular Signatures; QUADrATiC; QUB Accelerated Drug And Transcriptome Connectivity; SDTNBI, Substructure-Drug-Target Network-Based Inference.

---

repositioning is an important approach, as it can decrease the time/cost of drug approval because it takes into account issues of toxicity and specificity from early testing and, thereby, paves the way for future discoveries by categorization of drugs by physiologic proxy.[5] Purposeful drug repositioning is often called retooling, reprofiling, retasking, and even drug rescue.[6]

The field of drug repositioning has emerged over the past decade, driven by collaborations among structural scientists, physicians, medicinal chemists, animal model experts, geneticists, computational modelers, immunologists, artificial intelligence/machine learning experts, and bioinformaticians. There are 4 major approaches to drug repositioning that have been used over the years: computational modeling, disease mechanism of action–based approaches, genetic profiling, and translational bioinformatics. Some approaches, such as computational modeling, are most appropriate for small molecules, whereas other approaches can be used to reposition either biologics or small molecules. The focus here is on techniques that stem from genomic information gathered from patients with rheumatic autoimmune inflammatory disease (RAID) and compared with healthy individuals. Small molecules that bind protein products of differentially expressed genes (DEGs) identified following microarray or RNA-Seq can be predicted by computational modeling. Patterns of DEGs in a particular disease can be compared with those in a variety of databases composed of cells cultured in vitro with small molecules or with small hairpin RNAs (shRNAs) to identify either small molecules or biologics that may be effectively repositioned. Translational approaches use information from GWAS as well as phenome-wide association studies (PheWAS) to narrow down drug repositioning candidates. Machine learning can be a useful tool to assist in all approaches to drug repositioning, as the size and scope of the targets to potential drug repositioning candidates is not an issue.

PREDICTING DRUGS THAT BIND PROTEIN PRODUCTS OF GENES ABNORMALLY EXPRESSED IN DISEASE

Historically, there are a variety of approaches to predict drugs that bind and potentially interfere with the action of a target protein. *Molecular docking* approaches to drug repositioning use structural information related to drug:target interactions to predict additional novel targets for known drugs and can be useful when the specific target of interest is known. An example is PharmMAPPER (http://59.78.96.61/pharmmapper/help.php), which uses a database of solved crystal structures consisting of 7302 compounds that bind 2241 human proteins (generated from TargetBank, DrugBank, BindingDB, PDTD). This platform supports in silico virtual screening of potential drug repositioning targets for a given protein thought to be involved in disease pathogenesis using a reverse pharmacophore matching method, a type of machine learning.[7] *Computational modeling* approaches to drug repositioning are data driven and can explore multisystem targets based on activation site analysis and target validation (reviewed in Ref.[8]). An example is the BioGPS/FLAPdock system using a QSAR (Quantitative Structure-Activity Relationship) modeling and structural algorithm that clusters drugs into similar groups and then looks for target matches based on *disease mechanism*.[9] An obstacle in using *computational modeling* for drug repositioning in RAIDs is the lack of a singular agreed on mechanism or pathway for disease pathogenesis; computational modeling has been most successful for diseases such as cancer because of an abnormality in known oncogene products usually within a single cell type. These approaches do not incorporate genomic information into their predictions unlike the 2 algorithms highlighted in the next paragraph: CANDO (Computational Analysis of Novel Drug Opportunities) and SDTNBI (Substructure-Drug-Target Network-Based Inference).

CANDO goes a step further than these approaches by identifying all probable drugs that may interact with protein products of DEGs identified by microarray or RNA-Seq analyses.[10] The initial step is to reveal protein-protein interactions and potential drug-protein interactions using the interactome (http://interactome.dfci.harvard.edu/H_sapiens/) and STITCH (Search Tool for Interactions of Chemicals; (http://stitch.embl.de/). CANDO incorporates these results to predict and then rank the more than 180 million drug-target interactions possible between the 3733 drugs approved by the Food and Drug Administration (FDA) and 48,278 proteins in its database (http://ram.org/compbio/protinfo/cando/). Specifically, CANDO uses a fragment-based (48,278 structures of protein fragments) docking simulation of atomic interactions to determine binding affinities and thus potential inhibitory capacity of drug candidates for a particular protein (or set of proteins). Matrices (ie, heatmaps) are created to visualize putative interactions of proteins and compounds with pseudocolored confidence scores and clustering of drug-protein interaction predictions such as "on-target" (high-affinity agonist), "off-target" (low-affinity agonist) or "antitarget" (antagonist). Using retrospective identification of known drug-target interactions as the gold standard, machine learning accuracy of CANDO is approximately 50% for prediction of the top 10 protein candidates for a given drug.

Cross-referencing CANDO's results to 1439 disease indications with more than 2 FDA-approved compounds revealed some drug-target interactions relevant to RAID, including everolimus/Afinitor, riboflavin, digoxin, and imatinib. Similar to sirolimus, everolimus (a derivative of sirolimus), was predicted to be a polypharmaceutical with more than 150 protein targets. When CANDO cross-referenced everolimus to clinical indications, kidney diseases were identified confirming lupus nephritis as a possible off-label use of this drug.[3,4,11] Imatinib also was defined as a polypharmaceutical by CANDO with 46 protein targets. Glomerulonephritis and proteinuria were cross-referenced by CANDO with imatinib. This result confirms earlier reports suggesting that both sirolimus and imatinib are viable candidates for repositioning into lupus because they received drug repositioning Combined Lupus Treatment Scoring (CoLT) scores similar to or greater than lupus standard-of-care (SOC) drugs.[4]

By contrast, riboflavin/vitamin B2 and digoxin were predicted to have very few protein targets and to be effective in skin diseases and autoimmunity, respectively. An ongoing clinical trial is examining the effect of riboflavin/vitamin B2 on moderate to severe plaque psoriasis (NCT02622386; https://clinicaltrials.gov/ct2/show/NCT02622386). Interestingly, peptides from riboflavin presented in the context of nonclassical major histocompatibility complex class I–related molecules have been shown to interact with the T-cell receptor of interleukin (IL)-17A–secreting innate T cells ($CD8^+CD161^+ROR\gamma t^+$) called mucosal-associated invariant T cells, whose peripheral presence has been shown to correlate with disease activity in psoriasis.[12]

Another drug CANDO predicted to have very few protein targets is digoxin. Cross-referencing to clinical indications revealed digoxin's applicability for autoimmune disease. Digoxin binds the orphan nuclear receptor $ROR\gamma t$[13] and inhibits transcription of IL-17A, the hallmark cytokine of Th17 T cells that play a role in autoimmune diseases, such as systemic lupus erythematosus (SLE) and psoriasis.[14] Traditionally, digoxin has been used for congestive heart failure. CANDO's highlighting digoxin brings up an interesting question: is the standard use of digoxin that was discovered by serendipity an off-target effect and is the *on-target effect* inhibition of $ROR\gamma t$ and IL-17A production? These questions will become more common as bioinformatics approaches elicit novel drug-protein interactions pairs.

SDTNBI (http://lmmd.ecust.edu.cn/methods/bsdtnbi/)[15] has the ability to predict novel drug-target interactions based on known substructures of drug-protein families and connect them to known networks of associations between drugs-gene products, drugs-diseases, and diseases-genes. SDTNBI looks for novel drug-target interactions with potential binding based on chemical substructure. For SDTNBI, substructures must be in SMILE format (Simplified Molecular-Input Line-Entry) and candidate compounds must have the following attributes of optimal drugs: molecular weight ($\leq$500 Da), log p ($\leq$5) for optimal solubility in water and fat, number hydrogen bond donors (HBD$\leq$5), number HB acceptors (HBA$\leq$10), and a $K_i/K_D/IC_{50}/EC_{50} \leq 10$ μM.

Using SDTNBI, 6568 compounds with resolved structures from DrugBank were compared to test proteins to detect known interactions and predict novel interactions. DGIdb (Drug-Gene Interactions database; http://dgidb.genome.wustl.edu/) and DRAR-CPI (Drug Repositioning and Adverse Reaction–Chemical Protein Interactions; https://cpi.bio-x.cn/drar/) were used to predict drug-gene product interactions; the Comparative Toxicogenomics databases (http://ctdbase.org/) were used to predict drug-disease associations; and the DisGeNet was used to predict disease-gene (http://www.disgenet.org/web/DisGeNET/menu) associations. As a test relevant to RAID, proteins that bound celecoxib/Celebrex were queried by SDTNBI and new protein interactions were predicted. SDTNBI correctly predicted association of celecoxib, a coxib used as an anti-inflammatory/analgesic in many conditions with PTGS2 (cyclooxygenase 2) but also with the products of 5 other genes (MB/myoglobin, carbonic anhydrase family members-3/13/7 as well as the G-protein–coupled ADRA2B/adrenoreceptor α2b). Interaction between celecoxib and the ADRA2B gene product may contribute to the adverse events of water retention and salt sensitivity.[16]

USING MOLECULAR ACTIVITY SIMILARITY TO PREDICT DRUGS FROM DIFFERENTIALLY EXPRESSED GENE PROFILES

In 2006, Lamb and colleagues[17] used *"molecular activity similarity"* to characterize compounds based on their theorized impact on proteins expressed within a cell and connect them to disease state by comparison with a query microarray profile (ie, patients with SLE vs healthy individuals). "Molecular activity similarity" has evolved into phenomics, or the study of the phenotype of a cell or organism; in this case, the effect of drugs or gene manipulation (ie, knockout, overexpression). The main assumption behind the concept of a connectivity map is that a biological state, whether physiologic, pathologic, or induced with chemical or genomic perturbations, can be described in terms of a genomic signature (ie, the genome-wide mRNA levels as measured by microarray technologies). The closeness or connection between the reference gene-expression profile and a query disease signature is defined by a similarity metric called a "connectivity score." There are numerous algorithms that use molecular similarity to make drug repositioning predictions from a genomic signature, including Connectivity Map (cMAP)/Library of Integrated Network-Based Cellular Signatures (LINCS), D-GEX (Deep machine learning-Gene EXpression), Cogena (Co-expressed gene-set enrichment analysis), QUADrATiC (QUB Accelerated Drug And Transcriptome Connectivity), and DTome (Drug-Target Interactome).

The first iteration of cMAP consisted of 6100 gene-expression profiles for 1309 perturbagens (a substance that changes processes within a cell) in 5 cell lines[17] (https://www.ncbi.nlm.nih.gov/geo/query/acc.cgi?acc=GSE5258). cMAP is now part of the perturbagen database that is publically available at http://www.lincscloud.org/l1000/ called LINCS and consists of representative information linking gene expression to perturbagen profiles, generated from more than 1.3 million reference gene-expression profiles obtained from 25 cell types that were antagonized by 20,413 chemical perturbagens and 22,119 knockout or overexpression genetic perturbagens. LINCS was developed using a Luminex platform called the L1000 to measure the expression profile of 978 "landmark genes." Expression of the rest of the approximately 21,000 genes in the human transcriptome is computationally inferred using linear regression modeling. This work was based on the premise that relationships exist between genes and expression of genes within a cell is highly correlated. Using principal component analysis, the number of measurements needed to generate meaningful gene-expression data for the 21,305 AffyMetrix probes measuring human gene expression used in cMAP was reduced to 978 "landmark genes" that capture 80% of the gene relationships in the original cMAP database.[18]

In 2016, a few of the developers of the L1000 generated a novel method called D-GEX (https://github.com/uci-cbcl/D-GEX) with the goal of capturing 100% of the gene-expression relationships in the original cMAP database as well as exploring nonlinear complex relationships between genes that linear regression modeling may have missed.[19] D-GEX is a multitask, multilayer feed-forward neural network that uses general purpose graphics processing units to optimize the speed of training with good scalability as data size increases. Input data consists of the "LINCS landmark genes" and output data consists of the target genes (ie, the rest of the genes in the human transcriptome). D-GEX examines all relationships between the input and output using hierarchical layers of abstraction (ie, hidden layers), similar to machine learning algorithms for natural language processing. The developers of D-GEX noticed that landmark genes and target genes have connections in the hidden layers that are positively or negatively correlated (adjusted R^2) and can be represented by edges. Moreover, input and output layers are related through what the investigators call "hub units" in the hidden layers of abstraction that capture strong connections between landmark genes and target genes. Similar to LINCS, the results of D-GEX are available for query at https://cbcl.ics.uci.edu/public_data/D-GEX/; this dataset consists of 1,328,098 expression profiles generated from D-GEX training on 978 landmark genes and 21,290 target genes inferring expression values of unmeasured target genes from the L1000 dataset.

Three recent studies have examined the role of connectivity mapping in drug repositioning: 1 in SLE,[4] 1 in psoriasis,[20] and 1 in cystic fibrosis (CF).[21] All 3 articles analyzed publicly available microarray datasets for genes differentially expressed in disease compared with unaffected individuals and queried LINCS for potential targets for drug repositioning. The SLE article used LINCS to confirm 2 drug repositioning candidates, a biologic specific for IL-12/23 called ustekinumab and the small molecules (ruxolitinib or tofacitinib) directed against Janus Activated Kinases. The investigators of the psoriasis article developed an algorithm they call "Cogena" (https://bioconductor.org/packages/release/bioc/html/cogena.html). Initially, Cogena identifies the top 100 upregulated and downregulated DEGs by LIMMA (Linear Models of MicroArray) and queried cMAP corresponding gene-set drug libraries. To identify antagonists, Cogena focused on upregulated genes that generate a library of drugs with negative connectivity scores and vice-versa. Second, using a hypergeometric test for gene-set enrichment analysis, heatmaps were generated for drug-GeneCluster relationships with a significant false discovery rate (FDR) and the drugs were ranked by enrichment score. Proof-of-principle of "Cogena" was demonstrated because 3 SOC psoriasis drugs were identified (methotrexate, cyclosporine, and betamethasone). The CF article used cMAP but took a different approach, querying for what DEGs in their microarray datasets correlated with their hypothesized "seed gene" *A20/TNFAIP3* (inhibits nuclear factor [NF]-κB activation). They identified 6 genes (*ATF3, RAB5C, DENND44, POP121, ICAM1, PSEN1*) significantly correlated with A20 and 4 drug candidates targeting A20, 2 of which were ruled out because of toxicity. In vitro experiments compared the activity of the 2 candidates, ikarugamycin and quercetin, on CF cells and came to the conclusion that quercetin is a viable candidate for repositioning into CF to increase A20 expression and thus inhibit inflammation-induced NF-κB activity that causes damage in CF.

The investigators of a fourth article developed the "QUADrATiC" algorithm[22] (https://omictools.com/qub-accelerated-drug-and-transcriptomic-connectivity-tool) and used the HDAC (histone deacetylase) gene signature relevant to many RAIDs (including SLE)[4] as their proof-of-principle experiment to predict drugs. Similar to the other 3 articles, QUADrATiC queried LINCS for ranked drugs that correspond to a given DEG expression dataset. Unique compared with the other articles summarized previously is the extra step of using DrugBank (http://www.drugbank.ca/; http://www.ncbi.nlm.nih.gov/pubmed/24203711) in conjunction with FDA Parser (http://www.fda.gov/downloads/BiologicsBloodVaccines/NewsEvents/WorkshopsMeetings Conferences/UCM422055.pdf) to narrow down the LINCS drugs to those that are FDA-approved. This also decreased the more than 1.3 million reference gene-expression profiles to 83,939. Similar to Cogena, QUADrATiC queried LINCS with upregulated (and downregulated) DEGs generated by LIMMA to receive respective drug profiles with negative (or positive) connectivity scores representing ranking of potential antagonists of the gene signature. Similar to "Cogena," QUADrATiC has the added ability to provide estimated P values (FDR) for each connectivity score as well as to output a Comma Separated Variable (CSV) file of the normalized connection fractions with data sorted by drug (column) or by drug and treated cell line (row). To explore the mechanism of action of drugs, QUADrATiC determines the effect of each probe on the connection strength for a drug treatment set based on a value called the contribution factor of each probe, allowing for visualization by heatmap showing the relative contribution of each probe in the DEG signature to each drug prediction.

The QUADrATiC study compared and contrasted predicted FDA-approved drugs for the HDAC signature with those predicted using cMAP itself or sscMAP (statistically significant connections MAP), an algorithm from 2009.[23,24] QUADrATiC elucidated 447 significant positive connections to the HDAC signature representing 231 unique compounds. All 3 algorithms predicted 2 drugs: vorinostat and valproic acid. Of the 10 drugs predicted by sscMAP, QUADrATiC predicted 8 of them to be significant. QUADrATiC predicted 223 FDA-approved drugs that were not predicted by either cMAP or sscMAP; the top 4 were everolimus, perhexiline, topical crotamiton, and menadione/vitamin K3. Interestingly, everolimus, as well as HDAC inhibitors, are often used synergistically for several malignancies.[25] Relevant to RAIDs, everolimus is used off-label in SLE.[26] The relevance of menadione/vitamin K3 is emphasized by the finding that it may be an HDAC inhibitor.[27] These results indicate that QUADrATiC may be a useful tool to identify additional candidate drugs for a disease based on a "seed" signature, in this case the HDAC signature.

In vitro shRNAs or RNA inhibitors (RNAi), turn off genes in a reversible fashion. LINCS uses this technology to use reference gene-expression profiles of cell lines with or without shRNA knockdown to compare with a disease gene profile (ie, patients with SLE vs healthy controls) to predict gene products that could be targeted by a chemical inhibitor of the gene knocked down with shRNA. One study (https://www.cellecta.com/) used an RNAi-based screening approach coupled with computational network modeling to identify drugs that target regulators of apoptosis mediated by FAS/cluster of differentiation 95 (CD95)/tumor necrosis factor receptor super family 6 (TNFRSF6) and TNF/TNFSF2, each of which has been implicated in initiation and pathogenesis of RAIDs.[28,29] This study is part of the National Institutes of Health (NIH)-funded DECIPHER Project (http://www.decipherproject.net/) whose goal is to identify functionally validated shRNAs that can be used in mouse or human cells (120,000 validated as of 2016). This library of shRNAs called PathwayDecipher targets 24% of human protein-encoding genes (5046 genes with $\geq$5 unique shRNAs/gene) that are separated into annotated functional groups (eg, signaling molecules, transcription factors, nucleic acid binding). The 5046 genes represented in PathwayDecipher are associated with 2669 discrete disease processes and can be visualized in 602 pathways (402 manually curated, 200 canonical). Known drug targets are encoded by 19% of these 5046 genes (943 genes).

To determine candidate drugs that target apoptosis mediated by FAS/CD95/TNFRSF6 and TNF/TNFSF2, Komarov and colleagues[30] transfected cells with the pooled PathwayDecipher shRNA library and stimulated in the presence or absence of antibodies to the TNF-family members mentioned previously. Candidate genes were identified based on increased expression in cells that survived apoptosis, based on inhibition by discrete shRNAs. These potential suppressors of FAS-induced and TNF-induced apoptosis were prioritized using a feed-forward–based network approach to identify key upstream and downstream signaling nodes. Additionally, a bipartite graph composed of all FDA-approved drugs and gene-expression protein products was examined for drug-target candidate pairs using DTome[31] (https://

bioinfo.uth.edu/DTome/) and the subscription-based Thomas Reuters Integrity database (https://integrity.thomson-pharma.com/integrity/xmlxsl/). One of the drugs identified to be repositioned into diseases mediated by FAS-induced and/or TNF-induced apoptosis is cantharidin, a natural product secreted by blister beetles. The bipartite graph shown by Komarov and colleagues[30] matched up cantharidin with PPP2R5A (the regulatory subunit of the protein serine/threonine phosphatase PP2A). Topical cantharidin is commonly used to treat warts as well as molluscum contagiosum. There are positive case reports showing that topical cantharidin may be effective for some dermatologic autoimmune diseases, such as psoriasis.[32]

DRUG PREDICTIONS FROM TRANSLATIONAL BIOINFORMATICS (GENOME-WIDE ASSOCIATION STUDIES, PHENOME-WIDE ASSOCIATION STUDIES)

Translational bioinformatics is a combinatory approach that uses a variety of methods and disciplines to identify drug repositioning candidates. To be accurate and effective in their predictions, bioinformaticians need to work closely with experts in pharmacology and clinicians well versed in the disease for which they are seeking new drugs.[33] Key to successful drug repositioning is the identification of relationships between diseases and drugs. Emergence of GWAS has provided opportunities to look for disease-gene relationships that may indicate novel therapeutic targets. GWAS approaches these relationships by investigating the role of a particular genetic variant in a given disease or set of diseases. Phenomics is the study of the phenome in relationship to gene expression (genomics) and protein expression (proteomics). A tool to graphically represent how diseases are related genomically and phenotypically to each other is the Human Disease Network (HDN) (https://exploringdata.github.io/info/human-disease-network/). In the HDN, each node corresponds to a disease and its size indicates the number of genes associated with that disease. Diseases/nodes are connected to one another if they have associated genes in common.

In contrast to GWAS, PheWAS approaches disease-drug relationships by asking the question of what diseases are associated with a single change at the genetic/genomic/proteomic level. PheWAS examine the phenome, or the set of phenotypes observed in anything from a population of cells to an entire organism, such as a patient with RAID. HLA is an example of a gene family that was identified to associate with multiple RAIDs by PheWAS.[34] PheWAS are useful to identify association of a given gene (genetics, genomics) or gene product (proteomics) across multiple phenotypes (in this case, diseases). Although phenotype has a basis in genotype, several factors influence phenotype, such as germline variations (single nucleotide polymorphisms [SNPs]), somatic mutation (ie, initiates/propagates malignancies), epigenetics, or the regulatory influences on gene expression, as well as environmental factors.

One goal of PheWAS in drug repositioning to is identify a selected set of genes that are related to the phenotype of a disease and hypothesize candidate drugs for repositioning. One way to approach PheWAS-based drug repositioning draws on resources that relay information about a patient group at the clinical level, such as electronic medical/health records (EMRs/EHRs) as well as data about the cells and tissues of a patient group compared with unaffected individuals. There are several databases that include clinical information about patient groups, including clinical trial information (ClinicalTrials.gov), adverse event registries and EMRs. Newer databases focused on disease PheWAS combine genetic or genomic information with EMRs. The eMERGE database is funded by NIH and combines DNA biorepositories with EMRs from patient groups such as those with rheumatoid arthritis (RA) (https://www.genome.

gov/27540473/electronic-medical-records-and-genomics-emerge-network/; https://emerge.mc.vanderbilt.edu/). One offshoot of eMERGE is the knowledge-base called PheKB (https://phekb.org/) that identifies characteristics of patient groups, such as those with RA. Other databases similar to eMERGE are the Million Veteran Program (http://www.research.va.gov/mvp/veterans.cfm), the UK BioBank (http://www.ukbiobank.ac.uk/), and the University of California San Francisco–Kaiser Permanente Research Program on Genes, Environment, and Health (https://www.dor.kaiser.org/external/DORExternal/rpgeh/index.aspx). These 4 databases represent more than 1 million patients with dense genotype data and complete EMR information.

In 2013, proof-of-concept of eMERGE was demonstrated with 3144 SNPs implicated by GWAS to represent human traits and 1358 EMR phenotypes in 13,835 patients.[35] Two previously identified SNPs in RA (rs6910071, C6orf10; rs660895, HLA-DRB1) were "re-discovered" using this approach.[36] To visualize associations, the negative log of the P values of associations between symptomatic phenotypes and diseases for each SNP were graphed. Symptomatic phenotypes are coded in EMRs by International Classification of Diseases, Ninth Revision identifiers (https://cran.r-project.org/web/packages/icd9/vignettes/introduction.html) that are part of the Metathesaurus created by the National Library of Medicine (NLM; https://www.nlm.nih.gov/research/umls/). From 7945 disease-drug pairs identified in this study, 908 had strong support in the literature and 4837 were novel candidate diseases for repositioning of the identified compounds.

This original study was revisited when the Rastegar-Mojarad group extracted 212,851 SNP-disease associations from the database of Denny and colleagues[35] to perform PheWAS with additional information sources.[36] SNPs were narrowed down to those 1501 SNPs that mapped directly to a gene (dbSNP; http://www.ncbi.nlm.nih.gov/projects/SNP/) and these were retained to query DrugBank, yielding 52,966 unique disease-drug relationships. A total of 127 of these relationships were positive controls, in that they were previously documented experimentally. To extract paired disease-drug terms from PubMed abstracts, the "elasticsearch" engine Apache Lucene4 (https://lucene.apache.org/) was used in conjunction with MetaMap (https://metamap.nlm.nih.gov/), the foundation of the NLM's medical text indexer that uses natural language processing/computational linguistics to recognize disease names in PubMed abstracts. This MetaMap/ApacheLucene search identified 2583 drug indications (ie, disease-drug pairs) that had strong support in both PubMed as well as in (ClinicalTrials.gov/), more than 12,000 that had support from either of these resources, as well as 38,035 disease-drug relationships that were completely novel. An example of a positive control in this study was the demonstrated association between rs4795067 that contains the *NOS2* gene with the disease-drug relationship of RA and dexamethasone. A novel disease-drug relationship identified for autoimmunity was type1 diabetes with zidovudine, a nucleoside/nucleotide reverse-transcriptase inhibitor that was matched up with telomerase reverse transcriptase identified in the rs2736100 locus. Of interest, zidovudine was evaluated by Grammer and colleagues[4] for repositioning into SLE but was not considered a high-priority candidate because of an adverse event profile.

The approach described previously is now publicly available as the "RE:fineDrugs" algorithm (http://drug-repurposing.nationwidechildrens.org/search) that is user-friendly and integrates the 212,851 SNP-disease associations from the GWAS and PheWAS studies described previously.[37] The current version of RE:fineDrugs contains relationship information for 60,911 potential associations with 1770 diseases, 916 genes, and 567 drugs. The RE:fineDrugs database is completely searchable on these 3 parameters, and filters can be applied for strength of evidence from PubMed and/or the NIH Clinical Trials Registry (clinicaltrials.gov/). Using the advanced search function of RE:fineDrugs, users can filter and sort by odds ratio, P value, literature support, clinical trial evidence, disease name, and/or drug name. Searches can be visualized as a prioritized list of drug repositioning candidates for a given disease. The investigators use the *IL2RB* gene as an example that returns 12 pairs of disease-drug associations with an interesting candidate that has been validated in the literature for its predicted disease, the use of daclizumab for asthma.[38]

USING MACHINE LEARNING/DATABASES TO IDENTIFY DISEASE-DRUG AND GENE-DRUG RELATIONSHIPS

Drug repositioning candidates have been identified in a variety of ways using networks for protein-protein interactions to visualize where drugs may interrupt signaling cascades involved in disease states. One recent study looking for drug repositioning candidates for patients with SLE used a Big-Data approach that identified DEGs in patients with lupus compared with healthy individuals.[4] Network analysis of protein-protein interactions (PPIs) was performed with STRING (Search Tool for the Retrieval of Interacting Genes/Proteins;(http://string-db.org/), and potential drugs were identified by a variety of methods including the L1000 version of cMAP/LINCS. Another recent study independently looked for drug repositioning candidates in non–small-cell lung cancer in a similar manner[39] using BioGrid[40] (http://thebiogrid.org/), instead of STRING, to identify PPIs and then used machine learning to find additional candidate drug targets using the open-source WEKA (Waikato Environment for Knowledge Analysis) software (http://www.cs.waikato.ac.nz/ml/index.html). In essence, WEKA uses binary yes/no choices based on drug-target attributes in its Support Vector Machine (SVM) algorithm. Interactions, or DDIs (drug-drug interactions), between domains of proteins (ie, kinase-substrate interaction) were identified using PFam (http://pfam.xfam.org/). The likelihood a domain is located in a disease-associated gene product (ie, SNP or over-/under-DEG compared with normal) was calculated as the DFS (Domain Frequency Score). Disease Linker Degree (DLD) is a calculation that indicates the likelihood an interaction edge (ie, DDI) connects to many nodes (other DDIs) associated with disease. Both DFS and DLD were supplied to the SVM as a yes/no "voting" choice. The output of WEKA was compared with the genes identified by a pipeline similar to that of Grammer and colleagues,[4] but using different algorithms to determine a network of genes, also called topological parameter classification (BioGrid PPIs; ConsensusDB). ConsensusDB (http://consensuspathdb.org/) includes binary and complex protein-protein, genetic, metabolic, signaling, gene regulatory, and drug-target interactions, as well as biochemical pathways. Specifically, ConsensusDB can be used to identify all potential interactions of the products of DEGs with other proteins, as well as all signaling cascades, metabolic reactions, and binding to RNA/DNA. The list of genes identified by machine learning and by the traditional approach were used to query cMAP for potential drug repositioning candidates. Results were compared with the drugs suggested by ConsensusDB that interact with particular gene products.

There are 2 main types of machine learning algorithms that have been used to identify gene product targets for drugs: "similarity based" and "learning to rank (LTR)" feature-based. The main assumption of similarity-based methods is that similar drugs bind similar targets. LTR is best known for its use in ranking Web page usage based on multiuser queries (ie, the more often a Web page is queried, the more important it is considered to be). In LTR, each "instance" (in this case drug) is multiclassified, meaning it is represented by many labels (or targets defined in this case in DrugBank). Many drugs are polypharmaceuticals, meaning that they have multiple targets.

Ravindranath and colleagues[41] published a k-NN similarity-based machine learning algorithm that uses Naive Bayesian classification to predict targets for drugs. In short, this study used hierarchical clustering with k-NN analysis to group drugs by target similarity (Tanimoto coefficient >0.5). The investigators used the original GEO dataset cMAP to create their library of drug-gene signatures[17] (https://www.ncbi.nlm.nih.gov/geo/query/acc.cgi?acc=GSE5258). Following LIMMA DEG analysis, the 477 gene products known to bind 1 of the 1309 drugs in the original cMAP screen were grouped together by similarity (ie, the drugs with the most similar targets were grouped together). Similarity of targets was defined by gene ontology (GO) and kyoto encyclopedia of genes and genomes (KEGG) pathway analysis. An example relevant for RAID is that a cluster of drugs (rosiglitazone, trosiglitazone) organized with FABP4 and ANGPTL4, known targets of PPARγ.[4] The Ravindranath algorithm may be a useful addition to LINCS analysis of DEGs from patients with RAID compared with controls.

Finally, in collaboration with the NIH Cancer Genome Atlas project, Louhimo and colleagues[42] developed the GOPredict prioritization system (http://csblcanges.fimm.fi/GOPredict/) to rank candidate drugs for repositioning into cancer. Their scoring system is the first to integrate transcriptomically altered drug targets (DEGs), genomic-level point mutations/somatic copy number, and epigenetics (promoter hypomethylation) with interactome/pathway information to identify and rank potential drug repositioning candidates. The goal of their work was to identify precision therapy for a given cancer that would benefit most patients. The main input data were publically available gene-expression datasets from GEO. The investigators preferred to work with raw microarray data but incorporated previously normalized data when necessary. For each dataset, the investigators ranked the statistically significant DEG (patients vs healthy controls) based on LFC (Log_2-Fold Change) and organized them into "activating" (DE_UP_genes), "inactivating" (DE_DOWN_genes), and "survival-associated" based on univariate association of gene copy number increasing with survival. Gene ranking by "K-ranks" is important for GOPredict, so that all genes are considered to be potential drug targets, not just those genes that are most well-studied in the literature.

Ranked genes are connected to biology using GO-terms that define processes/pathways. Only those genes that clearly positively or negatively regulate a GO-process are retained. "K-ranks" of genes are summed up for each GO-term to produce a cancer-essentiality score (CE-score) with statistical significance assessed with a permutation test. These CE-scores are used to recalibrate gene "K-ranks" using the harmonic mean of the P values of the GO-processes a gene regulates so that highly connected GO-terms are not overrepresented in the data. An "activity matrix" (ie, table or heatmap) is created to summarize the data by denoting the status (UP, red; DOWN, blue; no change, white) of each ranked gene over several datasets; additional information such as status of methylation and "survival status" are indicated in the table or heatmap. Drugs for potential repositioning were identified using KEGGDrug (http://www.genome.jp/kegg/drug/) and DrugBank (https://www.drugbank.ca/) to find drug-target pairs. These pairs were prioritized based on recalibrated K-ranks and the priority rank of the drug is averaged over all genes so that there is a balance between number of targets a drug interacts with as well as the ranking of the gene based on DE expression and pathway information. GOPredict may be a useful algorithm to identify RAID drug repositioning candidates using transcriptomically regulated DE genes and Weighted Gene Coexpression Network Analysis of gene expression that identifies groups of genes correlated with disease activity (ie, for SLE, modules of genes positively or negatively correlated with SLE Disease Activity Index).

SUMMARY

The need for new drugs for patients with some RAIDs is monumental, and there is great promise for repositioning drugs into these diseases in the near future. Collaboration among scientists in a variety of fields is key for narrowing down potential targets and drugs that may be effective in RAIDs. The approaches described here all use publically available data generated by rheumatologists, immunologists, geneticists, and other scientists examining DEG in patients compared with controls as well as disease-associated SNP and disease-related hypomethylation patterns. In addition, a variety of techniques to identify optimal target-drug pairs spans scientific expertise that ranges from structural chemistry/pharmacology (molecular docking of drugs with proteins), computational modeling (using datasets generated from in vitro experiments with cells cultured with perturbagen with shRNAs), translational bioinformatics (finding relationships in EMRs, clinical trial data, and drug-target predictions from genomics and/or genetics), and artificial intelligence cognitive computer systems use machine learning to "put it all together" to find relationships that predict optimal drug repositioning candidates for RAIDs.

REFERENCES

1. Nosengo N. Can you teach old drugs new tricks? Nature 2016;534(7607):314–6.
2. Available at: http://www.the-scientist.com/?articles.view/articleNo/47744/title/Repurposing-Existing-Drugs-for-New-Indications/. Accessed January 1, 2017.
3. Grammer AC, Ryals MM, Catalina MD, et al. Repositioning drugs for SLE. In: Tsokos G, Buyon J, Koike T, et al, editors. Repositioning drugs for SLE. Systemic lupus erythematosus. 5th edition. Amsterdam: Elsevier Academic Press; 2016. p. 567–73.
4. Grammer AC, Ryals MM, Heuer SE, et al. Drug repositioning in SLE: crowdsourcing, literature-mining and big data analysis. Lupus 2016;25(10):1150–70.
5. Avorn J. The $2.6 billion pill–methodologic and policy considerations. N Engl J Med 2015;372:1877–9.
6. Lan Langedijk J, Mantel-Teeuwisse AK, Slijkerman DS, et al. Drug repositioning and repurposing: terminology and definitions in literature. Drug Discov Today 2015;20:1027–34.
7. Wang X, Pan C, Gong J, et al. Enhancing the enrichment of pharmacophore-based target prediction for the polypharmacological profiles of drugs. J Chem Inf Model 2016;56(6):1175–83.
8. Luo H, Mattes W, Mendrick DL, et al. Molecular docking for identification of potential targets for drug repurposing. Curr Top Med Chem 2016;16(30):3636–45.
9. Siragusa L, Luciani R, Borsari C, et al. Comparing drug images and repurposing drugs with BioGPS and FLAPdock: the thymidylate synthase case. ChemMedChem 2016;11(15):1653–66.
10. Chopra G, Samudrala R. Exploring polypharmacology in drug discovery and repurposing using the CANDO platform. Curr Pharm Des 2016;22(21):3109–23.
11. Chan TM. Treatment of severe lupus nephritis: the new horizon. Nat Rev Nephrol 2015;11(1):46–61.
12. Johnston A, Gudjonsson JE. Psoriasis and the MAITing game: a role for IL-17A+ invariant TCR CD8+ T cells in psoriasis? J Invest Dermatol 2014;134(12):2864–6.

13. Huh JR, Leung MW, Huang P, et al. Digoxin and its derivatives suppress TH17 cell differentiation by antagonizing RORγt activity. Nature 2011;472(7344): 486–90.

14. Fasching P, Stradner M, Graninger W, et al. Therapeutic potential of targeting the Th17/Treg axis in autoimmune disorders [Review]. Molecules 2017;22(1). http://dx.doi.org/10.3390/molecules22010134.

15. Wu Z, Cheng F, Li J, et al. An integrated network and chemoinformatics tool for systematic prediction of drug-target interactions and drug repositioning. Brief Bioinform 2017;18(2):333–47.

16. Makaritsis KP, Handy DE, Johns C, et al. Role of the alpha2B-adrenergic receptor in the development of salt-induced hypertension. Hypertension 1999;33(1):14–7.

17. Lamb J, Crawford ED, Peck D, et al. The connectivity map: using gene-expression signatures to connect small molecules, genes, and disease. Science 2006;313(5795):1929–35.

18. Available at: http://support.lincscloud.org/hc/en-us/articles/202092616-The-Landmark-Genes. Accessed January 1, 2013.

19. Chen Y, Li Y, Narayan R, et al. Gene expression inference with deep learning. Bioinformatics 2016;32(12):1832–9.

20. Jia Z, Liu Y, Guan N, et al. Cogena, a novel tool for co-expressed gene-set enrichment analysis, applied to drug repositioning and drug mode of action discovery. BMC Genomics 2016;17:414.

21. Malcomson B, Wilson H, Veglia E, et al. Connectivity mapping (ssCMap) to predict A20-inducing drugs and their antiinflammatory action in cystic fibrosis. Proc Natl Acad Sci U S A 2016;113(26):E3725–34.

22. O'Reilly PG, Wen Q, Bankhead P, et al. QUADrATiC: scalable gene expression connectivity mapping for repurposing FDA-approved therapeutics. BMC Bioinformatics 2016;17(1):198.

23. Zhang SD, Gant TW. sscMap: an extensible Java application for connecting small-molecule drugs using gene-expression signatures. BMC Bioinformatics 2009;10:236.

24. Zhang SD, Gant TW. A simple and robust method for connecting small-molecule drugs using gene-expression signatures. BMC Bioinformatics 2008;9:258.

25. Rodriguez-Cerdeira C, Sanchez-Blanco E, Molares-Vila A. Clinical application of development of nonantibiotic macrolides that correct inflammation-driven immune dysfunction in inflammatory skin diseases. Mediators Inflamm 2012;2012: 563709.

26. Oki Y, Buglio D, Fanale M, et al. Phase I study of panobinostat plus everolimus in patients with relapsed or refractory lymphoma. Clin Cancer Res 2013;19(24): 6882–90.

27. Lin C, Kang J, Zheng R. Vitamin K3 triggers human leukemia cell death through hydrogen peroxide generation and histone hyperacetylation. Pharmazie 2005; 60(10):765–71.

28. Nagata S, Tanaka M. Programmed cell death and the immune system [Review]. Nat Rev Immunol 2017. http://dx.doi.org/10.1038/nri.2016.153.

29. Wu DJ, Adamopoulos IE. Autophagy and autoimmunity. Clin Immunol 2017;176: 55–62.

30. Komarov AP, Komarova EA, Green K, et al. Functional genetics-directed identification of novel pharmacological inhibitors of FAS- and TNF-dependent apoptosis that protect mice from acute liver failure. Cell Death Dis 2016;7:e2145.

31. Sun J, Wu Y, Xu H, et al. DTome: a web-based tool for drug-target interactome construction. BMC Bioinformatics 2012;13(Suppl 9):S7.

32. Cherniack EP. Bugs as drugs, part 1: insects: the "new" alternative medicine for the 21st century? [Review]. Altern Med Rev 2010;15(2):124–35.
33. Readhead B, Dudley J. Translational bioinformatics approaches to drug development [Review]. Adv Wound Care (New Rochelle) 2013;2(9):470–89.
34. Ceccarelli F, Agmon-Levin N, Perricone C. Genetic factors of autoimmune diseases. J Immunol Res 2016;2016:3476023.
35. Denny JC, Bastarache L, Ritchie MD, et al. Systematic comparison of phenome-wide association study of electronic medical record data and genome-wide association study data. Nat Biotechnol 2013;31(12):1102–10.
36. Rastegar-Mojarad M, Ye Z, Kolesar JM, et al. Opportunities for drug repositioning from phenome-wide association studies. Nat Biotechnol 2015;33(4):342–5.
37. Moosavinasab S, Patterson J, Strouse R, et al. 'RE:fine drugs': an interactive dashboard to access drug repurposing opportunities. Database (Oxford) 2016; 2016. http://dx.doi.org/10.1093/database/baw083.
38. Menzella F, Lusuardi M, Galeone C, et al. Tailored therapy for severe asthma. Multidiscip Respir Med 2015;10(1):1.
39. Huang CH, Chang PM, Hsu CW, et al. Drug repositioning for non-small cell lung cancer by using machine learning algorithms and topological graph theory. BMC Bioinformatics 2016;17(Suppl 1):2.
40. Chatr-Aryamontri A, Oughtred R, Boucher L, et al. The BioGRID interaction database: 2017 update. Nucleic Acids Res 2017;45(D1):D369–79.
41. Ravindranath AC, Perualila-Tan N, Kasim A, et al, QSTAR Consortium. Connecting gene expression data from connectivity map and in silico target predictions for small molecule mechanism-of-action analysis. Mol Biosyst 2015;11(1):86–96.
42. Louhimo R, Laakso M, Belitskin D, et al. Data integration to prioritize drugs using genomics and curated data. BioData Min 2016;9:21.

Future Directions of Genomics Research in Rheumatic Diseases

Yukinori Okada, MD, PhD[a,*], Toshihiro Kishikawa, MD[a,b],
Saori Sakaue, MD[a,c], Jun Hirata, MS[a,d,e]

KEYWORDS

- Human genetics • Statistical genetics • Genome-wide association study
- Next-generation sequencing • Human leukocyte antigen

KEY POINTS

- Recent developments in human genome genotyping and sequencing technologies have successfully identified several risk genes of rheumatic diseases.
- Fine-mapping studies using the HLA imputation method revealed that both classic and nonclassic HLA genes contribute to the risk of rheumatic diseases.
- Integration of human disease genomics with biological, medical, and clinical databases should contribute to the elucidation of disease pathogenicity and novel drug discovery.
- Disease risk genes identified by large-scale genetic studies are considered to be promising resources for novel drug discovery, including drug repositioning (eg, CDK4/6 inhibitors), and biomarker microRNA screening (miR-4728-5p and its target gene of PADI2) for rheumatoid arthritis.

BACKGROUND

Rheumatic diseases are autoimmune diseases that are characterized by inflammation and destruction of joints, muscles, blood vessels, and organs. Both genetic and environmental factors typically contribute to the onset of rheumatic diseases. For example, familial and epidemiologic studies have demonstrated that approximately

Disclosure statement: J. Hirata is currently employed by Teijin Pharma Limited.
[a] Department of Statistical Genetics, Osaka University Graduate School of Medicine, 2-2 Yamadaoka, Suita, Osaka 565-0871, Japan; [b] Department of Otorhinolaryngology, Head and Neck Surgery, Osaka University Graduate School of Medicine, 2-2 Yamadaoka, Suita, Osaka 565-0871, Japan; [c] Department of Allergy and Rheumatology, Graduate School of Medicine, The University of Tokyo, 7-3-1 Hongo, Bunkyo-ku, Tokyo 113-0033, Japan; [d] Department of Human Genetics and Disease Diversity, Graduate School of Medical and Dental Sciences, Tokyo Medical and Dental University, 1-5-45 Yushima, Bunkyo-ku, Tokyo 113-8510, Japan; [e] Pharmaceutical Discovery Research Laboratories, Teijin Pharma Limited, 4-3-2, Asahigaoka, Hino-shi, Tokyo 191-8512, Japan
* Corresponding author.
E-mail address: yokada@sg.med.osaka-u.ac.jp

50% of the disease risk of rheumatoid arthritis (RA), one of the most common rheumatic diseases that affect synovial joints, is explained by genetic factors.[1] Recent developments in human genome sequencing technologies, such as high-density single nucleotide polymorphism (SNP) microarrays and next-generation sequencing (NGS), have substantially contributed to the elucidation of the genetic architecture of human complex traits. In particular, genome-wide association studies (GWAS), a method of statistical genetics that massively evaluates the disease risk of genome-wide SNPs, has successfully identified several human disease risk genes.[2] Specifically for RA, a large-scale transethnic GWAS identified more than 100 risk genetic loci, with implications for novel drug discovery.[3,4] In this review, the authors highlight recent findings on genomics of rheumatic diseases and their application to translational research.

ROLES OF THE MAJOR HISTOCOMPATIBILITY REGION TO RISK OF RHEUMATIC DISEASES

The major histocompatibility complex (MHC) region, a genetic locus located at chromosome 6p23, is known to have a strong impact on the genetic risk of rheumatic diseases. Although this region is only 0.1% of the length of the human genome, the MHC region confers most of the risk for most rheumatic diseases. The initial identification of the genetic risk loci was reported to be associated with the HLA genes located in the MHC region, such as *HLA-DRB1* for RA,[5] *HLA-C* for psoriasis,[6] *HLA-B* for ankylosing spondylitis,[7] and *HLA-DPB1* for Graves disease.[6] However, delineation of the detailed disease risk of HLA alleles has been challenging and controversial owing to the complex structures of the polymorphisms in the MHC region. For RA, the *HLA-DRB1* alleles, which share a conserved amino acid sequences at positions 70 to 74 and are called shared epitope (SE) alleles, confer strong risk in multiple populations,[5,8,9] but non-SE *HLA-DRB1* alleles contribute risk as well.[9]

Recently, the method of statistical genetics called HLA imputation was developed.[10] This approach computationally imputes (ie, estimates) HLA alleles of the individuals using SNP genotyping data and, therefore, allows comprehensive HLA allele risk assessment using existing large-scale GWAS data without additional genotyping costs.[10] Application of the HLA imputation method to GWAS data had facilitated successful fine-mapping of the risk HLA variants of multiple diseases.[11–21] HLA imputation-based analysis of GWAS data in autoantibody-positive RA revealed that most of the MHC risk was explained by amino acid sequence polymorphisms at positions 11 and 13 of HLA-DRβ1 molecule in multiple populations, including Europeans,[11,12] East Asians,[13] Japanese,[14] and African Americans (**Fig. 1**).[15] The

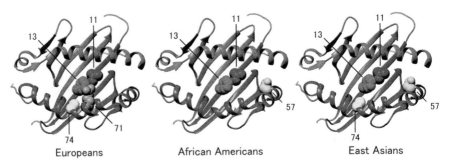

Fig. 1. Amino acid positions of RA risk on 3-dimensional structure of the HLA-DRβ1 molecule. HLA-DRβ1 amino acid sequence alterations at positions 11 and 13 confer strong risk of RA in multiple populations.[11–15]

HLA imputation method contributed to HLA allele fine-mapping of other rheumatic or immune-related diseases, including psoriasis,[16] Graves diseases,[17] type 1 diabetes,[18] systemic lupus erythematosus,[19] the subset of patients with lung adenocarcinoma with mutations in the epidermal growth factor receptor,[20] and natural killer T-cell lymphoma.[21]

Most of these HLA fine-mapping studies indicated that the amino acid sequence polymorphisms of the classic HLA genes were disease risk variants. However, the recent HLA imputation analysis of RA GWAS data in the Japanese populations reported that the synonymous variant of *HLA-DOA*, one of the nonclassic HLA genes, had risk independently from other classic HLA genes, including *HLA-DRB1*.[14] The *HLA-DOA* risk variant demonstrated an expression quantitative trait locus effect on *HLA-DOA* mRNA expressions, suggesting a dosage contribution of the nonclassic HLA genes to the disease biology.

GENOME-WIDE ASSOCIATION STUDIES IDENTIFIED MANY NON–MAJOR HISTOCOMPATIBILITY COMPLEX RISK GENES

Genetic variants outside of the MHC region confer relatively weaker disease risk compared with those in the MHC region, so many subjects and controls are required to have sufficient statistical power to identify these variants. Implementation of GWAS helped to address this issue, and this approach has successfully identified many disease risk genes of rheumatic diseases.[3,22,23] Initially, GWAS was performed for single populations; but currently, large-scale transethnic meta-analyses are routinely conducted.[3,24]

Although the GWAS strategy successfully identified disease risk genes, only a small fraction of the disease risk was explained by GWAS-identified risk variants. This problem is called missing heritability.[25] Multiple hypotheses have been proposed to explain missing heritability (also see Vincent A. Laufer and colleagues article, "Integrative Approaches to Understanding the Pathogenic Role of Genetic Variation in Rheumatic Diseases," in this issue), such as rare risk variants not represented on SNP genotyping panels. With the development of NGS technologies, rare risk variants could be identified[26,27]; it was discovered that these rare variants had small contributions to the genetic risk of common diseases in the populations,[28] so they did not contribute substantially to solving the problem of missing heritability. Assessment of the role of rare variant risks by whole-exome sequencing or whole-genome sequencing will require relatively larger sample sizes compared with evaluation of common variants by GWAS,[29] and further synthesis of the studies through international collaborative partnerships will be necessary. Although further analytical assessments may be warranted, polygenic effects from genome-wide common SNPs with very weak risk have also been considered to potentially explain missing heritability.[30,31] Other genetic factors not typically assessed in the GWAS approaches, such as a nonadditive effect of the genetic risk variants[32,33] and gene-gene interactions,[34] have also been suggested for filling in the unexplained missing heritability.

Another future goal of genetic studies is to identify the variants associated with disease prognosis or severity. Previous studies suggested that the genetic factors for diseases onset and prognosis may not be identical,[16,35] and genetic studies specifically focusing on clinical outcomes are warranted.

INSIGHTS INTO DISEASE BIOLOGY

The goal of genetic studies should not only be identification of disease risk genes but also elucidation of underlying disease biology and translation to novel clues to cure the diseases. Thus, establishment of the methodology to link disease genetics to disease biology are warranted. The authors propose that translational integration of disease genetics with a variety of existing biological and medical data would contribute to this link[3] (also see the article by Laufer and colleagues).

Pioneering application of this strategy to the genetics of RA has found several features relevant to the cause of this disease: (1) most genetic risk variants change amino acid sequences or expression of the genes, (2) the contribution of regulatory T-cells, (3) shared risk genes with lymphomas and primary immunodeficiency syndromes, and (4) the contribution of cytokine pathways (interleukin 10, granulocyte-macrophage colony-stimulating factor, and interferon).[3] Although most of the biological pathways implicated by the RA genetic studies were shared between the populations, it is of note that the several pathways showed ethnically heterogeneous impact.[36]

These successful examples may suggest that functional annotations of the risk genetic variants are critically important to fully understand disease pathogenesis. International projects, such as the Genotype-Tissue Expression[37] and ENCODE[38] projects, have provided comprehensive catalogs of epigenetic information in a cell-type specific manner, which should be pivotal resources for the interpretation of the human disease genetics. Genome-wide annotations of GWAS results suggest that noncoding variants located at sites with epigenetic modifications in immune-related cell types play important roles in rheumatic diseases.[39,40] Integration of the GWAS results of approximately 20 human complex traits from several millions of subjects and microRNA (miRNA)-target gene networks demonstrated the significant contribution of miRNA to the genetics of RA as well as the identification of novel biomarker candidates of *PADI2* and miR-4728-5p.[41]

Cognitive computing or machine-learning approaches could be effective methods to dissect genetic and biological features of the diseases. Application of machine-learning methods to both RA and schizophrenia GWAS data sets revealed that the negatively correlated risk genetic scores of the diseases could partially explain lower comorbidity between these two diseases.[42]

FUTURE DIRECTIONS TOWARD DRUG DISCOVERY

Another important goal of human genetics is novel drug discovery for disease treatment. Considering that success rate of novel drug discovery are becoming lower despite increases in the cost, improvement of the productivity of the drug discovery process is necessary.[43] Retrospective studies investigating drug discovery pipelines and clinical trial results suggested that utilization of disease-associated gene information should improve the productivity.[44,45]

As empirical evidence to support this hypothesis, the authors' in silico network-based analysis demonstrated that RA risk genes identified by GWAS were significantly strongly connected to the target genes of the drugs currently indicated for RA treatment.[3] Although several successful drug discoveries based on genetics of rare diseases exist (eg, *PCSK9* for familial hypercholesterolemia and *XOR* for hereditary xanthinuria), the authors' study is one of the initial examples that human genetics could be a guide for drug development of common diseases.[4] The authors' analysis also suggested the possibility of applying a network to find candidates of novel drug repositioning (eg, CDK4/6 inhibitors for RA and GSK3B inhibitors for type 2 diabetes).[3,46] Considering that drug repositioning is a promising method to reduce drug discovery costs, it should also be examined whether this human genetics-based drug repositioning approach is effective for other common diseases.

ACKNOWLEDGMENTS

The authors thank Dr Robert M. Plenge at Merck & Co, Dr Soumya Raychaudhuri at Harvard Medical School, Professor Hidenori Inohara at Osaka University, Professor Kazuhiko Yamamoto at the University of Tokyo, and Professor Toshihiro Tanaka at Tokyo Medical and Dental University for their kind mentorship and advice.

REFERENCES

1. Yamamoto K, Okada Y, Suzuki A, et al. Genetic studies of rheumatoid arthritis. Proc Jpn Acad Ser B Phys Biol Sci 2015;91:410–22.
2. Welter D, MacArthur J, Morales J, et al. The NHGRI GWAS catalog, a curated resource of SNP-trait associations. Nucleic Acids Res 2014;42:D1001–6.
3. Okada Y, Wu D, Trynka G, et al. Genetics of rheumatoid arthritis contributes to biology and drug discovery. Nature 2014;506:376–81.
4. Okada Y. From the era of genome analysis to the era of genomic drug discovery: a pioneering example of rheumatoid arthritis. Clin Genet 2014;86:432–40.
5. Gregersen PK, Silver J, Winchester RJ. The shared epitope hypothesis. An approach to understanding the molecular genetics of susceptibility to rheumatoid arthritis. Arthritis Rheum 1987;30:1205–13.
6. Onuma H, Ota M, Sugenoya A, et al. Association of HLA-DPB1*0501 with early-onset Graves' disease in Japanese. Hum Immunol 1994;39:195–201.
7. Sengupta S, Sehgal S, Aikat BK, et al. HLA B27 in ankylosing spondylitis in India. Lancet 1977;1:1209–10.
8. Kazkaz L, Marotte H, Hamwi M, et al. Rheumatoid arthritis and genetic markers in Syrian and French populations: different effect of the shared epitope. Ann Rheum Dis 2007;66:195–201.
9. Okada Y, Yamada R, Suzuki A, et al. Contribution of a haplotype in the HLA region to anti-cyclic citrullinated peptide antibody positivity in rheumatoid arthritis, independently of HLA-DRB1. Arthritis Rheum 2009;60:3582–90.
10. Jia X, Han B, Onengut-Gumuscu S, et al. Imputing amino acid polymorphisms in human leukocyte antigens. PLoS One 2013;8:e64683.
11. Raychaudhuri S, Sandor C, Stahl EA, et al. Five amino acids in three HLA proteins explain most of the association between MHC and seropositive rheumatoid arthritis. Nat Genet 2012;44:291–6.
12. Han B, Diogo D, Eyre S, et al. Fine mapping seronegative and seropositive rheumatoid arthritis to shared and distinct HLA alleles by adjusting for the effects of heterogeneity. Am J Hum Genet 2014;94:522–32.
13. Okada Y, Kim K, Han B, et al. Risk for ACPA-positive rheumatoid arthritis is driven by shared HLA amino acid polymorphisms in Asian and European populations. Hum Mol Genet 2014;23:6916–26.
14. Okada Y, Suzuki A, Ikari K, et al. Contribution of a non-classical HLA gene, HLA-DOA, to the risk of rheumatoid arthritis. Am J Hum Genet 2016;99:366–74.
15. Reynolds RJ, Ahmed AF, Danila MI, et al. HLA-DRB1-associated rheumatoid arthritis risk at multiple levels in African Americans: hierarchical classification systems, amino acid positions, and residues. Arthritis Rheum 2014;66:3274–82.
16. Okada Y, Han B, Tsoi LC, et al. Fine mapping major histocompatibility complex associations in psoriasis and its clinical subtypes. Am J Hum Genet 2014;95:162–72.
17. Okada Y, Momozawa Y, Ashikawa K, et al. Construction of a population-specific HLA imputation reference panel and its application to Graves' disease risk in Japanese. Nat Genet 2015;47:798–802.

18. Hu X, Deutsch AJ, Lenz TL, et al. Additive and interaction effects at three amino acid positions in HLA-DQ and HLA-DR molecules drive type 1 diabetes risk. Nat Genet 2015;47:898–905.

19. Kim K, Bang SY, Lee HS, et al. The HLA-DRbeta1 amino acid positions 11-13-26 explain the majority of SLE-MHC associations. Nat Commun 2014;5:5902.

20. Shiraishi K, Okada Y, Takahashi A, et al. Association of variations in HLA class II and other loci with susceptibility to EGFR-mutated lung adenocarcinoma. Nat Commun 2016;7:12451.

21. Li Z, Xia Y, Feng LN, et al. Genetic risk of extranodal natural killer T-cell lymphoma: a genome-wide association study. Lancet Oncol 2016;17:1240–7.

22. Liu JZ, van, Sommeren S, Huang H, et al. Association analyses identify 38 susceptibility loci for inflammatory bowel disease and highlight shared genetic risk across populations. Nat Genet 2015;47:979–86.

23. Bentham J, Morris DL, Cunninghame Graham DS, et al. Genetic association analyses implicate aberrant regulation of innate and adaptive immunity genes in the pathogenesis of systemic lupus erythematosus. Nat Genet 2015;47:1457–64.

24. Kanai M, Tanaka T, Okada Y. Empirical estimation of genome-wide significance thresholds based on the 1000 Genomes Project data set. J Hum Genet 2016; 61(10):861–6.

25. Maher B. Personal genomes: the case of the missing heritability. Nature 2008; 456:18–21.

26. Okada Y, Plenge RM. Entering the age of whole-exome sequencing in rheumatic diseases: novel insights into disease pathogenicity. Arthritis Rheum 2013;65: 1975–9.

27. Okada Y, Diogo D, Greenberg JD, et al. Integration of sequence data from a consanguineous family with genetic data from an outbred population identifies PLB1 as a candidate rheumatoid arthritis risk gene. PLoS One 2014;9:e87645.

28. Hunt KA, Mistry V, Bockett NA, et al. Negligible impact of rare autoimmune-locus coding-region variants on missing heritability. Nature 2013;498:232–5.

29. Fuchsberger C, Flannick J, Teslovich TM, et al. The genetic architecture of type 2 diabetes. Nature 2016;536(7614):41–7.

30. Stahl EA, Wegmann D, Trynka G, et al. Bayesian inference analyses of the polygenic architecture of rheumatoid arthritis. Nat Genet 2012;44:483–9.

31. Finucane HK, Bulik-Sullivan B, Gusev A, et al. Partitioning heritability by functional annotation using genome-wide association summary statistics. Nat Genet 2015; 47:1228–35.

32. Lenz TL, Deutsch AJ, Han B, et al. Widespread non-additive and interaction effects within HLA loci modulate the risk of autoimmune diseases. Nat Genet 2015;47:1085–90.

33. Joshi PK, Esko T, Mattsson H, et al. Directional dominance on stature and cognition in diverse human populations. Nature 2015;523:459–62.

34. Zuk O, Hechter E, Sunyaev SR, et al. The mystery of missing heritability: genetic interactions create phantom heritability. Proc Natl Acad Sci U S A 2012;109: 1193–8.

35. Scott IC, Rijsdijk F, Walker J, et al. Do genetic susceptibility variants associate with disease severity in early active rheumatoid arthritis? J Rheumatol 2015;42: 1131–40.

36. Okada Y, Raj T, Yamamot T. Ethnically shared and heterogeneous impacts of molecular pathways suggested by the genome-wide meta-analysis of rheumatoid arthritis. Rheumatology (Oxford) 2016;55:186–9.

37. GTEx Consortium. Human genomics. The Genotype-Tissue Expression (GTEx) pilot analysis: multi-tissue gene regulation in humans. Science 2015;348:648–60.
38. ENCODE Project Consortium. An integrated encyclopedia of DNA elements in the human genome. Nature 2012;489:57–74.
39. Raj T, Rothamel K, Mostafavi S, et al. Polarization of the effects of autoimmune and neurodegenerative risk alleles in leukocytes. Science 2014;344:519–23.
40. Trynka G, Sandor C, Han B, et al. Chromatin marks identify critical cell types for fine mapping complex trait variants. Nat Genet 2013;45:124–30.
41. Okada Y, Muramatsu T, Suita N, et al. Significant impact of miRNA-target gene networks on genetics of human complex traits. Sci Rep 2016;6:22223.
42. Lee SH, Byrne EM, Hultman CM, et al. New data and an old puzzle: the negative association between schizophrenia and rheumatoid arthritis. Int J Epidemiol 2015;44:1706–21.
43. Sanseau P, Agarwal P, Barnes MR, et al. Use of genome-wide association studies for drug repositioning. Nat Biotechnol 2012;30:317–20.
44. Nelson MR, Tipney H, Painter JL, et al. The support of human genetic evidence for approved drug indications. Nat Genet 2015;47:856–60.
45. Cook D, Brown D, Alexander R, et al. Lessons learned from the fate of AstraZeneca's drug pipeline: a five-dimensional framework. Nat Rev Drug Discov 2014; 13:419–31.
46. Imamura M, Takahashi A, Yamauchi T, et al. Genome-wide association studies in the Japanese population identify seven novel loci for type 2 diabetes. Nat Commun 2016;7:10531.

Special Article

A Review of Systemic Corticosteroid Use in Pregnancy and the Risk of Select Pregnancy and Birth Outcomes

CrossMark

Gretchen Bandoli, PhD[a,*], Kristin Palmsten, ScD[a],
Chelsey J. Forbess Smith, MD[b], Christina D. Chambers, PhD, MPH[a]

KEYWORDS

- Pregnancy • Corticosteroids • Adverse pregnancy and birth outcomes • Review

KEY POINTS

- Corticosteroids are often necessary to control the symptoms of various medical conditions in pregnancy, including rheumatoid arthritis, systemic lupus erythematosus, and inflammatory bowel disease.
- Investigations into adverse pregnancy and birth outcomes following corticosteroid exposure have lacked adequate exploration into confounding by disease or disease severity.
- There may be a small increased risk of cleft lip with or without cleft palate associated with first-trimester corticosteroid use. This review does not find sufficient evidence to support an increased risk of preterm birth, low birth weight, or preeclampsia following systemic corticosteroid use in pregnancy. There is insufficient evidence to determine whether systemic corticosteroids are linked to gestational diabetes mellitus.

INTRODUCTION

Corticosteroids are administered in pregnancy for their immunosuppressive and anti-inflammatory effects.[1] They are used to treat symptoms of autoimmune conditions, because many standard immunosuppressive drugs and biologic agents are regarded

Disclosure: The authors report no conflicts of interest or financial disclosures.
Funding: G. Bandoli is supported by the National Institutes of Health (NIH) Grant TL1TR001443. K. Palmsten is supported by a career development award from the Eunice Kennedy Shriver National Institute of Child Health and Human Development, National Institutes of Health Grant K99HD082412. The content is solely the responsibility of the authors and does not necessarily represent the official views of the NIH.

[a] Department of Pediatrics, University of California, San Diego, 9500 Gilman Drive, Mail Code 0828, La Jolla, CA 92093-0412, USA; [b] Department of Rheumatology, University of California, San Diego, 9500 Gilman Drive, Mail Code 0656, La Jolla, CA 92093-0412, USA
* Corresponding author.
E-mail address: gbandoli@ucsd.edu

as riskier in pregnancy or as having unknown effects on fetal development.[2] Synthetic corticosteroids are often used to manage patients' disease severity and flares. These corticosteroids were developed to have amplified glucocorticoid activity and reduced mineralocorticoid activity compared with naturally occurring cortisol and have significantly more potent anti-inflammatory activity.[3] Although it is considered optimal to use prednisone at less than 20 mg/d in pregnancy, it is generally accepted that higher doses are allowable for aggressive disease.[4] Inflammation from uncontrolled autoimmune activity is potentially more harmful to maternal and fetal health than high-dose steroids.[4]

CORTICOSTEROIDS AND THE PLACENTA

Cortisol, a naturally occurring glucocorticoid in humans, is critical for embryogenesis. However, in most species, maternal glucocorticoid levels are much higher than those in the developing fetus.[5] The passage of natural and synthetic glucocorticoids is regulated primarily by 11β-hydroxysteroid dehydrogenase type 2 (11βHSD2). This enzyme is expressed in aldosterone-selective tissues and the placenta and encoded by the HSD11B2 gene. 11βHSD2 converts active glucocorticoids such as cortisol and prednisolone to their inactive metabolites: cortisone and prednisone.[5,6] Approximately 90% of cortisol is converted into cortisone. However, 11βHSD2 is less efficient at metabolizing synthetic corticosteroids, resulting in greater fetal exposure to active corticosteroids.[6] There remains, however, a significant conversion of synthetic short-acting corticosteroids to inactive metabolites. Clinical studies have reported 8- to 10-fold lower concentrations of fetal prednisolone to maternal prednisolone following maternal intravenous administration.[3] Endogenous fetal glucocorticoid levels are maintained at significantly lower levels than maternal levels; thus, even small transfers of synthetic corticosteroids across the placenta could have adverse developmental effects. It is important to evaluate the potential for adverse pregnancy or birth outcomes during this critical time in human development.

ADVERSE PREGNANCY AND BIRTH OUTCOMES

Autoimmune conditions are more prevalent in women than men and often occur during a woman's reproductive years.[7] Generally, autoimmune conditions are not thought to substantially affect fertility,[4] and thus, many women and their clinicians are confronted with concerns about how autoimmune disease and the associated treatments may affect pregnancy and birth outcomes. Concerns about the safety of corticosteroids in pregnancy arose in the 1950s following reports of oral clefts in the offspring of pregnant mice treated with corticosteroids.[8] The association between corticosteroids and oral clefts was also observed in epidemiologic studies, although estimates have varied widely and results have been inconsistent.[9] Additional findings suggested that oral corticosteroids (specifically prednisone) were associated with intrauterine growth restriction in humans and mice; these outcomes were reported to be independent of maternal disease.[10] Finally, a parallel body of literature has noted the increased risks for numerous adverse pregnancy and birth outcomes in women with autoimmune diseases, including preterm birth, preeclampsia, and gestational diabetes mellitus.[4,11–13] These articles generally conclude with an unanswered question: is the increased risk for adverse outcomes associated with the disease or the treatment?

In an effort to address this question, this review focuses on systemic corticosteroids and the associations with oral clefts, low birth weight (<2500 g), preterm birth (<37 weeks' gestation), preeclampsia, and gestational diabetes mellitus. This review focuses on systemic corticosteroids, rather than inhaled or topical treatments, given the greater systemic bioavailability and systemic effects of these forms,[14–18] and consequently, the potential for greater fetal exposure. Careful consideration is given to study design and statistical analysis, with emphasis on the comparison group and mitigation of confounding by disease indication or severity.

LITERATURE REVIEW

Studies for this narrative review were identified from PubMed, with the search terms "glucocorticoids" or "corticosteroids" or "prednisone" and "pregnancy outcomes," "birth outcomes," "oral clefts," "preeclampsia," "preterm birth," "birth weight," or "gestational diabetes." Additional searches were performed for "pregnancy or birth outcomes" and "rheumatoid arthritis," "Crohn disease," "inflammatory bowel disease," "systemic lupus erythematosus," "autoimmune disease," and "rheumatic diseases." Search results were narrowed to focus on oral or systemic corticosteroids, and whenever possible, limited to indications for autoimmune conditions.

ORAL CLEFTS

Clefts of the lip and palate affect approximately 1.7 in 1000 live births, with lifelong effects on speech and hearing.[19] Development of the lip and palate require a highly coordinated series of events that are completed by the fifth or sixth week for closure of the lip and the eighth or ninth week for closure of the palate.[20,21] Typically, the causes of disruption in this process are unknown.[19] Oral clefts can be categorized into those that affect the palate only, the lip only, or the lip and the palate.[20,22] Given the low prevalence, researchers often group the latter 2 into one category (cleft lip with or without cleft palate).[20] Cleft palate alone has a lower prevalence than cleft lip (with or without cleft palate) and the 2 are thought to have different genetic and etiologic risk factors.[20,22] Following earlier findings that corticosteroids caused cleft palate in mice,[8] several epidemiologic studies have investigated the association in humans (**Table 1**).

Because of the low prevalence of oral clefts, most studies of systemic corticosteroids have been case-control,[9,23–27] although at least 2 were retrospective cohort studies.[28] All case-control studies relied on recall of medication exposure by parents after the birth,[9,23–27] potentially biasing associations if parents of offspring with clefts report medication use with more or less accuracy than controls. Several case-control studies stratified exposure into oral or systemic corticosteroids,[9,23,24,26,27] and a few focused on systemic use[24,26] reported statistically significant associations of approximately 2- to 9-fold greater risk for cleft lip with or without cleft palate. Others found similar increases in odds with confidence intervals (CIs) slightly crossing the null (resulting in $P>.05$).[9,23,27]

In general, early case-control studies (before 2000) reported stronger odds of cleft lip with or without cleft palate following corticosteroid exposure as summarized in a meta-analysis in 2000 (odds ratio [OR] any corticosteroid use during the first trimester: 3.4, 95% CI 2.0, 5.7).[29] Of note, although previous studies separately estimated cleft lip and cleft palate, the meta-analysis grouped all outcomes into "oral clefts." In more recent studies, the strength of the associations of corticosteroids and oral clefts has reduced to nonsignificant findings. Analyzing data from the National Birth Defect Prevention Study (NBDPS) in the time periods of 1997 to 2002 and 2003 to 2009, Skuladottir and colleagues[9] reported weaker associations between systemic corticosteroids and cleft lip and palate in the latter years. The study followed the same protocol and procedures, case ascertainment, and recruitment practices during both time periods. The investigators note the increased use of corticosteroids among mothers of controls and the decreased use among mothers of cleft lip and palate

Table 1
Studies of oral or systemic corticosteroids and the risk of oral clefts (organized chronologically)

Author, Year	Study Population	Study Design	Number of Cases	Odds Ratio, 95% CI	Corticosteroid Use During 1st Trimester
Czeizel & Rockenbauer,[23] 1997	Hungarian Case-Control Surveillance of Congenital Abnormalities (Hungary)	Population-based case-control	n = 1223 CLP	CLP: 1.3 (0.8, 2.0)	Oral[a]
Rodriguez-Pinilla & Martinez-Frías,[24] 1998	Spanish Collaborative Study of Congenital Malformations (Spain)	Hospital-based case-control	n = 631 CLP	CLP: 8.9 (2.0, 37.9)	Systemic use
Carmichael & Shaw,[25] 1999	California Birth Defects Monitoring Program (US)	Population-based case-control	n = 348 CLP\nn = 141 CP	CLP: 4.3 (1.1, 17.2)\nCP: 5.3 (1.1, 26.5)	Any use\nAny use
Pradat et al,[26] 2003	MADRE project (worldwide)	Case-control	n = 645 CLP	CLP: 1.9 (1.2, 3.0)	Systemic use
Carmichael et al,[27] 2007	National Birth Defects Prevention Study (US)	Population-based case-control	n = 1141 CLP\nn = 628 CP	CLP: 2.1 (0.9, 4.7)\nCP: 0.8 (0.2, 3.6)	Systemic use\nSystemic use
Hviid & Mølgaard-Nielsen,[28] 2011	Danish Medical Birth Registry (Denmark)	Population-based retrospective cohort	n = 875 CLP\nn = 357 CP	CLP: 1.1 (0.8, 1.4)\nCP: 1.2 (0.8, 1.8)	Any use\nAny use
Skuladottir et al,[9] 2014	National Birth Defects Prevention Study (US)	Population-based case-control	n = 2680 CLP\nn = 1415 CP	CLP: 1.6 (0.9, 2.8)\nCP: 0.8 (0.3, 2.1)	Systemic use\nSystemic use
Bay Bjørn et al,[30] 2014	Danish Medical Birth Registry (Denmark)	Population-based retrospective cohort	n = 147 oral clefts	CLP: 0.4 (0.1, 2.8)	Any use
Park-Wyllie et al,[29] 2000	Meta-analysis focusing on oral clefts	Meta-analysis of case-control studies[b]	n = 2551 oral clefts	Summary OR: 3.4 (2.0, 5.7)	Any use

Abbreviations: CLP, cleft lip with or without cleft palate; CP, cleft palate.
[a] Estimate for corticosteroids at any time in pregnancy.
[b] Robert (1994), Czeizel (1997), Rodriguez-Pinilla (1998), Carmichael (1999).

cases in the latter time period. Overall, it is unclear what is driving the observed reduction in risk, but some possibilities include a temporal trend toward shorter durations or lower doses of systemic corticosteroids in favor of alternative treatments. In addition, the underlying medical conditions necessitating corticosteroid use may change over time, resulting in different risk estimates.

Two retrospective population-based cohorts have been reported.[28,30] Both studies relied on medical records of corticosteroid exposure, mitigating risk of recall bias. Unfortunately, in both studies, the investigators were unable to estimate the risk of oral corticosteroids, specifically, because of no observed exposed cases. In the study by Hviid and Mølgaard-Nielsen[28] using all live births in Denmark from 1996 to 2008 (n = 832,636), estimates for exposure to any corticosteroids during the first trimester did not correlate with increased risk for cleft lip or cleft palate. Only those exposed to topical corticosteroids had a higher risk of cleft lip with or without cleft palate (OR 1.45 [1.03, 2.05]), although it is unclear if the increased risk is due to systemic absorption from the topical treatment, the dermatologic condition for which the topical steroids were used (ie, eczema or psoriasis), or disease severity. Another study by Bay Bjørn and colleagues[30] relied on live births from primiparous women in northern Denmark from 1999 to 2009 (n = 83,043). The unadjusted odds of oral clefts following exposure to any corticosteroids (inhaled or oral) in the first trimester was also null (OR 0.4 [0.1, 2.8]). Because of the relatively small sample, cleft lip and cleft palate were analyzed together.

A serious methodologic consideration for all studies in **Table 1** is that none adjusted for underlying disease or disease severity. Confounding by disease or disease severity occurs when the underlying disease or severity of the disease is associated with the exposure, is not a result of the exposure, and is associated with the outcome. In the case of corticosteroids, the first 2 points are undisputable, that is, corticosteroids are taken as a result of the underlying disease and associated flares.[2,3] Whether maternal disease or disease activity is associated with oral clefts, directly or through common causes, such as smoking, alcohol, interpregnancy interval, or obesity,[31,32] remains unanswered. Consequently, studies that group any underlying indication for corticosteroids without statistical adjustment for the disease or severity are difficult to interpret. Furthermore, none of the studies considered systemic corticosteroid dose, which is necessary to evaluate potential teratogenicity.

Another methodologic consideration for the body of evidence is temporality of the corticosteroid exposure relative to the oral cleft. Several studies of oral clefts count exposure from a few weeks before estimated conception through the end of the first trimester.[9,24–28,30] However, the critical periods for formation of the lip and palate encompass only specific weeks in the first trimester.[20,21] This practice could lead to potential exposure misclassification, that is, for those exposures that took place only outside the biologically relevant time period in early gestation. This bias from misclassification would result in smaller effect estimates. Skuladottir and colleagues[9] attempted to look at any corticosteroid use by small time intervals (1–4 weeks preconception, and 1–4 weeks, 5–8 weeks, and 9–12 weeks postconception). Even with 2372 cases of clefts, the number of pregnancies exposed to corticosteroids within specific gestational windows were very small. The small sample available for analysis led to inconsistent results, demonstrating the difficulty of defining risk periods for corticosteroid use in epidemiologic studies.

In summary, the evidence for cleft palate alone is not sufficient to summarize. The estimated risk of cleft lip with or without cleft palate from corticosteroid exposure has weakened over time, and no study published after 2003 has reported a statistically significant risk estimate. The largest case-control study to date (NBDPS) has estimated a modest (60%) increase in the odds of cleft lip with or without cleft palate, although the CI did slightly cross 1.0.[9] Cohort studies, which are not subject to recall bias, have been limited by insufficient sample sizes to differentiate between routes of administration[28,30] or type of oral cleft.[30] Examining the evidence and methodological limitations in totality, systemic corticosteroids may be associated with small increases in the risk of cleft lip with or without palate. Assuming a causal OR of 1.6 (from the NBDPS), the risk of cleft lip with or without cleft palate among women using corticosteroids in the relevant time frame would increase from 1.7 per 1000 live births to 2.7 per 1000 live births. Ultimately, the sample sizes required to detect a relatively small risk of cleft lip and to address the contribution of specific maternal diseases, dose, and timing, are challenging to obtain.

PRETERM BIRTH AND LOW BIRTH WEIGHT

After reports that corticosteroids were teratogenic in mice, researchers reported that prednisone use in pregnancy was associated with low birth weight in the full-term offspring of both humans and mice.[10,33] Researchers studying rodent models concluded that corticosteroids, not underlying maternal disease, were the cause of the findings.[10] Many epidemiologic studies of pregnancies complicated by autoimmune diseases, including rheumatoid arthritis (RA), inflammatory bowel disease (IBD), and systemic lupus erythematosus (SLE), have noted the increased risk of low birth weight and preterm birth.[11–13,34] Although most such studies have not attempted to isolate the effects of corticosteroids from underlying maternal disease, some have as summarized in **Table 2**.

LOW BIRTH WEIGHT

A few studies have reported birth weight or intrauterine growth restriction (IUGR) as an outcome. Among women with Crohn disease in Denmark, corticosteroids (local and/or systemic) were not associated with birth weight after adjusting for gestational age and disease activity (adjusted risk ratio [aRR]: 1.1 [0.2, 5.7]). Of note, although neither the crude nor the adjusted effect estimates were statistically significant, the risk ratio was reduced by 21% after adjustment for maternal age and parity.[35] Similarly, in a study of pregnant women with RA,[36] although birth weight was associated with prednisone use, upon adjustment to a standard deviation score accounting for gestational age at delivery and sex of the newborn, the results were no longer statistically significant. A study in a cohort of pregnant women with SLE reported elevated odds of IUGR following prednisone use, although CIs were wide and crossed the null.[37] It was not apparent that the estimates were adjusted for gestational age or disease severity. Finally, although Gur and colleagues[38] found a univariate association between lower birth weight and any corticosteroid use among premature births, the results are difficult to interpret as there was no adjustment for maternal disease.

PRETERM BIRTH

Studies have examined the use of prednisone or prednisolone in pregnant women with SLE and the odds of preterm birth.[37,39] Two reports of increased risk in women with SLE appear to be univariate comparisons unadjusted for disease severity or any other maternal characteristics and are therefore not easy to interpret.[37,39] A third univariate association in a population-based study was not adjusted for underlying maternal disease.[38] From the Danish cohort of pregnant women with Crohn disease, Nørgård and colleagues[35] reported that after adjusting for mothers' age, parity, and disease

Table 2
Studies of oral or systemic corticosteroids and the risk of preterm birth, low birth weight, or intrauterine growth retardation (organized chronologically)

Author, Year	Study Population or Location	Study Design	Outcome	Measure of Association with Corticosteroid Use	Corticosteroid	Indication for Use
Gur et al,[38] 2003	Israeli Teratogen Information Service	Retrospective cohort of 311 pregnant women exposed to glucocorticoids and 790 unexposed women	Preterm birth Birth weight (among PTBs)	26.9% vs 10.8% ($P = .001$) 2300 g vs 2550 g ($P = .003$)	Prednisone Any corticosteroids	Multiple Multiple
Chakravarty et al,[39] 2005	Stanford University (US)	Retrospective cohort of 63 pregnancies in 48 women with SLE between 1991 and 2001	Preterm birth	OR: 1.8 (1.1, 3.0)	Prednisone	SLE
Norgård et al,[35] 2007	Danish National Registry of Patients (Denmark)	Retrospective cohort study of 900 children born to CD women between 1996 and 2004	Low birth weight Preterm birth	RR: 1.1 (0.2, 5.7) RR: 1.4 (0.6, 3.3)	Local or systemic corticosteroids Local or systemic corticosteroids	CD CD
de Man et al,[36] 2009	PARA study (Netherlands)	Population-based cohort study of 152 women with RA	Birth weight SDS Gestational age	Beta estimate: −0.2 (−0.6, 0.2) 38.8 wk vs 39.9 wk ($P = .001$)	Prednisone Prednisone	RA RA
Al Arfaj & Khalil,[37] 2010	King Khalid University Hospital (Saudi Arabia)	Retrospective cohort of 383 pregnancies exposed to SLE between 1980 and 2006	Preterm birth IUGR	OR: 5.7 (1.3, 25.1) OR: 2.6 (0.9, 8.0)	Prednisolone Prednisolone	SLE SLE
Boyd et al,[40] 2015	Danish National Birth Cohort (Denmark)	86,591 women with live births (666 with IBD) enrolled between 1996 and 2003	Preterm birth	HR: 6.3 (3.1, 12.7)	Systemic corticosteroids	IBD

Abbreviations: CD, Crohn disease; HR, hazard ratio; RR, risk ratio; SDS, standard deviation score (adjusted for gestational age).

activity, there was no association between prednisolone and preterm birth. Finally, from a separate Danish cohort of pregnant women with IBD, there was an increased risk of preterm delivery following systemic corticosteroid use compared with women without IBD (adjusted hazard ratio [aHR]: 6.3 [3.1, 12.7]).[40] The hazard ratio was adjusted for maternal characteristics (including age, smoking, and alcohol use) but not underlying disease or disease severity. Of note, among women with IBD without medication use, there was a 50% increase in the risk of preterm birth relative to women without IBD (aHR: 1.5 [1.0, 2.4]).[40] This finding suggests that IBD itself contributes to the increased risk of preterm birth. Furthermore, the investigators note that associations with preterm birth were strongest in the women who used corticosteroid medication, which is a marker of active disease and is also associated with preeclampsia. Thus, they conclude that early delivery may have been necessitated by severe disease activity or preeclampsia as opposed to a direct effect from corticosteroids.[40]

Compared with the previous studies examining the risk of oral clefts, these studies tended to be conducted in women with a specific disease, removing the potential for confounding by indication. However, as noted, only one study[35] adjusted for disease activity, and upon adjustment, estimates for preterm birth were not statistically significant. A few investigators noted positive associations between disease[40] or disease severity[36,40] and preterm birth or birth weight. Interestingly, in the cohort of pregnant women with RA, disease severity remained a significant predictor of birth weight after adjusting for gestational age and prednisone use.[36] These findings, and the attenuation of associations after accounting for disease severity, highlight the great likelihood for confounding by disease severity in this body of research. Although it is difficult to tease apart disease severity and corticosteroid use, measuring disease activity and adjusting for it in multivariate analyses will better inform clinical decision making.

To summarize, it appears that disease severity, not corticosteroids, is responsible for reported associations with preterm birth. Furthermore, one can surmise that any association between corticosteroids and low birth weight is most likely mediated by gestational age, with little evidence of a direct effect on birth weight.

PREECLAMPSIA

Preeclampsia, a pregnancy disorder characterized by high blood pressure and proteinuria, is a serious pregnancy complication associated with both maternal and fetal morbidity and mortality.[41] Preeclampsia is histologically described by restrained trophoblast invasion, vasculitis, thrombosis, and ischemia of the placenta.[42] Although specific mechanisms are not understood, it is hypothesized that preeclampsia may have an autoimmune contribution.[42] Indeed, preeclampsia has been associated with both RA and SLE.[13,34]

At least 3 studies have reported effects of corticosteroids on the risk of preeclampsia (**Table 3**). One study analyzing perinatal outcomes in patients with SLE was not adjusted for any potential confounders, thus making interpretation difficult.[39] Investigators analyzing the Danish National Birth Cohort reported an increased risk of preeclampsia from systemic corticosteroid use when compared with women without IBD (aHR: 3.5 [1.4, 9.1]), which was adjusted for maternal characteristics but not disease or disease severity.[40] Finally, relying on a large health care database in British Columbia, Palmsten and colleagues[43] found that women who used corticosteroids for the first time during pregnancy had an elevated (although not statistically significant) risk of preeclampsia relative to those who used corticosteroids in the past year before pregnancy (aRR 1.4 [0.9, 1.9]). Continuous use of corticosteroids in this

Table 3
Studies of oral or systemic corticosteroids and the risk of gestational diabetes or preeclampsia (organized chronologically)

Author, Year	Study Population or Location	Study Design	Outcome	Measure of Association with Corticosteroid Use	Corticosteroid	Indication for Use
Chakravarty et al,[39] 2005	Stanford University (US)	Retrospective cohort of 63 pregnancies in 48 women with SLE between 1991 and 2001	Preeclampsia	OR: 1.8 (0.7, 5.0)	Prednisone	SLE
Yildirim et al,[45] 2006	Aegean Obstetrics and Gynecology Training and Research Hospital (Turkey)	Retrospective cohort of 25 pregnant women with ITP and 108 pregnant women without ITP	Gestational diabetes	24.0% vs 2.8% ($P = .01$)	>4 wk of corticosteroid vs no use	ITP
Palmsten et al,[43] 2012	Health care database British Columbia (Canada)	306,831 pregnancies with live birth between 1997 and 2006	Preeclampsia Preeclampsia	RR: 0.9 (0.5, 1.6) RR: 1.4 (0.9, 1.9)	Continuous use vs past use corticosteroid First use vs past use corticosteroid	Multiple Multiple
Boyd et al,[40] 2015	Danish National Birth Cohort (Denmark)	86,792 women with live-births (666 with IBD) enrolled between 1996 and 2003	Preeclampsia	HR: 3.5 (1.4, 9.1)	Systemic corticosteroids	IBD
Leung et al,[46] 2015	Alberta Health Services (Canada)	Retrospective cohort of 116 live births to women with IBD between 2006 and 2009; 381 matched women without IBD	Gestational diabetes Gestational diabetes	OR: 4.5 (1.2, 16.8) (IBD on steroids vs controls) OR: 2.0 (0.0, 15.3) (IBD on steroids vs IBD not on steroids)	Oral prednisone or intravenous corticosteroids Oral prednisone or intravenous corticosteroids	IBD IBD

population was not associated with preeclampsia relative to past users. These results were adjusted for underlying disease and proxy measures for disease severity. The investigators noted dissimilarities in factors related to autoimmune characteristics at baseline between first-time users and past users, hypothesizing that residual confounding by disease severity may bias estimates of first-time users.[43]

The only study that adjusted for disease and a proxy of disease severity did not find evidence of an association between corticosteroid use and preeclampsia.[43] Any increased risk associated with autoimmune conditions is most likely confounded by the disease severity. In addition, previous studies of preeclampsia have not evaluated the dose of corticosteroids, which is important because prednisone at high doses can cause sodium retention and high blood pressure.

GESTATIONAL DIABETES MELLITUS

The risk of gestational diabetes mellitus from corticosteroid use has received little attention to date (see **Table 3**). This condition, characterized by high blood glucose levels in pregnancy in women without previously diagnosed diabetes, is associated with adverse outcomes in the developing fetus.[44] The rationale for studying corticosteroids with gestational diabetes mellitus follows reports in humans and animal models of higher plasma cortisol levels in individuals with gestational diabetes mellitus.[45]

In a retrospective cohort study of 25 pregnancies with idiopathic thrombocytopenic purpura (ITP) and 108 pregnancies without ITP, greater than 4 weeks of prednisone use was associated with gestational diabetes mellitus (24% vs 2.8%, $P = .01$).[45] These results were not adjusted for any maternal conditions, and it was suggested that all ITP subjects were exposed to greater than 4 weeks of prednisone, prohibiting disentanglement of underlying disease and medication.[45] The second study was conducted within a retrospective cohort of 116 women with IBD and 381 women without IBD.[46] Leung and colleagues[46] reported an increase odds of gestational diabetes mellitus from oral prednisone or intravenous corticosteroids relative to women without IBD (OR: 4.5 [1.2, 16.8]). These results were only adjusted for age and smoking. When women with IBD without corticosteroid use were compared, there was no longer a statistically significant finding (OR: 2.0 [0.0, 15.3]). Because of the low prevalence of gestational diabetes mellitus, only 15 women experienced the outcome (7 with IBD and 8 without IBD), resulting in very wide CIs and precluding further statistical adjustment.

In summary, neither study is of sufficient methodologic quality to rule out an effect of systemic corticosteroid use on the development of gestational diabetes mellitus. As noted in previous sections, confounding by disease and disease severity must be addressed to support the hypothesized association.

SUMMARY AND CONSIDERATIONS FOR FURTHER RESEARCH

As summarized in **Tables 1–3**, many researchers have investigated the effects of corticosteroids on adverse pregnancy and birth outcomes. This type of research informs clinicians and pregnant women when assessing risk:benefit ratios. Foregoing treatment of an autoimmune condition is not an option for many pregnant women, because active disease can pose threats to both maternal and fetal health.[4] Because of ethical concerns, randomized clinical trials are rarely possible, and investigations must rely on observational data. One of the greatest threats to internal validity in observational studies results from confounding. In pharmacoepidemiologic studies, confounding by indication is one of the most difficult to address.[47] Disease and disease severity are often related to pharmacologic exposure and to adverse outcomes. Investigations that do not account for this systematic bias are largely incapable of estimating the independent effects of the pharmacologic agent. Therefore, studies that compare oral corticosteroids with alternative treatments in women with autoimmune disease would reduce confounding by underlying disease and would provide clinically relevant risk information. In addition, the threat of recall bias inherent to case-control studies can be mitigated by relying on medical or pharmacy dispensing records for exposure assessment.

Another concern when interpreting results for all outcomes is whether timing of exposure or dose was accounted for. This concern was discussed specifically for oral cleft formation earlier, but also applies to the other outcomes investigated. For example, for preterm birth, corticosteroid use should not be considered after 37 gestational weeks because the outcome is no longer possible. Furthermore, when exposure is dichotomized as use any time during pregnancy versus no use, bias can arise when corticosteroid use occurs after the onset of the outcome (eg, preeclampsia, gestational diabetes mellitus). Finally, it is particularly useful to examine the daily and cumulative dose of pharmacologic agents, especially in patients with autoimmune conditions in which disease severity alters the course of therapy. Recent work examining the daily and cumulative dose of prednisone in pregnant women with autoimmune disease revealed variability in amount and pattern of use, which can be linked with perinatal outcomes.[48]

As a final consideration, it has been shown that placentas from female fetuses born within 72 hours of betamethasone administration had higher 11βHSD2 activity levels compared with placentas from male fetuses, suggesting female offspring may be more protected from corticosteroid exposure.[6] In addition, maternal psychological factors may downregulate 11βHSD2 activity, resulting in greater corticosteroid exposure to the developing fetus.[49] Future research on the effects of corticosteroids in pregnancy and birth outcomes may benefit from investigation into offspring sex, maternal psychological stress, and other potential modifiers.

In summary, there may be a modest increase in the risk of cleft lip with or without palate from systemic corticosteroid use, but data are conflicting, and it is unknown to what extent maternal disease itself could contribute. There is little evidence that systemic corticosteroid use in pregnancy independently increases risks of preterm birth, low birth weight, or preeclampsia. Currently, there is not enough evidence to determine whether systemic corticosteroids could contribute to gestational diabetes mellitus. Future studies would benefit from more rigorous evaluation of confounding by disease or disease severity. Further inquiry into the impacts of dose and timing of corticosteroid use, as well as potential effect modifiers, could identify subgroups whose pregnancies are adversely affected by corticosteroids.

Despite the lack of direct evidence supporting causal associations between antenatal systemic corticosteroid exposure and adverse pregnancy outcomes, clinicians should follow similar principles when prescribing corticosteroids for the pregnant woman with autoimmune disease as for nonpregnant patients with rheumatic disease: to use the minimal dose and duration of corticosteroid to safely treat active disease manifestations. As always, the overall risks of corticosteroid use, which are dose and duration dependent, must be balanced with the necessity of treating active underlying disease.

REFERENCES

1. McGee DC. Steroid use during pregnancy. J Perinat Neonatal Nurs 2002;16(2): 26–39.

2. Ostensen M, Forger F. Management of RA medications in pregnant patients. Nat Rev Rheumatol 2009;5(7):382–90.

3. van Runnard Heimel PJ, Franx A, Schobben AF, et al. Corticosteroids, pregnancy, and HELLP syndrome: a review. Obstet Gynecol Surv 2005;60(1):57–70, 74.

4. Mitchell K, Kaul M, Clowse M. The management of rheumatic diseases in pregnancy. Scand J Rheumatol 2010;39(2):99–108.

5. Fowden AL, Forhead AJ, Coan PM, et al. The placenta and intrauterine programming. J Neuroendocrinol 2008;20(4):439–50.

6. Singh RR, Cuffe JS, Moritz KM. Short- and long-term effects of exposure to natural and synthetic glucocorticoids during development. Clin Exp Pharmacol Physiol 2012;39(11):979–89.

7. Borchers AT, Naguwa SM, Keen CL, et al. The implications of autoimmunity and pregnancy. J Autoimmun 2010;34(3):J287–99.

8. Fraser FC, Fainstat TD. Production of congenital defects in the offspring of pregnant mice treated with cortisone. Pediatrics 1951;8(4):527–33.

9. Skuladottir H, Wilcox AJ, Ma C, et al. Corticosteroid use and risk of orofacial clefts. Birth Defects Res A Clin Mol Teratol 2014;100(6):499–506.

10. Reinisch JM, Simon NG, Karow WG, et al. Prenatal exposure to prednisone in humans and animals retards intrauterine growth. Science 1978;202(4366):436–8.

11. Rom A, Wu CS, Olsen J, et al. Fetal growth and preterm birth in children exposed to maternal or paternal rheumatoid arthritis. A nationwide cohort study. Arthritis Rheum 2014;66(12):3265–73.

12. Broms G, Granath F, Linder M, et al. Birth outcomes in women with inflammatory bowel disease: effects of disease activity and drug exposure. Inflamm Bowel Dis 2014;20(6):1091–8.

13. Reed SD, Vollan TA, Svec MA. Pregnancy outcomes in women with rheumatoid arthritis in Washington State. Matern Child Health J 2006;10(4):361–6.

14. Barnes P, Pedersen S, Busse WW. Efficacy and safety of inhaled corticosteroids. New developments. Am J Respir Crit Care Med 1998;157:S1–53.

15. Frey BM, Frey FJ. Clinical pharmacokinetics of prednisone and prednisolone. Clin Pharmacokinet 1990;19(2):126–46.

16. Korting HC, Kerscher MJ, Schäfer-Korting M. Topical glucocorticoids with improved benefit/risk ratio: do they exist? J Am Acad Dermatol 1992;27(1):87–92.

17. Li JTC, Goldstein MF, Gross GN, et al. Effects of fluticasone propionate, triamcinolone acetonide, prednisone, and placebo on the hypothalamic-pituitary-adrenal axis. J Allergy Clin Immunol 1999;103(4):622–9.

18. Roeder A, Schaller M, Schäfer-Korting M, et al. Safety and efficacy of fluticasone propionate in the topical treatment of skin diseases. Skin Pharmacol Physiol 2005;18(1):3–11.

19. Mossey PA, Little J, Munger RG, et al. Cleft lip and palate. Lancet 2009; 374(9703):1773–85.

20. Jugessur A, Farlie P, Kilpatrick N. The genetics of isolated orofacial clefts: from genotypes to subphenotypes. Oral Dis 2009;15(7):437–53.

21. Jones KL, Jones MC, Del Campo M. Smith's recognizable patterns of human malformation. 7th edition. Philadelphia: Saunders; 2013.

22. Ludwig KU, Böhmer AC, Bowes J, et al. Imputation of orofacial clefting data identifies novel risk loci and sheds light on the genetic background of cleft lip ± cleft palate and cleft palate only. Hum Mol Genet 2017. http://dx.doi.org/10.1093/hmg/ddx012.

23. Czeizel AE, Rockenbauer M. Population-based case-control study of teratogenic potential of corticosteroids. Teratology 1997;56(5):335–40.

24. Rodríguez-Pinilla E, Martínez-Frías ML. Corticosteroids during pregnancy and oral clefts: a case-control study. Teratology 1998;58(1):2–5.

25. Carmichael SL, Shaw GM. Maternal corticosteroid use and risk of selected congenital anomalies. Am J Med Genet 1999;86(3):242–4.
26. Pradat P, Robert-Gnansia E, Di Tanna GL, et al. First trimester exposure to corticosteroids and oral clefts. Birth Defects Res A Clin Mol Teratol 2003;67(12): 968–70.
27. Carmichael SL, Shaw GM, Ma C, et al. Maternal corticosteroid use and orofacial clefts. Am J Obstet Gynecol 2007;197(6):585.e1-7.
28. Hviid A, Mølgaard-Nielsen D. Corticosteroid use during pregnancy and risk of orofacial clefts. CMAJ 2011;183(7):796–804.
29. Park-Wyllie L, Mazzotta P, Pastuszak A, et al. Birth defects after maternal exposure to corticosteroids: prospective cohort study and meta-analysis of epidemiological studies. Teratology 2000;62(6):385–92.
30. Bay Bjørn AM, Ehrenstein V, Hundborg HH, et al. Use of corticosteroids in early pregnancy is not associated with risk of oral clefts and other congenital malformations in offspring. Am J Ther 2014;21(2):73–80.
31. Bille C, Olsen J, Vach W, et al. Oral clefts and life style factors - a case-cohort study based on prospective Danish data. Eur J Epidemiol 2007;22(3):173–81.
32. Villamor E, Sparén P, Cnattingius S. Risk of oral clefts in relation to prepregnancy weight change and interpregnancy interval. Am J Epidemiol 2008;167(11): 1305–11.
33. Reinisch JM, Simon NG, Gandelman R. Prenatal exposure to prednisone permanently alters fighting behavior of female mice. Pharmacol Biochem Behav 1980; 12:213–6.
34. Lateef A, Petri M. Managing lupus patients during pregnancy. Best Pract Res Clin Rheumatol 2013;27(3):435–47.
35. Nørgård B, Pedersen L, Christensen LA, et al. Therapeutic drug use in women with Crohn's disease and birth outcomes: a Danish nationwide cohort study. Am J Gastroenterol 2007;102(7):1406–13.
36. De Man YA, Hazes JMW, Van Der Heide H, et al. Association of higher rheumatoid arthritis disease activity during pregnancy with lower birth weight: results of a national prospective study. Arthritis Rheum 2009;60(11):3196–206.
37. Al Arfaj AS, Khalil N. Pregnancy outcome in 396 pregnancies in patients with SLE in Saudi Arabia. Lupus 2010;19(14):1665–73.
38. Gur C, Diav-Citrin O, Shechtman S, et al. Pregnancy outcome after first trimester exposure to corticosteroids: a prospective controlled study. Reprod Toxicol 2004; 18(1):93–101.
39. Chakravarty EF, Colón I, Langen ES, et al. Factors that predict prematurity and preeclampsia in pregnancies that are complicated by systemic lupus erythematosus. Am J Obstet Gynecol 2005;192(6):1897–904.
40. Boyd HA, Basit S, Harpsøe MC, et al. Inflammatory bowel disease and risk of adverse pregnancy outcomes. PLoS One 2015;10(6):e0129567.
41. Shih T, Peneva D, Xu X, et al. The rising burden of preeclampsia in the United States impacts both maternal and child health. Am J Perinatol 2016;33(4): 329–38.
42. Páez MC, Matsuura E, Díaz LA, et al. Laminin-1 (LM-111) in preeclampsia and systemic lupus erythematosus. Autoimmunity 2013;46(1):14–20.
43. Palmsten K, Hernández-Diaz S, Kuriya B, et al. Use of disease-modifying antirheumatic drugs during pregnancy and risk of preeclampsia. Arthritis Care Res 2012;64(11):1730–8.
44. Reece EA. The fetal and maternal consequences of gestational diabetes mellitus. J Matern Fetal Neonatal Med 2010;23(3):199–203.

45. Yildirim Y, Tinar S, Oner RS, et al. Gestational diabetes mellitus in patients receiving long-term corticosteroid therapy during pregnancy. J Perinat Med 2006;34(4):280–4.

46. Leung YPY, Kaplan GG, Coward S, et al. Intrapartum corticosteroid use significantly increases the risk of gestational diabetes in women with inflammatory bowel disease. J Crohns Colitis 2015;9(3):223–30.

47. Bosco JLF, Silliman RA, Thwin SS, et al. A most stubborn bias: no adjustment method fully resolves confounding by indication in observational studies. J Clin Epidemiol 2010;63(1):64–74.

48. Palmsten K, Rolland M, Hebert M, et al. Patterns of prednisone use during pregnancy: daily and cumulative dose [Abstract]. San Diego (CA): Health Care Systems Research Network; 2017.

49. Bronson SL, Bale TL. The placenta as a mediator of stress effects on neurodevelopmental reprogramming. Neuropsychopharmacology 2015;41(1):1–12.

Printed and bound by CPI Group (UK) Ltd, Croydon, CR0 4YY

08/05/2025

01864701-0005